Springer

Berlin
Heidelberg
New York
Hong Kong
London
Milan
Paris
Tokyo

Nalin Gupta
Anuradha Banerjee
Daphne Haas-Kogan
(Editors)

Pediatric CNS Tumors

With 153 Figures and 33 Tables

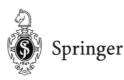 Springer

ISBN 3-540-00294-4
Springer-Verlag Berlin Heidelberg New York

Nalin Gupta, MD, PhD
Assistant Professor
Chief, Division of Pediatric Neurosurgery
Departments of Neurological Surgery
and Pediatrics
University of California, San Francisco

Anuradha Banerjee, MD, MPH
Assistant Professor
Division of Neuro-Oncology
Departments of Neurological Surgery
and Pediatrics
University of California, San Francisco

Daphne Haas-Kogan, MD
Associate Professor
Department of Radiation Oncology
University of California, San Francisco

Library of Congress Cataloging-in-Publication Data
Pediatric CNS tumors/N.Gupta, A. Banerjee, D. Haas-Kogan
(eds.) p. ; cm. Includes bibliographical references and index.
ISBN 3-540-00294-4 (alk. paper) 1. Central nervous system–
Tumors. 2. Tumors in children. I. Title: Title on contents p.: Central nervous system tumors in children. II. Gupta, N. (Nalin),
1964– III. Banerjee, A. (Anuradha), 1964– IV. Haas-Kogan, D.
(Daphne), 1964– [DNLM: 1. Central Nervous System Neoplasms–Child. WL 358 P3703 2004] RC280.N43P37 2004 618.
92'9928–dc21

Springer-Verlag is a part of Springer Science + Business Media

springeronline.com

© Springer-Verlag Berlin Heidelberg 2004
Printed in Germany

Cover design: E. Kirchner, Heidelberg
Product management and layout: B. Wieland, Heidelberg
Reproduction and typesetting: AM-production, Wiesloch
Printing and bookbinding: Appl, Wemding

21/3150 – 5 4 3 2 1 0
Printed on acid-free paper

Dedication

We dedicate this book to
Heather, Willi and Scott,
as well as to our colleagues and patients.

Preface

Pediatric brain tumors present a tremendous challenge to the physician. Their diverse biological behaviors, in the unique context of the developing nervous system, require flexible and tailored treatment plans. Exponential expansion in our understanding of the molecular and genetic basis of human malignancies has led to the introduction of biologically based therapeutic agents and their incorporation into multimodality approaches to brain tumors. The next 10 years promise great excitement as these agents enter clinical trials and are brought into everyday practice. The goal of this textbook is to provide a concise, current, scientifically based description of the management of central nervous system tumors in children. The epidemiology, pathology, clinical presentation, diagnostic evaluation, treatment, and outcome are provided for selected tumor types in the initial 11 chapters. In the final 4 chapters, many of the diagnostic and treatment modalities common to all tumors are discussed with an emphasis on emerging and experimental techniques. For the interested reader, additional information is available in other general textbooks [1, 2]. The World Health Organization classification is a particularly valuable resource [3].

For the most part, this book outlines the general principles used for management of brain and spinal cord tumors at the University of California, San Francisco. Although this may underemphasize other equally valid approaches, we believe that a consistent management philosophy offers some advantages to the reader. We fully recognize that a variety of effective treatment strategies are utilized by other practitioners and institutions. Finally, we strongly believe that improvements in clinical outcomes for our patients can only happen through participation in well-designed clinical trials. The results from such trials in the past have led to the validation of successful treatment strategies used for many other childhood malignancies.

The editors would like to acknowledge the contribution of the authors, our colleagues at the University of California, San Francisco, the editorial staff at Springer-Verlag, and our many mentors in the preparation of this book. We are indebted to Judi Chesler, who provided endless administrative assistance, and Sharon Reynolds, who carefully edited the various versions of the text.

Nalin Gupta, MD, PhD
Anu Banerjee, MD, MPH
Daphne Haas-Kogan, MD

References
1. Keating RF, Goodrich JT, Packer RJ (eds) (2001) Tumors of the pediatric central nervous system. Thieme, New York
2. Kaye AH, Laws ER (eds) (2001) Brain tumors: an encyclopedic approach. Churchill Livingstone, London
3. Kleihues P, Cavenee WK (eds) (2000) Pathology and genetics of tumors of central nervous system. IARC Press, Lyon

Contributors

Arthur R. Ablin, MD
Professor Emeritus
Division of Pediatric Hematology and Oncology
Department of Pediatrics
University of California, San Francisco
505 Parnassus Ave., Box 0106
San Francisco, California 94143-0106
USA
aablin@itsa.ucsf.edu

Anuradha Banerjee, MD, MPH
Assistant Professor
Division of Neuro-Oncology
Departments of Neurological Surgery and Pediatrics
University of California, San Francisco
400 Parnassus Ave., Box 0372
San Francisco, California 94143-0372
USA
banerjee@neurosurg.ucsf.edu

A. James Barkovich, MD
Professor
Division of Neuroradiology
Departments of Neuroradiology, Neurology,
and Pediatrics
University of California, San Francisco
505 Parnassus Ave., L 371, Box 0628
San Francisco, California 94143-0628
USA
jim.barkovich@radiology.ucsf.edu

Mitchel S. Berger, MD
Professor and Chairman
Department of Neurological Surgery
Director, Brain Tumor Research Center
University of California, San Francisco
505 Parnassus Ave., Rm M779, Box 0112
San Francisco, California 94143-0112
USA
bergerm@neurosurg.ucsf.edu

Sean O. Bryant, MD
Staff Neuroradiologist
Diversified Radiology of Colorado
3900 South Wadsworth Blvd, Suite 210
Lakewood, Colorado 80235
USA
sbryant@divrad.com

Soonmee Cha, MD
Assistant Professor
Division of Neuroradiology
Department of Radiology
University of California, San Francisco
505 Parnassus Ave., L 371, Box 0628
San Francisco, California 94143-0628
USA
soonmee.cha@radiology.ucsf.edu

John H. Chi, MD, MPH
Resident
Department of Neurological Surgery
University of California, San Francisco
505 Parnassus Ave., Box 0112
San Francisco, California 94143-0112
USA
chijo@neurosurg.ucsf.edu

Rose Du, MD, PhD
Resident
Department of Neurological Surgery
University of California, San Francisco
505 Parnassus Ave., Box 0112
San Francisco, California 94143-0112
USA
durose@neurosurg.ucsf.edu

Benjamin M. Fisch, MD
Staff Physician
Alameda Radiation Oncology
27204 Calaroga Avenue
Hayward, California 94545
USA
bfisch@alamedaradonc.com

Paul G. Fisher, MD
Associate Professor
Departments of Neurology, Pediatrics,
and Neurosurgery and Human Biology
Beirne Family Director of Neuro-Oncology
at Packard Children's Hospital
Stanford University
300 Pasteur Drive, Rm A343
Palo Alto, California 94305-5235
USA
pfisher@stanford.edu

Mittul Gulati, MD
Resident
Department of Urology
University of California, Los Angeles
10833 Le Conte Blvd
Los Angeles, California 90095
USA
mgulati@mednet.ucla.edu

Nalin Gupta, MD, PhD
Assistant Professor
Departments of Neurological Surgery and Pediatrics
University of California, San Francisco
505 Parnassus Ave., Rm M779, Box 0112
San Francisco, California 94143-0112
USA
guptan@neurosurg.ucsf.edu

Daphne Haas-Kogan, MD
Associate Professor
Department of Radiation Oncology
University of California, San Francisco
UCSF Comprehensive Cancer Center
1600 Divisidero St., Suite H1031, Box 1708
San Francisco, California 94115-1708
USA
hkogan@radonc17.ucsf.edu

Biljana N. Horn, MD
Assistant Clinical Professor
Division of Pediatric Hematology and Oncology
Department of Pediatrics
University of California, San Francisco
505 Parnassus Ave., Rm M647, Box 0106
San Francisco, California 94143-0106
USA
hornb@peds.ucsf.edu

G. Evren Keles, MD
Assistant Professor
Department of Neurological Surgery
University of California, San Francisco
505 Parnassus Ave, Rm M779, Box 0112
San Francisco, California 94143-0112
USA
kelese@neurosurg.ucsf.edu

Cornelia S. von Koch, MD, PhD
Chief Resident
Department of Neurological Surgery
University of California, San Francisco
505 Parnassus Ave., Rm M779, Box 0112
San Francisco, California 94143-0112
USA
vonkochc@neurosurg.ucsf.edu

Kenneth H. Lieuw, MD, PhD
Clinical Fellow
Division of Pediatric Hematology and Oncology
Department of Pediatrics
University of California, San Francisco
505 Parnassus Ave., Rm M647, Box 0106
San Francisco, California 94143-0106
USA
khlieuw@itsa.ucsf.edu

Robert H. Lustig, MD
Professor
Division of Pediatric Endocrinology
Department of Pediatrics
University of California, San Francisco
513 Parnassus Ave., Rm S679, Box 0434
San Francisco, California 94143-0434
USA
rlustig@peds.ucsf.edu

Katherine K. Matthay, MD
Professor
Chief, Division of Pediatric Hematology
and Oncology
Department of Pediatrics
University of California, San Francisco
505 Parnassus Ave., Rm M647, Box 0106
San Francisco, CA 94143-0106
USA
matthayk@peds.ucsf.edu

Michael W. McDermott, MD, FRCSC
Associate Professor and Vice-Chairman
Department of Neurological Surgery
University of California, San Francisco
505 Parnassus Ave., Rm M779, Box 0112
San Francisco, California 94143-0112
USA
mcdermottm@neurosurg.ucsf.edu

Edward Pan, MD
Co-Medical Director, Neuro-Oncology Center
Florida Hospital Cancer Institute
390 Lakeview St.
Orlando, Florida 32804
USA

Victor L. Perry, MD
Assistant Professor
Division of Pediatric Neurosurgery
Department of Neurological Surgery
University of California, San Francisco
505 Parnassus Ave., Rm M779, Box 0112
San Francisco, California 94143-0112
USA
perryv@neurosurg.ucsf.edu

Michael D. Prados, MD
Professor
Department of Neurological Surgery
Chief, Neuro-Oncology Service
University of California, San Francisco
400 Parnassus Ave., Box 0372
San Francisco, California 94143-0372
USA
pradosm@neurosurg.ucsf.edu

Dev Puri, MD
Resident
School of Radiation Therapy
Memorial Sloan-Kettering Cancer Center
1275 York Avenue
New York City, New York 10021
USA
purid@mskcc.org

Alfredo Quinones-Hinojosa, MD
Resident
Department of Neurological Surgery
University of California, San Francisco
505 Parnassus Ave., Rm M779, Box 0112
San Francisco, California 94143-0112
USA
quinones@neurosurg.ucsf.edu

Meic H. Schmidt, MD
Assistant Professor
Department of Neurological Surgery
Director, Spinal Oncology
University of Utah Medical Center
30 North 1900 East, Suite 3B409
Salt Lake City, Utah 84132
USA
meic.schmidt@hsc.utah.edu

Matthew D. Smyth, MD
Assistant Professor
Department of Neurosurgery
Director, Pediatric Epilepsy Surgery Program
Washington University
and St. Louis Children's Hospital
One Children's Place
St. Louis, Missouri 63110-1077
USA
smythm@nsurg.wustl.edu

Brian S. Tseng, MD, PhD
Assistant Professor
Division of Pediatric Neurology
Department of Pediatrics
University of Colorado and The Children's Hospital
1056 East 19th Ave.
Denver, Colorado 80218
USA

Contents

8   Neuronal Tumors
C. S. von Koch · M. H. Schmidt · V. Perry

9   Choroid Plexus Tumors
N. Gupta

10   Intramedullary Spinal Cord Tumors
A. Quinones-Hinojosa · M. Gulati
M. H. Schmidt

11   Neurocutaneous Syndromes and Associated CNS Tumors

B. S. Tseng · D. Haas-Kogan

12   Modern Neuroimaging of Pediatric CNS Tumors

S. O. Bryant · S. Cha · A. J. Barkovich

Introduction

N. Gupta · D. Haas-Kogan · A. Banerjee

Central nervous system (CNS) tumors are the most common solid tumors of childhood and are second only to leukemia and lymphoma in overall incidence of neoplasia in this age group. Reflecting the cytologic complexity of the CNS, a bewildering variety of tumors are encountered in the brain and spinal cord. Similarly, outcomes range from curable (cerebellar astrocytoma) to those with a uniformly dismal prognosis (diffuse pontine glioma). In the past 20 years, mortality from leukemia has declined faster than from CNS tumors. Consequently, deaths from CNS tumors (0.8 per 100,000 in 1995) now exceed those from acute lymphoblastic leukemia (0.4 per 100,000 in 1995; Bleyer 1999). For these reasons, management of CNS tumors is likely to remain a challenge for the near future.

The evaluation and treatment of these tumors is also complex, given the difficulty of their surgical removal, complications related to treatment, and poor response to therapy in certain situations. For this reason, the management of pediatric CNS tumors has evolved to require a multi-disciplinary effort with participation of subspecialists in pediatric oncology, radiation oncology, and neurosurgery. Although individual practitioners can provide excellent care, the complete spectrum of treatment options can only be delivered in a team environment. In addition, active participation of other members of the health care team such as physical therapists, child life specialists, social workers, and general pediatricians contributes to the optimal care of these patients and their families.

Etiology of Central Nervous System Tumors

Despite the wealth of biologic information available, specific etiologic agents or events responsible for the majority of brain tumors remain unknown. Known risk factors include heritable genetic syndromes (such as neurofibromatosis types 1 and 2, basal cell nevus, tuberous sclerosis, and those of Gorlin, Turcot, Li-Fraumeni, and von Hippel-Lindau), and exposure to therapeutic ionizing radiation. With regard to the latter group, ionizing radiation was used in the early and mid-20th century to treat tinea capitis and thyroid diseases (Ron et al. 1988). Long-term sequelae included meningiomas, gliomas, and nerve sheath tumors. There has been concern regarding potential risks from low-level electromagnetic radiation such as those occurring from high-tension power lines. Ongoing studies over many years have failed to show conclusive evidence for a causative role (Gurney and van Wijngaarden 1999). Similarly, no evidence exists for a linkage between cellular phone use and cancer (Johansen et al. 2001). Except for medulloblastoma and germ cell tumors (occurring more often in males), the incidence is equal in boys and girls. Other risk factors such as maternal consumption of cured meats, and a first degree relative with a brain tumor have been implicated but conclusive evidence is lacking.

Table 1. WHO classification of tumors of the nervous system (Kleihues and Cavenee 2000)

TUMORS OF NEUROEPITHELIAL TISSUE

Astrocytic tumors

Diffuse astrocytoma	9400/3[a]
Fibrillary astrocytoma	9420/3
Protoplasmic astrocytoma	9410/3
Gemistocytic astrocytoma	9411/3
Anaplastic astrocytoma	9401/3
Glioblastoma	9440/3
Giant cell glioblastoma	9441/3
Gliosarcoma	9442/3
Pilocytic astrocytoma	9421/1
Pleomorphic xanthoastrocytoma	9424/3
Subependymal giant cell astrocytoma	9384/1

Oligodendroglial tumors

Oligodendroglioma	9450/3
Anaplastic oligodendroglioma	9451/3

Mixed gliomas

Oligoastrocytoma	9382/3
Anaplastic oligoastrocytoma	9382/3[b]

Ependymal tumors

Ependymoma	9391/3
Cellular	9391/3
Papillary	9393/3
Clear cell	9391/3
Tanycytic	9391/3
Anaplastic ependymoma	9392/3
Myxopapillary ependymoma	9394/1
Subependymoma	9383/1

Choroid plexus tumors

Choroid plexus papilloma	9390/0
Choroid plexus carcinoma	9390/3

Glial tumors of uncertain origin

Astroblastoma	9430/3
Gliomatosis cerebri	9381/3
Chordoid glioma of 3rd ventricle	9444/1

Neuronal and mixed neuronal-glial tumors

Gangliocytoma	9492/0
Dysplastic gangliocytoma of cerebellum (Lhermitte-Duclos)	9493/0

Desmoplastic infantile astrocytoma / ganglioglioma	9412/1
Dysembryoplastic neuroepithelial tumor	9413/0
Ganglioglioma	9505/1
Anaplastic ganglioglioma	9505/3
Central neurocytoma	9506/1
Cerebellar liponeurocytoma	9506/1
Paraganglioma of filum terminale	8680/1

Neuroblastic tumors

Olfactory neuroblastoma (Esthesioneuroblastoma)	9522/3
Olfactory neuroepithelioma	9523/3
Neuroblastomas of the adrenal gland and sympathetic nervous system	9500/3

Pineal parenchymal tumors

Pineocytoma	9361/1
Pineoblastoma	9362/3
Pineal parenchymal tumor of intermediate differentiation	9362/3

Embryonal tumors

Medulloepithelioma	9501/3
Ependymoblastoma	9392/3
Medulloblastoma	9470/3
Desmoplastic medulloblastoma	9471/3
Large cell medulloblastoma	9474/3
Medullomyoblastoma	9472/3
Melanotic medulloblastoma	9470/3
Supratentorial primitive neuroectodermal tumor (PNET)	9473/3
Neuroblastoma	9500/3
Ganglioneuroblastoma	9490/3
Atypical teratoid/rhabdoid tumor	9508/3

TUMORS OF PERIPHERAL NERVES

Schwannoma

(neurilemmoma, neurinoma)	9560/0
Cellular	9560/0
Plexiform	9560/0
Melanotic	9560/0

[a] Morphology code of the International Classification of Diseases for Oncology (ICD-O) and the Systematized Nomenclature of Medicine (SNOMED). Behavior is coded /0 for benign tumors, /1 for low or uncertain malignant potential or borderline malignancy, /2 for in situ lesions and /3 for malignant tumors.

[b] The italicized numbers are provisional codes proposed for the third edition of ICD-O. They should, for the most part, be incorporated into the next edition of ICD-O, but they are subject to changeNeuronal and mixed neuronal-glial tumors

Table 1. (Continued)

Neurofibroma	9540/0	Chondrosarcoma	9220/3
Plexiform	9550/0	Osteoma	9180/0
		Osteosarcoma	9180/3
Perineurioma	*9571/0*	Osteochondroma	9210/0
Intraneural perineurioma	*9571/0*	Hemangioma	9120/0
Soft tissue perineurioma	*9571/0*	Epithelioid hemangioendothelioma	9133/1
		Hemangiopericytoma	9150/1
Malignant peripheral nerve sheath tumor		Angiosarcoma	9120/3
(MPNST)	*9540/3*	Kaposi sarcoma	9140/3
Epithelioid	*9540/3*		
MPNST with divergent mesenchymal		**Primary melanocytic lesions**	
and / or epithelial differentiation	*9540/3*	Diffuse melanocytosis	*8728/0*
Melanotic	*9540/3*	Melanocytoma	*8728/1*
Melanotic psammomatous	*9540/3*	Malignant melanoma	8720/3
		Meningeal melanomatosis	*8728/3*
TUMORS OF THE MENINGES		**Tumors of uncertain histogenesis**	
		Haemangioblastoma	9161/1
Tumors of meningothelial cells			
Meningioma	9530/0		
Meningothelial	9531/0	**LYMPHOMAS AND HAEMOPOIETIC NEOPLASMS**	
Fibrous (fibroblastic)	9532/0		
Transitional (mixed)	9537/0	Malignant lymphomas	9590/3
Psammomatous	9533/0	Plasmacytoma	9731/3
Angiomatous	9534/0	Granulocytic sarcoma	9930/3
Microcystic	*9530/0*		
Secretory	*9530/0*		
Lymphoplasmacyte-rich	*9530/0*	**GERM CELL TUMORS**	
Metaplastic	*9530/0*		
Clear cell	*9538/1*	Germinoma	9064/3
Chordoid	*9538/1*	Embryonal carcinoma	9070/3
Atypical	*9539/1*	Yolk sac tumor	9071/3
Papillary	*9538/3*	Choriocarcinoma	9100/3
Rhabdoid	*9538/3*	Teratoma	9080/1
Anaplastic meningioma	9530/3	Mature	9080/0
		Immature	9080/3
Mesenchymal, non-meningothelial tumors		Teratoma with malignant transformation	9084/3
Lipoma	8850/0	Mixed germ cell tumors	9085/3
Angiolipoma	8861/0		
Hibernoma	8880/0		
Liposarcoma (intracranial)	8850/3	**TUMORS OF THE SELLAR REGION**	
Solitary fibrous tumor	*8815/0*	Craniopharyngioma	9350/1
Fibrosarcoma	8810/3	Adamantinomatous	*9351/1*
Malignant fibrous histiocytoma	8830/3	Papillary	*9352/1*
Leiomyoma	8890/0	Granular cell tumor	*9582/0*
Leiomyosarcoma	8890/3		
Rhabdomyoma	8900/0		
Rhabdomyosarcoma	8900/3	**METASTATIC TUMORS**	
Chondroma	9220/0		

Classification of CNS Tumors

The nomenclature and classification of all brain tumors has evolved over the past few decades. Common tumor types such as astrocytoma, pituitary adenoma, and meningioma are readily recognized by standard histopathology. Most tumors within these groups can be diagnosed with reasonable consistency by most neuropathologists. Beyond the initial diagnosis, great controversy has arisen over matters such as grading of astrocytomas, immunophenotype of pituitary adenoma, and classification of primitive undifferentiated tumors, to name a few examples. The overall trend is toward greater standardization in the diagnosis and classification.

The most commonly used classification of CNS tumors is the one developed and adopted by the World Health Organization (WHO; Table 1; Kleihues and Cavenee 2000). This classification is still rooted in the tradition of histologic appearance that is the basis of virtually all modern pathology. It should be appreciated that the expanding impact of molecular classification will likely change how tumors are both divided and treated in the near future (Pollack et al. 2002). Two recent publications suggest how molecular features are likely to improve prognostication and treatment planning. Pollack et al. (2002) noted a marked difference in survival in a group of children with high-grade astrocytomas whose tumors had low expression of p53 protein. This group had a progression-free survival of approximately 44 months compared to patients with increased expression of p53 whose survival was 17 months. It should be noted that conventional histology would not have identified this subgroup from the overall group of patients with high-grade astrocytomas. In another example, Pomeroy et al. (2002) using gene expression arrays, stated that medulloblastoma tumors differ from other embryonal tumors, and furthermore, subgroups defined by patterns of gene expression predict clinical outcome. Although standardization and widespread acceptance are limited, these types of molecular classification are likely to change how we view and treat tumors within histology-based categories.

Epidemiology of Childhood CNS Tumors

In both the popular and scientific literature, the incidence of childhood brain tumors is reported to be increasing. The epidemiologic data do suggest such a trend but the actual details are unclear. Two fundamental problems exist. First is a lack of consistent definitions and pathologic criteria for various tumor types over time. This remains a problem despite the availability of the WHO classification system. Second is the lack of truly inclusive tumor registries by organ site. In the United States, comprehensive national data for cancer incidence are not available. Rather, data from nine registries have been compiled since 1973 by the National Cancer Institute as the Surveillance, Epidemiology, and End Results (SEER) program and extrapolated to represent national data. These data demonstrate an overall incidence of CNS cancer to be 3.5 per 100,000 children <15 years of age (Ries et al. 2000). If all CNS neoplasms are included, the SEER incidence data may be low. One report suggests that if benign tumors were accurately included in the SEER database, the overall incidence of brain tumors might be 72% higher (Gurney and Kadan-Lottick 2001). An additional source of information is a report from the Central Brain Tumor Registry of the United States (CBTRUS), a non-profit agency organized for the purpose of collecting and publishing epidemiologic data for brain tumors (CBTRUS 2002). The incidence data published by this group are similar to those published by other groups (Table 2).

Some of the most robust data is reported from countries with small homogeneous populations. In a population-based study from Sweden, the overall incidence of primary brain tumors in children was 35.9/million children; with 29.6/million of the overall group being malignant (Hjalmars et al. 1999). An advantage of this study, besides a homogeneous data base, is pathological confirmation for the majority of registered cases. Over the twenty year study period, a small but measurable increase in malignant tumors was reported. A few limitations are noted. The authors include Grade I and II astrocytomas in the malignant group, which creates the impression that the majority of childhood tumors are malignant and skews incidence data for this subgroup. If Grade I and II astrocytomas are included in the benign category, as some authors would, the majority of tumors would be considered benign. Whether an increase in the incidence of malignant tumors would still be observed is unclear. Another national study from Denmark examined the incidence of intracranial brain tumor from 1960–1984. The annual incidence was 32.5/million children <15 years of age. The incidence increased slightly over the time period studied. This study is limited because it came prior to modern imaging techniques, before the "jump" in incidence noted in other registries in the mid to late 1980s (see below).

A recent report examining incidence of childhood cancer based on SEER data revealed that while there was a modest increase in CNS tumors, most of the increase was clustered in the early 1980s with stability thereafter (Gurney and Kadan-Lottick 2001). Another analysis suggested that increases in this time period, the "jump", could be best explained by improved detection and imaging (Smith et al. 1998). The difficulty with this conclusion is that if improved diagnosis created an artificial increase in incidence, then incidence should return to the previous levels once the prevalent cases are detected. This correction has not occurred. Data from the CBTRUS appear to confirm that overall incidence of brain tumors (adult and pediatric) has increased; however, when the diagnosis of primary CNS lymphoma was excluded, a statistically significant change was not observed (Jukich et al. 2001). Presumably, this was due to the effect of AIDS-related CNS lymphoma, and lymphoma occurring in the elderly population impacting overall brain tumor incidence.

McNeil et al. (2002) observe that as a group, the incidence of medulloblastoma and primitive neuroectodermal tumor (PNET) rose 23% from 1973 to 1998. This report appears to be convincing but a closer examination of the data reveals that the rates of medulloblastoma have remained unchanged while those of PNET have risen from virtually zero in 1982 to 2/million by 1998. The authors recognize that changes in diagnostic criteria have occurred and that the "nosology have been under revision." Changes in nomenclature are likely to account at least in part for

the increase reported. Furthermore, a selected review of the SEER data by diagnosis cannot exclude the possibility that PNET tumors were being attributed to other categories before 1982.

As measured by survival, the impact of CNS tumors on the population affected is substantial. These tumors are exceedingly heterogeneous and survival is affected by factors such as age, histology, size, stage, and location within the CNS. From the SEER data, between 1985–1994 the 5 year survival for all CNS tumors was 45% for children <1 year of age, 59% for 1 to 4 years, 64% for 5 to 9 years, 70% for 10 to 14 years, and 77% for 15 to 19 years. Astrocytoma carries the best prognosis, with PNET next, followed by ependymoma, and then brainstem glioma.

In conclusion, although the majority of data suggest a slight increase in the incidence of CNS tumors, this finding is not accepted by all investigators. Some suggest that changing diagnostic criteria and classification account for the increased incidence.

Future Directions

The primary areas of research in the diagnosis and treatment of pediatric brain tumors are molecular phenotyping, development of biologically directed therapies, and application of functional data to increase the safety and extent of surgical resection. As described in the various chapters of this monograph, the molecular and genetic profiles of various tumors are much better defined through the use of established techniques such as comparative genomic hybridization, gene sequencing, and in situ hybridization. Newer technologies such as gene, protein, and chromosome arrays will lead to an improved classification system of tumors based on genotype and phenotype correlations, rather than on histopathology alone. Identification of molecular alterations should lead to more refined and effective agents that can be used in multimodality settings. The ultimate goal, not yet realized, is to prescribe therapy tailored to the exact biologic features of a given tumor.

From a practical perspective, rapid advances are being made in the diagnostic and therapeutic specialties and these are defined in greater detail in

Chapters 12–15. Advanced imaging techniques coupled with surgery, radiation, and chemotherapy should further improve results. Specific future surgical goals include delivery of local agents using new techniques such as direct convection-enhanced delivery, and mapping of functional cortex to allow increased extent of resection.

References

Bleyer WA (1999) Epidemiologic impact of children with brain tumors. Childs Nerv Syst 15:758–763

CBTRUS (2002) Statistical report: primary brain tumors in the United States, 1995–1999. Central Brain Tumor Registry of the United States

Gurney JG, Kadan-Lottick N (2001) Brain and other central nervous system tumors: rates, trends, and epidemiology. Curr Opin Oncol 13:160–166

Gurney JG, van Wijngaarden E (1999) Extremely low frequency electromagnetic fields (EMF) and brain cancer in adults and children: review and comment. Neuro-oncol 1:212–220

Hjalmars U, Kulldorff M, Wahlqvist Y et al (1999) Increased incidence rates but no space-time clustering of childhood astrocytoma in Sweden, 1973–1992: a population-based study of pediatric brain tumors. Cancer 85:2077–2090

Johansen C, Boice J Jr, McLaughlin J et al (2001) Cellular telephones and cancer–a nationwide cohort study in Denmark. J Natl Cancer Inst 93:203–207

Jukich PJ, McCarthy BJ, Surawicz TS et al (2001) Trends in incidence of primary brain tumors in the United States, 1985–1994. Neuro-oncol 3:141–151

Kleihues P. Cavenee WK eds. (2000). Pathology and genetics of tumours of the nervous system. Lyon, IARC Press

McNeil DE, Cote TR, Clegg L et al (2002) Incidence and trends in pediatric malignancies medulloblastoma/primitive neuroectodermal tumor: a SEER update. Surveillance epidemiology and end results. Med Pediatr Oncol 39:190–194

Pollack IF, Biegel J, Yates A et al (2002) Risk assignment in childhood brain tumors: the emerging role of molecular and biologic classification. Curr Oncol Rep 4:114–122

Pollack IF, Finkelstein SD, Woods J et al (2002) Expression of p53 and prognosis in children with malignant gliomas. N Engl J Med 346:420–427

Pomeroy SL, Tamayo P, Gaasenbeek M et al (2002) Prediction of central nervous system embryonal tumour outcome based on gene expression. Nature 415:436–442

Ries LAG, Eisner MP, Kosary CL et al eds. (2000) SEER cancer statistics review 1975–2000. Bethesda, National Cancer Institute

Ron E, Modan B, Boice JDJr et al (1988) Tumors of the brain and nervous system after radiotherapy in childhood. N Engl J Med 319:1033–1039

Smith MA, Freidlin B, Ries LA et al (1998) Trends in reported incidence of primary malignant brain tumors in children in the United States. J Natl Cancer Inst 90:1269–1277

Supratentorial Gliomas

G. Evren Keles · A. Banerjee
D. Puri · M. S. Berger

Contents

1.1 Introduction

Astrocytomas constitute approximately half of all pediatric supratentorial tumors. The most common histologic subtypes are pilocytic and fibrillary astrocytomas, which are considered low-grade astrocytomas. A variety of other, less common glial tumors are also seen in this region, including pleomorphic xanthoastrocytoma, subependymal giant cell astrocytoma, high-grade gliomas, ganglioglioma and desmoplastic infantile ganglioglioma, astroblastoma, ependymoma, and oligodendroglioma. This chapter will focus on low-grade and high-grade astrocytomas, optic pathway gliomas, and oligodendrogliomas. The majority of the other tumor types are discussed in other sections of this text.

1.2 Astrocytomas

1.2.1 Epidemiology

Supratentorial tumors account for 40–60 % of all pediatric brain tumors, and are almost twice as common in infants as in older children (Dohrmann et al. 1985; Dropcho et al. 1987; Farwell et al. 1977). The majority of supratentorial tumors are gliomas (astrocytoma, oligodendroglioma, and ependymoma) with the most common subtype being low-grade gliomas, which constitute approximately half of this group. In contrast to the distribution of gliomas in adults, malignant gliomas account for only 20 % of all childhood supratentorial gliomas.

For the majority of gliomas, the etiology is unknown. Children with familial cancer predisposition syndromes have an increased risk of developing both low-grade and high-grade glioma. In particular, children with neurofibromatosis type 1 (NF1) have an increased risk of developing astrocytomas (see Chap. 11). Although the usual location of astrocytomas in patients with NF1 are the optic nerves, optic chiasm, hypothalamus, and/or brainstem, astrocytomas may also occur within the cerebral hemispheres (Listernick et al. 1999). For unknown reasons, the incidence is higher in females (Airewele et al. 2001). Patients with Li-Fraumeni syndrome, arising from a germline mutation in the p53 tumor suppressor gene, have an increased risk of developing a heterogeneous group of tumors, including malignant astrocytoma and glioblastoma multiforme. Primary CNS malignancies typically present in young adulthood in patients with Li-Fraumeni syndrome (Kleihues et al. 1997; Varley et al. 1997).

The only environmental agent clearly associated with increased risk of developing glioma is exposure to ionizing radiation, which results in a 2.6-fold increased risk of developing glioma (Ron et al. 1988). Recent case reports have implied that radiation-induced mutagen sensitivity of lymphocytes may be associated with an increased risk for glioma (Bondy et al. 2001).

1.2.2 Pathology

1.2.2.1 Low-Grade Astrocytoma

According to the World Health Organization classification, grade I astrocytomas are limited to non-infiltrating pilocytic tumors (also known as juvenile pilocytic astrocytoma, or JPA). The most common location for JPA is within the cerebellar hemispheres (see Chap. 2), although they also occur within the cerebral hemispheres, brainstem, and spinal cord. In general, JPAs tend to be well circumscribed and do not infiltrate into the surrounding brain. The one exception is optic pathway glioma, a subtype of JPA that arises within the visual pathways and typically presents with visual loss. These gliomas can infiltrate widely, even into the visual cortex. This subtype is discussed in greater detail in Sect. 1.3.

Grade II astrocytomas are distinct from pilocytic tumors in their location, degree of infiltration, and presence of genetic aberrations (Kleihues and Cavenee 2000). Grossly, grade II astrocytomas are ill-defined lesions which tend to enlarge and distort involved structures. Destruction of brain tissue, however, is more characteristic of higher-grade tumors. Microscopic examination of resected tumor specimens invariably shows diffuse infiltration of the surrounding gray and white matter. Low-power microscopy may show a subtle increase in overall cellularity, and disruption of the orderly pattern of glial cells along myelinated fibers. Higher-power examination demonstrates neoplastic astrocytes with indistinct cytoplasmic features. The diagnosis is often based on the appearance of the nuclei, which are characteristically elongated. Nuclear atypia is minimal in low-grade astrocytomas and mitotic activity is infrequent.

1.2.2.2 Other Low-Grade Subtypes

Low-grade astrocytomas can be further subdivided on the basis of their microscopic appearance. The prognostic value of these subgroups is not entirely clear. While the diffuse fibrillary astrocytoma is the most common grade II astrocytoma, a number of other variants are described. Gemistocytic astrocytomas are composed of neoplastic astrocytes with abundant eosinophilic, glial fibrillary acidic protein (GFAP)-positive cytoplasm. The WHO recognizes the gemistocytic subtype as low-grade astrocytoma, as long as cellularity and nuclear atypia remain mild (Kleihues and Cavenee 2000). Pleomorphic xanthoastrocytoma (PXA), a newly described subtype, is a rare, GFAP-positive astrocytic tumor typically occurring in the cerebral hemispheres of children and young adults (Kepes et al. 1973). Histologically, PXA is characterized by extreme pleomorphism with large, neoplastic astrocytic cells. The neoplastic astrocytes display substantial nuclear pleomorphism and very atypical nuclei. The borders are often infiltrative, and tumor cells may display clustering in an epitheliod fashion (Lindboe et al. 1992; Powell et al. 1996). Desmoplastic infantile astrocytoma (DIA) is a rare tumor occurring in infants of up to 18 months of age. Grossly, these tumors are typically large, cystic, supratentorial in location, and have a dural attachment. The histologic appearance demonstrates loose to dense collagenous stroma with wavy fascicles of spindle cells (Taratuto et al. 1984). The rarest subtype is the protoplasmic astrocytoma, which has prominent microcysts, mucoid degeneration, and a paucity of GFAP positivity. Some consider this a histological pattern of fibrillary astrocytoma, rather than a true variant. Regardless of subtype, all low-grade astrocytomas have low cellularity, limited nuclear atypia, and rare mitotic activity. Low-grade astrocytomas with a single mitotic figure behave more like a low-grade tumor with respect to prognosis (Giannini et al. 1999). If confirmed, this suggests that the finding of isolated mitoses may not be sufficient to upgrade an otherwise low-grade astrocytoma to a higher-grade lesion.

1.2.2.3 Anaplastic Astrocytoma and Glioblastoma Multiforme

Anaplastic astrocytoma (WHO grade III) and glioblastoma multiforme (GBM, WHO grade IV) are both diffusely infiltrative, malignant gliomas. In addition to high mitotic activity, the main cellular feature of malignant glial cells is local tissue invasion, which typically occurs along the path of deep white matter tracts, e.g., corpus callosum, anterior commissure, fornix, and internal capsule. When malignant astrocytomas demonstrate diffuse infiltration as the primary feature from the outset, often throughout the entire hemisphere, the condition is termed gliomatosis cerebri.

Compared to grade II astrocytoma, anaplastic astrocytoma exhibits greater cellularity, nuclear atypia, a high degree of cellular pleomorphism, and the presence of multiple mitotic figures. The diagnosis of GBM is usually made by the additional presence of necrosis or microvascular proliferation. GBMs are usually circumscribed in appearance but the borders are poorly defined. As the name implies, the character of the tumor is heterogeneous; firm areas alternate with soft or cystic regions, and mottled areas of hemorrhage and necrosis give the gross specimen an overall moth-eaten appearance. The central area of low attenuation on neuroimaging studies corresponds to confluent areas of tissue necrosis and degeneration. This central area is often surrounded by an irregular zone of denser, more vascular tissue that corresponds to the area of higher attenuation and contrast enhancement. Finally, there is a peripheral zone of lesser cell density, edema, and microscopic tumor infiltration. This peripheral zone may vary in contour, with finger-like projections extending from the main tumor bulk. Significant variation in cellularity is often seen in different parts of the tumor, which can lead to misdiagnosis if the tumor is sampled incompletely.

1.2.2.4 Genetics

Cytogenetic abnormalities occur less frequently and with different patterns in children when compared to adult patients (Cheng et al. 1999). As expected, lower-grade tumors have fewer abnormalities compared to higher-grade tumors. In a recent study of 58 pediatric patients, 70% of grade I astrocytomas had a normal cytogenetic profile (Roberts et al. 2001). In another study of 109 pediatric brain tumors, low-grade astrocytomas showed mostly changes in chromosome copy number (Neumann et al. 1993). Higher-grade tumors in this study, especially ependymomas, demonstrated cytogenetic alterations that differed from abnormalities reported in adult cases. Molecular alterations in pediatric astrocytomas also differ from adult tumors. Mutation of p53, which is the only molecular genetic alteration consistently observed in otherwise healthy adult patients with low-grade astrocytomas, is not a frequent finding in the pediatric age group (Felix et al. 1995; Litofsky et al. 1994). Molecular characteristics of pediatric high-grade astrocytomas, however, include defects similar to those seen in adult high-grade astrocytomas. Pollack et al. in a study of 148 children with high-grade gliomas recently identified a subgroup of patients in whom overexpression of p53 correlated with a poorer overall prognosis (Pollack et al. 2002).

1.2.3 Clinical Features

Exact symptoms and signs caused by supratentorial gliomas depend upon the anatomic location, biologic aggressiveness of the tumor, and age of the patient. These signs and symptoms may be nonspecific, such as those associated with increased intracranial pressure (ICP), or may be focal and related to the location of the tumor. Nonspecific symptoms include headache, nausea and vomiting, subtle developmental delay, and behavioral changes. Some of the behavioral changes associated with slow-growing tumors in children include alterations in personality, irritability, altered psychomotor function, apathy, and declining school performance. It is not uncommon for symptoms to have been present for months or years prior to diagnosis. In infants with open cranial sutures, a tumor may reach a massive size with a gradual increase in head circumference without signs of increased ICP or any other symptoms. Focal symptoms depending on the location of the tumor include hemiparesis, monoparesis, hemisensory loss, dysphasia, aphasia, and impairment of recent memory. Tumors involving the optic pathways can present with quadrantanopsia or homonymous hemianopsia, and in cases with bilateral occipital lobe involvement, cortical blindness may result.

Epilepsy is the major presenting feature of pediatric patients with brain tumors; seizures occur in more than 50 % of children with hemispheric tumors (Keles and Berger 2000). The majority of patients with tumor-associated epilepsy harbor slow-growing, indolent neoplasms such as low-grade gliomas. Other relatively slow-growing tumors, e.g., astrocytomas, gangliogliomas, and oligodendrogliomas, may also present with a history of generalized seizures. Rapidly growing lesions are more likely to produce complex partial motor or sensory seizures, although generalized tonic–clonic seizures are also common. Malignant gliomas are less frequently associated with seizures and are more likely to cause focal neurologic deficits, mainly due to infiltration of normal tissue or local mass effect.

1.2.4 Diagnostic Imaging

Magnetic resonance imaging (MRI) and computerized tomography (CT) are essential tools in the diagnosis and treatment of brain tumors. Although CT is more commonly available, MRI provides higher sensitivity in differentiating tumor tissue from normal brain, allowing more detailed anatomic characterization of the lesion, and should be obtained in all children with a diagnosis of a brain tumor. A complete series should include the following sequences: T1-weighted axial and coronal (both before and after gadolinium), T2-weighted axial and coronal, and fluid attenuated inversion recovery (FLAIR). In addition, sagittal plane sequences are helpful in defining the anatomy of suprasellar and midline tumors. Other sequences such as fat suppression and MR angiography may also be required in specific situations. Newer techniques, such as MR spectroscopy, functional MRI, and perfusion measurements offer the potential of obtaining biochemical and functional information noninvasively (see Chap. 12). It is possible that in the future a pathologic diagnosis may be reached with substantial confidence without the need for open biopsy.

Although low-grade gliomas may produce considerable mass effect upon surrounding structures, neurological deficits may be minimal due to the slow growth of these tumors and the absence of tissue destruction. Low-grade astrocytomas typically appear as a non-enhancing iso- or hypodense mass on CT scan. Calcification may be detected in 15–20 % of cases, and mild to moderate inhomogeneous contrast enhancement can be seen in up to 40 % of all cases (Scott et al. 2002; Roberts et al. 2000; Bauman et al. 1999; Lote et al. 1998). Some tumors, characteristically JPAs, may have cystic changes. On MRI, T1-weighted images show a iso- to hypointense non-enhancing mass which is hyperintense on T2-weighted images. Low-grade astrocytomas have minimal to no contrast enhancement following gadolinium administration (Fig. 1.1c,d). For this reason, the tumor boundary is difficult to determine with any T1-weighted sequence. Fortunately, the FLAIR sequence is ideal for defining the extent of tumor infiltration (Fig. 1.1a,bd).

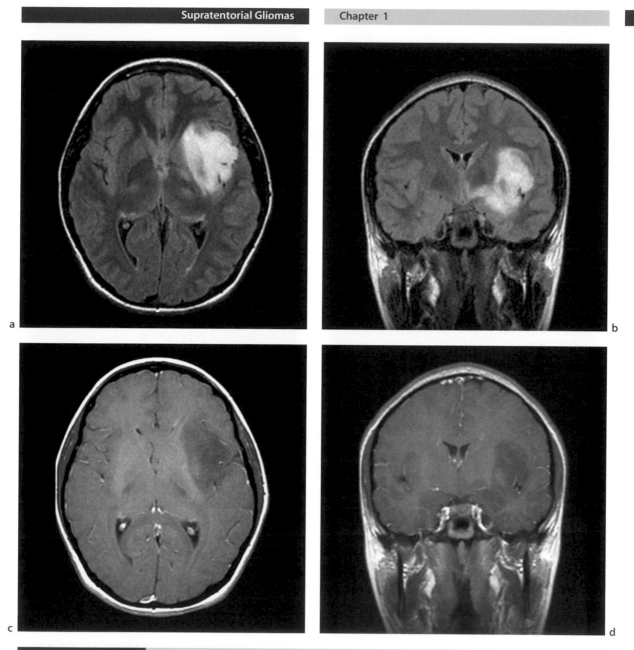

Figure 1.1 a–d

MR images from a teenage girl with a low-grade astrocytoma of the insula who presented with a single seizure. Her neurologic exam was normal. a, b Axial and coronal FLAIR images showing the extent of involvement. Note the tumor infiltration medially under the lentiform nucleus towards the hypothalamus. c, d Corresponding T1-weighted post-gadolinium images showing no appreciable enhancement

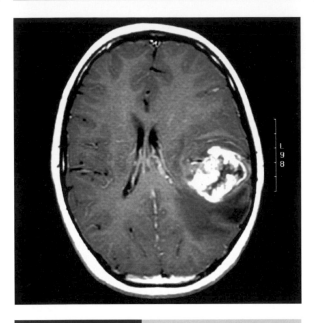

Figure 1.2

A post-gadolinium T1-weighted MR image of a teenage boy with a GBM who presented with dysphasia. A large tumor in the left frontoparietal area is visible. The margin of the tumor enhances, a central necrotic area is visible, and the low-signal region surrounding the mass represents tumor-associated edema

On T1-weighted images, GBM often demonstrates a central area of low density corresponding to necrosis. This area is surrounded by an area of high density that enhances with contrast and corresponds to actively dividing, proliferating tumor cells. A third low-attenuation area around the tumor is often seen, representing tumor-associated vasogenic edema but also containing infiltrating tumor cells (Fig. 1.2). Peritumoral edema surrounding most high-grade astrocytomas is easily seen as a hyperintense region of signal abnormality on T2-weighted images. The extent of peritumoral edema is underestimated on T1-weighted images.

Recurrence is an unavoidable feature of most glial neoplasms. For this reason, serial imaging over time is often the only method of determining whether tumor progression has occurred. For low-grade astro-cytomas, high-quality MRI scans should be obtained every six months. If there is concern that any changes have occurred, the interval should be decreased to three months. In general, for Grade II astrocytoma, the two most important features are an increase in the volume of T2-weighted abnormality, and/or new enhancement on post-gadolinium T1-weighted images. These features are also observed in patients who have received radiation treatment; differentiating tumor recurrence from radiation necrosis continues to present a challenge. Additional information can be obtained from MR spectroscopy and PET scans, but at times a surgical biopsy to obtain tissue is only way to confirm the diagnosis.

1.2.5 Treatment

1.2.5.1 Surgical Indications

A surgical procedure is usually the initial step in the management of supratentorial astrocytomas. The primary objective is to obtain tissue for pathological diagnosis. (The exception to this would be location-specific tumors such as optic pathway/chiasmatic gliomas.) For deep lesions or those in eloquent cortex, a stereotactic needle biopsy may be the only surgical option. The secondary objective is to perform as extensive a resection as possible with acceptable neurologic outcome for the patient. The two variables that must be considered are the extent and timing of resection. The prognostic importance of radical resection is documented for high-grade lesions, but the role of aggressive resection remains unclear for low-grade astrocytomas (Pollack et al. 1995; Campbell et al. 1996; Wisoff et al. 1998; Finlay and Wisoff 1999). In adults, there is evidence that the greater the extent of resection, the more favorable the outcome (Keles et al. 2001). The feasibility of an open surgical approach depends upon several factors. The most important is the exact location of the tumor. Lesions within the basal ganglia, thalamus, motor cortex, or brainstem are not amenable to open surgical resection, while tumors in other locations can be accessed through various standard approaches. Other factors that modify the decision to attempt a resective procedure are the patient's clinical condition, age, associated hydro-cephalus, and the surgeon's assessment of risk of neu-rologic sequelae. Technical adjuncts that allow safer resections in the supratentorial compartment are de-scribed in Chap. 13.

A second variable, aside from the decision to re-sect, is the timing of the procedure. This is a contro-versial topic and few conclusive studies have been published. There are reports questioning the value of immediate treatment when an imaging study sug-gests a low-grade glioma, as no definitive evidence exists demonstrating improvement in long-term sur-vival following early intervention (Cairncross and Laperriere 1989; Recht et al. 1992).

In addition to reduction of tumor burden and pro-viding a tissue diagnosis, resection permits manage-ment of increased ICP, prevention of an irreversible neurological deficit, decompression of adjacent brain structures, and control of seizures (Berger et al. 1991, 1993; Haglund et al. 1992; Keles and Berger 2000). For patients with discrete JPAs (WHO grade I), gross to-tal resection, when possible, is curative (see Chap. 2). Contemporary neurosurgical methods, including ul-trasonography, functional mapping, frameless navi-gational resection devices, and intraoperative imag-ing techniques enable more extensive resections with less morbidity. These techniques and intraoperative considerations specific to the pediatric age group are discussed in detail in Chap. 13.

1.2.5.2 Chemotherapy for Low-Grade Astrocytoma

Overall 5-year survival rates for patients with dien-cephalic and hemispheric tumors who have received radiation therapy range from 40% to 70%. Addition-ally, the morbidity associated with radiation treat-ment can be substantial, prompting numerous inves-tigators to explore chemotherapy as an alternative adjuvant treatment to control tumor progression. Chemotherapy effectively provides disease control in many optic pathway tumors (see section 1.3), and may improve prognosis for vision. Studies of early combination chemotherapy regimens with vincris-tine and actinomycin D, used in children less than

6 years of age, reported 62% progression-free surviv-al (PFS) without further therapy; those who did progress did so at a median of 3 years from start of therapy. The median post-treatment IQ in this group was 103 (Packer et al. 1988). It is important to recog-nize that prolonged periods of stable tumor size is considered a treatment "response" by many investi-gators. Alternative combination chemotherapy regi-mens have also been found to be associated with tu-mor responses in pilot studies. Other drug combina-tions that have been reported include lomustine and vincristine; procarbazine, lomustine, and vincristine (TPCV); and combinations using cisplatin (Edwards et al. 1980; Gajjar et al. 1993). The combination regi-men of carboplatin and vincristine has been associ-ated with objective response rates (stable disease as well as tumor shrinkage) in the range 60 to 70% (Packer et al. 1997). The combination of 6-thiogua-nine, procarbazine, lomustine, and vincristine (TPCV) has also been associated with a substantial response rate in a small cohort of patients (Prados et al. 1997). The relative effectiveness of carboplatin and vincristine versus TPCV is currently being evaluated in a randomized, phase III multi-institutional clinical trial conducted by the Children's Oncology group.

1.2.5.3 Chemotherapy for High-Grade Glioma

The effectiveness of adjuvant chemotherapy in con-junction with radiation for high-grade glioma is un-certain. A Phase III, randomized trial conducted by the Children's Cancer Group (CCG) established the role of chemotherapy. Children with high-grade glio-ma were randomized postoperatively to receive radi-ation therapy with or without chemotherapy with prednisone, lomustine, and vincristine. Children who had received postradiation chemotherapy had im-proved progression-free survival (46%) over those who did not (26%; Sposto et al. 1989). This benefit was most apparent in patients with glioblastoma multiforme who had at least partial resection of their tumor. A subsequent CCG study compared an inten-sive "eight drugs in one day" regimen to the more standard regimen of prednisone, vincristine, and lo-mustine. No difference in progression-free survival was seen between these regimens (5 year PFS 33% vs. 36%; Finlay et al. 1995). Based on these data, addition of adjuvant chemotherapy in addition to radiation appears to provide a small improvement in survival, and standard agents are lomustine and vincristine, in combination with procarbazine (PCV). Other drugs that have been investigated in single agent trials include cisplatin, carboplatin, cylophosphamide, ifosfamide, etoposide, and topotecan. Few have shown enough promise to warrant further investigation in phase III trials (Longee et al. 1990; Phuphanich et al. 1984; Walker et al. 1978; Chintagumpala et al. 2000). A recently published trial in adult patients with glioblastoma multiforme showed improved survival with the addition of temozolomide to radiation therapy (Stupp et al. 2002), and a recently reported phase II trial from the UK Children's Cancer Study Group showed modest response rates to temozolomide in children with recurrent and refractory malignant glioma (Lashford et al. 2002). Irinotecan has also been reported to have promising response rates in a small sample of patients with recurrent or refractory malignant glioma (Turner et al. 2002). These agents continue to undergo investigation. High-dose, myeloablative chemotherapy with autologous hematopoietic stem-cell rescue has been explored, with the intent to defer or delay radiation therapy. While this strategy has shown tumor responses, no convincing evidence exists to date showing improved survival over standard regimens (Mason et al. 1998; Heideman et al. 1993; Finley et al. 1996; Grovas et al. 1999; Bouffet et al. 1997). Notably, however, these trials typically enroll a heterogeneous group of patients, and the number of patients with high-grade glioma in these trials remains small. Strategies incorporating both myeloablative therapy and radiation therapy are currently under investigation.

1.2.5.4 Radiation Therapy

As discussed above, low-grade astrocytoma may be curable with gross total resection. For those patients with incompletely resected or unresectable disease, the use of radiation therapy is controversial. There is some evidence to suggest that while radiation therapy may prolong PFS, it has little impact on overall survival (Pollack et al. 1995). Its use is largely limited to patients with progressive or recurrent disease, or in the setting of a highly symptomatic patient who requires tumor stabilization to avert progression of symptoms.

Children treated with postoperative radiation therapy for incompletely resected, supratentorial high-grade glioma have a median survival of 18 months (Bloom et al. 1990; Dropcho et al. 1987; Marchese et al. 1990). Numerous questions about the optimal use of radiation for these patients remain, including the radiation field, and the utility of dose "boosting" techniques such as brachytherapy and stereotactic radiosurgery to increase the dose delivered to the tumor bed.

1.2.6 Outcome

Age and histological type are significant prognostic predictors. Although patients appear to benefit from more extensive resections, this issue remains controversial. In the majority of patients with tumor-associated epilepsy, including those patients with malignant astrocytomas, the seizures are infrequent and easily controlled with one antiepileptic drug. In this setting, removal of the tumor alone usually controls the epilepsy without the need for additional anticonvulsants. Children with indolent tumors, however, may have seizure activity that is refractory to medical therapy. Optimal control of the epilepsy without postoperative anticonvulsants in this situation is provided when extraoperative or intraoperative electrocorticographic mapping of separate seizure foci accompanies the tumor resection. When mapping is not utilized and a radical tumor resection is carried out with adjacent brain, the occurrence of seizures will be lessened, but most patients will have to remain on antiepileptic drugs (Berger et al. 1991/1992).

Dedifferentiation or malignant transformation is a well-described phenomenon in low-grade gliomas (Fig. 1.3). The incidence of recurrence at a higher histological grade ranges from 13% to 86% of tumors initially diagnosed as low grade (Keles et al. 2001). Similar to its broad range of incidence, the time to malignant differentiation is also variable, ranging

Figure 1.3 a,b

Low-grade astrocytoma can recur at higher grade. **a** Initial MRI
demonstrates a non-enhancing
mass in the left parietal lobe. Pathology was consistent with
Grade II astrocytoma. **b** Five
years later, follow-up imaging
demonstrates a new area of enhancement posterior to the
original tumor. Pathology of the
enhancing component was consistent with GBM

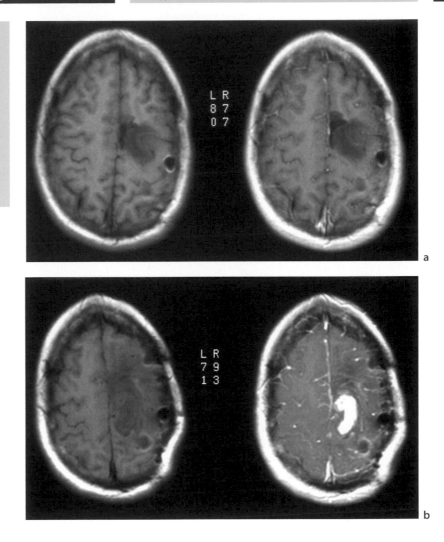

from 28 to 60 months. However, the factors resulting in the change to a malignant phenotype remain unclear. In a recent study investigating the relationship between anaplastic transformation and patient's age, a strong inverse relationship was found between age at initial diagnosis and time to progression to a higher-grade glioma (Shafqat et al. 1999).

For both low- and high-grade astrocytomas, the degree of cytoreduction achieved as measured by extent of resection appears to correlate with outcome and quality of life (Campbell et al. 1996; Keles et al. 2001; Pollack et al. 1995; Wolff et al. 2002). Patients with gross total resection live longer than those with partial resection, who in turn live longer than those who have biopsy only. A further consideration is that partial resection is often accompanied by significant postoperative edema surrounding residual tumor tissue along with increased neurological morbidity. However, the literature regarding the prognostic impact of surgery is controversial, and the controversy is mainly due to the lack of randomized studies addressing the issue. An additional complicating factor is the inconsistent and subjective methodology used in determining extent of resection.

Overall, PFS at 3 years ranges from 61% to 75% for patients with low-grade gliomas (Packer et al. 1997; Gururangan et al. 2002). These patients have a 10-year survival rate of 70 to 90%. Children with anaplastic gliomas who receive a gross total resection followed by local radiation therapy have a 40 to 50% 5-year survival rate (Sposto et al. 1989). Those patients with glioblastoma multiforme have a 20% survival rate after total resection and adjuvant therapy. Patients with subtotally resected glioblastoma multiforme rarely survive (Finlay et al. 1995).

1.3 Optic Pathway Gliomas

Optic pathway gliomas are a fascinating subset of low-grade astrocytomas that occur in some or all anatomical compartments of the optic pathway (optic nerve, chiasm, tract, or radiations). They grow as infiltrative lesions although large, expansile masses are also noted. Their borders are often poorly defined radiologically and a surgical plane is rarely observed. Because of their infiltrative nature, these tumors are often not confined to a single anatomic area and can extend into adjacent structures, most commonly into the hypothalamus. For this reason, naming these lesions according to their exact anatomical location may be misleading especially for tumors with radiologically ill-defined borders. As only 10% of optic nerve gliomas are confined to one optic nerve, and approximately 30% are bilateral, the majority of optic nerve gliomas involve the chiasm or the hypothalamus (Hoffman and Rutka 1999). Optic chiasmatic and hypothalamic gliomas are often considered as a single entity because of their potential to infiltrate both anatomical sites regardless of the original location of the tumor.

1.3.1 Epidemiology

Optic pathway gliomas account for 4 to 6% of all central nervous system tumors in the pediatric age group, 2% in adults, and 20 to 30% of all pediatric gliomas (Packer et al. 1999; Alvord and Lofton 1988; Borit and Richardson 1982; Farwell et al. 1977). The peak incidence is during the first decade with no sex predilection. Overall, neurofibromatosis (NF) is present in approximately one third of patients with optic pathway tumors. Approximately 15 to 20% of patients with neurofibromatosis type 1 (NF1) will have an optic glioma on MR scan, but only 1 to 5% become symptomatic (Ruggieri 1999). There is a higher likelihood of NF in patients who have multicentric optic gliomas, and a relatively lower incidence of NF in patients with chiasmatic tumors (Housepian 1977). The natural history of optic pathway gliomas is related to the presence of NF and to the location of the tumor. Patients with optic pathway gliomas who have NF1 seem to have a better overall prognosis than those without NF (Rush et al. 1982). However, this view is opposed by other studies showing that patients with NF have a similar prognosis to patients without NF following irradiation for chiasmatic glioma (Alvord and Lofton 1988). A more recent study showed a significantly favorable difference in time to tumor progression, i.e., time to recurrence of optic glioma, in the presence of NF (Deliganis et al. 1996). Approximately two thirds of optic gliomas associated with NF1 are indolent lesions with minimal progression. Although any location within the optic pathway from the retrobulbar area to the optic radiation may be affected, chiasmatic gliomas tend to have a more aggressive course both by invading the hypothalamus and by causing obstructive hydrocephalus by occluding the foramen of Munro. It is also known that optic and hypothalamic gliomas are more aggressive in children younger than 5 years of age (Dirks et al. 1994; Oxenhandler and Sayers 1978).

1.3.2 Pathology

Most tumors of the diencephalon and the optic pathways are histopathologically low-grade gliomas, typically pilocytic or fibrillary astrocytomas (Daumas-Duport et al. 1988; Ito et al. 1992). Histologically, optic nerve gliomas demonstrate two different patterns of growth. In non-NF patients progression tends to be confined to the optic nerve without significant involvement of the meninges. In patients with neurofibromatosis, tumor cells invade the subarachnoid space causing proliferative fibroblastic response and meningothelial hyperplasia (Stern et al. 1980). Locally, hypothalamic and optic gliomas may extend laterally, invading the perivascular space along the arteries of the circle of Willis, as well as expanding posteriorly toward the brainstem with rostral invagination into the third ventricle. Patients with chiasmatic–hypothalamic gliomas have an increased risk for disease dissemination along the neuraxis (Gajjar et al. 1995). It has been reported that the risk of multicentric dissemination is increased approximately 20-fold in this group of patients when compared to those with low-grade gliomas located elsewhere (Mamelak et al. 1994).

1.3.3 Clinical Features

Most optic pathway gliomas will present with some form of visual loss. Identifying the exact type of visual loss may be difficult early in the course of the disease, especially in very young children. The typical deficits are incongruent field deficits, at times restricted to one eye. Optic atrophy is commonly seen with large tumors. Children under 3 years of age are usually first brought to medical attention because of strabismus, proptosis, or nystagmus, or failure to meet developmental milestones. Tumors which involve the hypothalamus will often result in excessive growth or other associated endocrinologic disturbances, including precocious puberty. Hypothalamic tumors may reach a large size before diagnosis, and may result in diencephalic syndrome, characterized by failure to thrive despite apparent normal appetite in an otherwise healthy child. Tumors that extend upward into the third ventricle can cause hydrocephalus. Tumors with thalamic involvement may cause motor deficits on the side contralateral to the lesion.

1.3.4 Diagnostic Imaging

Optic pathway gliomas are usually well visualized on MRI. In children with NF1, there is often extensive streaking along the optic pathway and/or involvement of the optic nerve at the time of diagnosis, in addition to nonspecific white-matter abnormalities on T2-weighted sequences (see Chap. 11 for additional details). Optic pathway gliomas in children without NF1 tend to be more globular and somewhat more restricted to one anatomic location. The mass itself enhances homogeneously following gadolinium administration, although cysts are frequently seen. On FLAIR sequences, the infiltrative component of the tumor can be seen extending along the optic tracts (Fig. 1.4). Detailed fine cuts through the sella should be obtained. In these sequences, the optic nerve becomes continuous with the mass, a finding which helps to establish the radiologic diagnosis.

1.3.5 Treatment

1.3.5.1 Surgical Indications

Regardless of whether a patient has neurofibromatosis, a biopsy is not needed for an intrinsic chiasmatic/hypothalamic mass if the appearance on MR imaging is typical, i.e., involvement of the chiasm, optic nerve(s), and/or optic tracts. For patients without neurofibromatosis who present with an atypical chiasmatic hypothalamic mass, surgical biopsy may be needed to a diagnosis. If mass effect is present with neurologic symptoms, debulking of a large tumor may be the initial approach. Some neurosurgeons limit surgical indications to a subset of exophytic or cystic tumors with significant mass effect and hydrocephalus. However, a progressive visual deficit or progression on serial MR scans will necessitate intervention if there is an exophytic or cystic component. As 10 to 20% of children younger than 10 years of age with NF may have a low-grade glioma of the optic pathways, biopsy is not considered mandatory for asymptomatic patients with a chiasmatic/hypothalamic tumor (Lewis et al. 1984; Ruggieri 1999). Asymptomatic patients may be followed with serial clinical

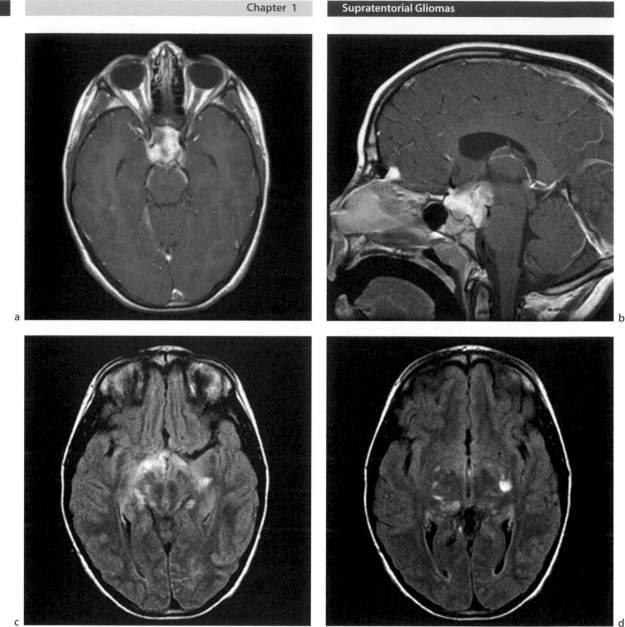

Figure 1.4 a–d

A chiasmatic/hypothalamic pilocytic astrocytoma in a 10-year-old girl with headaches. **a** The axial T1-weighted image shows the right optic nerve entering the enhancing portion of the tumor. A distinct boundary does not exist between the nerve and tumor. **b** The sagittal plane image clearly shows that the enhancing portion of the tumor is continuous with the hypothalamus. **c** FLAIR image shows indistinct increased signal intensity along the optic tracts extending posteriorly from the chiasm. **d** FLAIR image slightly superior to c shows additional abnormalities along the optic tract with a localized area of signal abnormality likely within the lateral geniculate nucleus on the left side

and visual examinations, MRI scans, endocrine replacement, and CSF shunting if necessary.

The only indication for resection of a unilateral optic nerve tumor is when vision is absent or significantly impaired. A relative indication is extreme proptosis with exposure keratitis caused by a large intraorbital optic nerve tumor. In addition, it is generally agreed that the exophytic portion of the lesion should be removed if vision is reasonable, and that nonresectable unilateral optic nerve lesions should be decompressed. Any surgery that may result in permanent neurological morbidity should be compared with alternative treatment modalities, in terms of potential benefits and risks. For instance, although a limited resection on an optic nerve glioma extending to the optic chiasm may be indicated, a major chiasmatic resection resulting in visual compromise is virtually never indicated.

For optic and diencephalic gliomas, none of these treatment modalities have been proven to be more effective in terms of time to tumor progression and survival. It is known that extensive surgical resections increase time to tumor progression and decrease the risk of malignant differentiation in patients harboring hemispheric low-grade gliomas (Berger et al. 1994). Although optic and diencephalic gliomas are almost always histologically low grade (WHO grade I), no study has addressed the issue of extent of resection as it affects tumor progression or overall survival in this patient population. Therefore, in addition to obtaining histological diagnosis if there is doubt based on MR scans, the goal in surgical resection is to achieve a transient control of the disease and to alleviate symptoms caused by the tumor mass.

1.3.5.2 Surgical Technique

For tumors involving one optic nerve, a frontal or frontotemporal approach may be used. With either technique, intraorbital and intracranial portions of the affected nerve as well as the chiasm are exposed. The optic chiasm and the intracranial portion of the affected optic nerve are inspected to determine a site for division, which should be more than 6 mm from the chiasm so as to avoid a contralateral superior temporal field defect. The orbital canal is drilled open, allowing decompression of the optic nerve. After closure of the annulus and periorbita, the orbital roof and supraorbital rim are reconstructed if needed. If the orbital roof is not repaired, one associated complication is pulsatile exophthalmos.

For chiasmatic-hypothalamic tumors, surgical goals should be balanced with the risks of increased visual loss and increased hypothalamic dysfunction. Improved visual and neurological outcomes following surgery have been reported for chiasmatic–hypothalamic gliomas (Bynke et al. 1977; Baram et al. 1986; Wisoff et al. 1990). Meticulous tumor debulking from the exophytic portion of a chiasmatic tumor may improve vision by relieving external pressure on the adjacent optic nerve (Oakes 1990). There are several surgical approaches to the chiasmatic hypothalamic region, each with certain advantages (Hoffman and Rutka 1999; Apuzzo and Litofsky 1993). Regardless of the approach, the aim is tumor debulking without causing additional deficit.

1.3.5.3 Radiation Therapy

There are several alternative treatment options: follow-up without intervention until clinical deterioration is evident, irradiation of all lesions with or without biopsy, biopsy for all lesions followed by radiation only for those located in the hypothalamus or posterior chiasm, or chemotherapy. Each of these options can be considered for certain subgroups of patients. For example, low-grade diencephalic tumors not involving the optic tracts may be treated with local field radiotherapy of 5,400 to 6,000 cGy, achieving a tumor response in the majority of patients. However, in the early postradiation period some patients may experience worsening of their symptoms reflected in a transient increase in the size of their lesion. Standard initial treatment for patients with chiasmatic gliomas who have progressive visual symptoms is regional radiotherapy, although these tumors are chemotherapy sensitive, and this modality is commonly used in infants and children prior to or instead of radiation therapy. An option for NF1 patients with optic pathway gliomas is follow-up with no treatment as long as the tumor remains quiescent on serial imaging studies and visual function is stable.

1.3.5.4 Chemotherapy

As the risk for late sequelae of cranial radiation decreases with age, chemotherapy prior to cranial radiotherapy as a means of delaying the use of radiation in children younger than 5 years of age has been proposed (Packer et al. 1988). In a study on children with newly-diagnosed, progressive low-grade gliomas, including 58 children with diencephalic tumors, 56% of the patients showed an objective response to treatment with combined carboplatin and vincristine chemotherapy (Packer et al. 1997).

1.3.6 Outcome

Radiologically, gross total resection is often impossible due to the eloquent location of diencephalic and optic gliomas. In addition to surgical morbidity, endocrine dysfunction in this patient population may also result from radiotherapy, and its reported incidence is highly variable, ranging from 10% to 70%. The most common manifestation of hypopituitarism following radiotherapy is growth hormone deficiency or growth retardation (Wong et al. 1987; Bataini et al. 1991; Tao et al. 1997). Diabetes insipidus, precocious puberty, and testosterone deficiency are also reported. Furthermore, radiotherapy can result in significant cognitive deficits, the severity of which may be inversely proportional to age at diagnosis (Ellenberg et al. 1987). Patients with unilateral intraorbital optic nerve gliomas have a good postoperative prognosis following appropriately timed surgery. However, regardless of their histologically benign features, chiasmatic–diencephalic gliomas carry a worse prognosis.

The operative procedures for chiasmatic/hypothalamic gliomas carry significant morbidity. Surgical morbidity may be in the form of immediate endocrinologic or neurologic deficits. Resulting sequelae may include hypothalamic/hypophyseal dysfunction,

increased visual impairment, memory loss, altered consciousness, and coma (Wisoff et al. 1990). Following an intraorbital approach, CSF leak may occur if the frontal sinus or any opened ethmoid sinuses have not been adequately reconstructed. Inadequate reconstruction of the orbital roof may result in pulsatile proptosis. Failure to repair a sectioned levator origin will result in ptosis. Surgical injury to the superior ophthalmic vein and to the nerves supplying the extraocular muscles will result in functional deficits (Housepian 1993). These complications are avoidable with appropriate surgical technique. In a large series of patients treated with intraorbital procedures, no significant CSF leaks, proptosis, infection, or extraocular problems were reported (Maroon and Kennerdell 1976).

Several studies have questioned whether the presence of NF1 has a prognostic effect for patients with optic pathway gliomas. Although Rush et al. (1982) reported a better outcome for optic glioma patients with NF, later studies failed to show a difference in terms of survival (Imes and Hoyt 1986; Alvord and Lofton 1988; Kovalic et al. 1990). In our experience, there was not a significant difference in survival based on the presence or absence of NF1. The 5- and 10-year survival rates for patients with optic gliomas and NF1 were 93% and 81%, respectively, as opposed to 83% and 76%, respectively, for patients without NF (Deliganis et al. 1996). However, a significant difference in the time to tumor progression (first relapse) was observed in favor of patients with neurofibromatosis. In a study including mostly diencephalic low-grade gliomas, Packer et al. did not find any prognostic benefit related to the presence of NF (Packer et al. 1997). In this study, the only statistically significant prognostic factor was age, and children 5 years old and younger had a 3-year progression-free survival rate of 74% compared with a rate of 39% in older children.

Another study examining clinical characteristics and consequences of treatment of children with hypothalamic/chiasmatic gliomas showed significant tumor progression despite a high survival rate (Janss et al. 1995). Although the 5-year survival rate was 93%, more than 80% of the children required surgery, chemotherapy, or radiotherapy within 2 years of diagnosis, and all but 9% eventually required radiation or chemotherapy within a median follow-up period of 6 years. In a recent multivariate analysis of potential prognostic factors in children with optic pathway gliomas, older age, presence of NF1, chemotherapy, and radiotherapy were found to have statistically significant effect on outcome (Chan et al. 1998). Overall, 5-year survival for patients with chiasmatic-hypothalamic gliomas is around 85% with a continuous decline over the subsequent years (Garvey and Packer 1996).

1.4 Oligodendroglioma

1.4.1 Epidemiology

Definitive data regarding the incidence of oligodendrogliomas relative to all intracranial gliomas is lacking, mainly due to significant differences in diagnostic criteria among neuropathologists. In the general population, the relative incidence of oligodendrogliomas ranges from 4% to 7% (Rubinstein 1972; Mork et al. 1985) to 18.8% and 33% in other series (Zulch 1986; Daumas-Duport et al. 1997). Oligodendrogliomas are rare in children and constitute approximately 1% of pediatric brain tumors (Razak et al. 1998).

Unlike in low-grade astrocytomas, p53 is only rarely mutated in oligodendrogliomas. However, over half of these tumors show a characteristic loss of the long arm of chromosome 1 and the short arm of chromosome 19. As 1p/19q loss is not seen in astrocytic tumors, the combination of p53 and 1p/19q analysis may serve in the future to distinguish an astrocytic (p53-mutant, 1p/19q intact) from an oligodendroglial (p53-wild type, 1p/19q deleted) genotype in cases that are difficult to distinguish histologically (Reifenberger et al. 1994)

1.4.2 Pathology

Oligodendrogliomas arise primarily in the white matter but tend to infiltrate the cerebral cortex more than do astrocytomas of a similar grade of malignancy. Oligodendrogliomas tend to form clusters of neoplastic cells in the subpial region, around neurons and blood vessels. Microscopically, classic oligodendrogliomas show uniform cell density at low power. Higher power reveals uniform round nuclei and distinctive perinuclear halos. This histologic appearance has been referred to as "fried eggs." However, frozen sections of oligodendroglioma fail to show the diagnostically helpful perinuclear halos; formalin-fixed material that has been previously frozen also fails to show these. Most oligodendrocytes show positive reactivity for S-100 protein. Low-grade oligodendrogliomas are distinguished from high-grade tumors on the basis of lower cellularity, inconspicuous mitotic activity, minimal nuclear atypia, and an absence of endothelial proliferation and necrosis.

1.4.3 Clinical Features

Similar to those of supratentorial astrocytomas, symptoms and signs of childhood oligodendrogliomas are dependent on the anatomic location of the tumor and the age of the patient. General nonspecific symptoms associated with increased intracranial pressure, and focal symptoms related to the location of the tumor have been outlined earlier in this chapter. Oligodendrogliomas have a slight predilection for the frontal lobes. Grey matter involvement is common, giving them on average a more superficial location than astrocytomas.

1.4.4 Diagnostic Imaging

The diagnosis of oligodendroglioma may be suggested on imaging studies by its location and presence of calcification. Although nonspecific, a fronto–temporal location, involvement including the superficial cortex, and intrinsic calcification are characteristic of oligodendrogliomas. Oligodendroglioma is the most common intracranial tumor to calcify (60–90 % are calcified), and CT has the advantage of better visualizing the calcium content of the tumor. Therefore CT and MR imaging are complementary methods to characterize the tumor and evaluate its extension. Approximately half of oligodendrogliomas moderately enhance, and enhancement is typically patchy.

1.4.5 Treatment

As with most gliomas, surgery is usually the initial therapeutic modality in the management of children with supratentorial oligodendroglioma, and may range from a stereotactic biopsy to an extensive resection with seizure surgery in patients with tumor-associated intractable epilepsy. The general surgical management principles discussed in reference to low-grade astrocytoma apply to supratentorial oligodendrogliomas. The surgical strategy should favor radical tumor removal when feasible.

The role of postoperative irradiation in the management of patients with oligodendrogliomas is controversial, and conclusions regarding the value of radiotherapy are contradictory. Some authors recommend immediate postoperative irradiation for patients with incompletely resected lesions (Lindegaard et al. 1987), whereas other studies failed to show any survival benefit with this approach (Bullard et al. 1987; Sun et al. 1988). Sufficient data are not available to support the recommendation that all patients with oligodendrogliomas should receive radiation therapy. Its efficacy has not been demonstrated, especially in children (Hirsch et al. 1989). Postoperative irradiation may be beneficial for patients with incompletely resected tumors, especially when unfavorable clinical or pathological characteristics are present. It is reasonable, however, to defer treatment in children until progression occurs.

Aggressive oligodendrogliomas have been shown to respond especially well to PCV chemotherapy (Glass et al. 1992; Cairncross et al. 1992). It has also been demonstrated that the allelic loss of chromosomes 1p and 19q predict response to chemotherapy and longer survival in patients with anaplastic oligo-

dendrogliomas (Cairncross et al. 1998), establishing a molecular marker for chemosensitivity in these tumors. Increasingly, preradiation chemotherapy with PCV is being used in treating anaplastic oligodendrogliomas since up to 70 % of patients may respond (Streffer et al. 2000; Paleologos et al. 1999). In addition, salvage therapy with PCV may be effective in patients who progress after radiotherapy (Streffer et al. 2000).

1.4.6 Outcome

For oligodendrogliomas, the most promising prognostic marker is combined loss of chromosomes 1p and 19q. The initial finding in anaplastic oligodendrogliomas was recently extended to low-grade tumors, and a similar relationship of 1p/19q loss with improved survival was found (Smith et al. 2000). Furthermore, 1p loss of heterozygosity (LOH) appears to be a stronger predictor of survival than the well-established prognostic factors of age and performance status (Bauman et al. 2000).

Limited data exist on the predictive role of surgery regarding outcome of patients with oligodendroglioma. Although most major series with statistical analysis show a favorable outcome associated with more extensive resections, the effect of extent of resection appears to be less prominent in oligodendrogliomas than in astrocytomas (Keles et al. 2001).

Although supported by a limited number of studies, oligodendrogliomas have a different natural history and a better overall prognosis than astrocytomas. Similar to epidemiological figures, survival data for oligodendrogliomas depend on the histological criteria used for diagnosis, and show significant variability. Survival rates are also affected by the inclusion of higher-grade oligodendrogliomas in some series and analysis of the data without adjusting for this variable. Five-year survival rates ranging from 27 % to 85 % have been reported, and are generally accepted to be at the higher end of this spectrum for the pediatric population.

1.5 Conclusion

Supratentorial low- and high-grade gliomas represent a significant disease burden in the pediatric population. High-grade tumors are treated aggressively with surgery, radiation, and adjunctive chemotherapy. Similar to results with adult high-grade gliomas, the long term outcome remains poor. Although gross total resection is associated with better long-term survival for lower-grade tumors, many infiltrative astrocytomas cannot be resected completely. For these tumors, the role of radiation and/or chemotherapy remains controversial and is the subject of ongoing clinical trials. Certain glioma subtypes such as optic pathway gliomas are being successfully treated with a variety of chemotherapy regimens.

References

Airewele GE, Sigurdson AJ, Wiley KJ, Frieden BE, Caldarera LW, Riccardi VM, Lewis RA, Chintagumpala MM, Ater JL, Plon SE, Bondy ML (2001) Neoplasms in neurofibromatosis 1 are related to gender but not to family history of cancer. Genet Epidemiol 20:75–86

Alvord EC, Lofton S (1988) Gliomas of the optic nerve or chiasm: Outcome by patient's age, tumor site, and treatment. J Neurosurg 68:85–98

Apuzzo MLJ, Litofsky NS (1993) Surgery in and around the anterior third ventricle. In: Apuzzo MLJ (ed) Brain surgery: complication avoidance and management, vol 1. Churchill Livingstone, New York, p 541

Baram TZ, Moser RP, van Eyes J (1986) Surgical management of progressive visual loss in optic gliomas of childhood. Ann Neurol 20:398

Bataini JP, Delanian S, Ponvert D (1991) Chiasmal gliomas. Results of irradiation management in 57 patients and review of the literature. Int J Radiat Oncol Biol Phys 21:615–623

Bauman G, Lote K, Larson D, Stalpers L, Leighton C, Fisher B, Wara W, MacDonald D, Stitt L, Cairncross JG (1999) Pretreatment factors predict overall survival for patients with low-grade glioma: a recursive partitioning analysis. Int J Radiat Oncol Biol Phys 45:923–929

Bauman GS, Ino Y, Ueki K et al (2000) Allelic loss of chromosome 1p and radiotherapy plus chemotherapy in patients with oligodendrogliomas. Int J Radiat Oncol Biol Phys 48:825–830

Berger MS, Ghatan S, Geyer JR et al (1991/1992) Seizure outcome in children with hemispheric tumors and associated intractable epilepsy: the role of tumor removal combined with seizure foci resection. Pediatr Neurosurg 17:185–191

Berger MS, Ghatan S, Haglund MM, Dobbins J, Ojemann GA (1993) Low-grade gliomas associated with intractable epilepsy: seizure outcome utilizing electrocorticography during tumor resection. J Neurosurg 79:62–69

Berger MS, Deliganis AV, Dobbins J, Keles GE (1994) The effect of extent of resection on recurrence in patients with low grade cerebral hemisphere gliomas. Cancer 74:1784–1791

Bloom HJ, Glees J, Bell J, Ashley SE, Gorman C (1990) The treatment and long-term prognosis of children with intracranial tumors: a study of 610 cases, 1950-1981. Int J Radiat Oncol Biol Phys 18:723–745

Borit A, Richardson EP Jr (1982) The biological and clinical behaviour of pilocytic astrocytomas of the optic pathways. Brain 105:161–187

Bondy ML, Wang LE, El-Zein R, de Andrade M et al (2001) Gamma-radiation sensitivity and risk of glioma. J Natl Cancer Inst 93:1553–1557

Bouffett E, Mottolese C, Jouvet A et al (1997) Etoposide and thiotepa followed by ABMT (autologous bone marrow transplantation) in children and young adults with high-grade gliomas. Eur J Cancer 33:91–95

Bullard DE, Rawlings CE, Phillips B et al (1987) Oligodendroglioma. An analysis of the value of radiation therapy. Cancer 60:2179–2188

Bynke H, Kagstrom E, Tjernstrom K (1997) Aspects on the treatment of gliomas of the anterior visual pathways. Acta Ophthalmol 55:269–280

Cairncross JG, Laperriere NJ (1989) Low-grade glioma. To treat or not to treat? Arch Neurol 46:1238–1239

Cairncross JG, Macdonald DR, Ramsay DA (1992) Aggressive oligodendroglioma: a chemosensitive tumour. Neurosurgery 31:78–82

Cairncross JG, Ueki K, Zlatescu MC et al (1998) Specific genetic predictors of chemotherapeutic response and survival in patients with anaplastic oligodendrogliomas. J Natl Cancer Inst 90:1473–1479

Campbell JW, Pollack IF, Martinez AJ et al (1996) High-grade astrocytomas in children: radiologically complete resection is associated with an excellent long-term prognosis. Neurosurgery 38:258–264

Chan MY, Foong AP, Heisey DM et al (1998) Potential prognostic factors of relapse-free survival in childhood optic pathway glioma: a multivariate analysis. Pediatr Neurosurg 29:23–28

Cheng Y, Ho-Keung NG, Zhang S-F, Pang JS-F, Zheng J, Poon W-S (1999) Genetic alterations in pediatric high grade astrocytomas. Hum Pathol 30:1284–1290

Chintagumpala M, Stewart C, Burger P et al. (2000) Responses to topotecan in newly diagnosed patients with high grade glioma – a Pediatric Oncology Group (POG) study. The 9th international symposium on pediatric neuro-oncology, 11–14 June 2000. San Francisco, CA, abstract

Daumas-Duport C, Scheithauer BW, O'Fallon J et al (1988) Grading of astrocytomas: a simple and reproducible method. Cancer 62:2152–2165

Daumas-Duport C, Varlet P, Tucker ML et al (1997) Oligodendrogliomas, part I. Patterns of growth, histological diagnosis, clinical and imaging correlations: a study of 153 cases. J Neuro Oncol 34:37–59

Deliganis AV, Geyer JR, Berger MS (1996) Prognostic significance of type 1 neurofibromatosis (von Recklinghausen's disease) in childhood optic glioma. Neurosurgery 38:1114–1119

Dirks PB, Jay V, Becker LE et al (1994) Development of anaplastic changes in low grade astrocytomas in children. Neurosurgery 34:68–78

Dohrmann GJ, Farwell JR, Flannery JT (1985) Astrocytomas in childhood: a population-based study. Surg Neurol 23:64–68

Dropcho EJ, Wisoff JH, Walker RW, Allen JC (1987) Supratentorial malignant gliomas in childhood: a review of fifty cases. Ann Neurol 22:355–364

Edwards MS, Levin VA, Wilson CB (1980) Brain tumor chemotherapy: an evaluation of agents in current use in phase II and III trials. Cancer Treat Rep 64:1179–1205

Ellenberg L, McComb JG, Siegel SE et al (1987) Factors affecting intellectual outcome in pediatric brain tumor patients. Neurosurgery 21:638–644

Farwell JR, Dohrmann GJ, Flannery JT (1977) Central nervous system tumors in children. Cancer 40:3123–3132

Felix CA, Slavc I, Dunn M, Strauss EA, Phillips PC, Rorke LB, Sutton L, Bunin GR, Biegel JA (1995) p53 gene mutations in pediatric brain tumors. Med Pediatr Oncol 25:431–436

Finlay JL, Wisoff JH (1999) The impact of extent of resection in the management of malignant gliomas of childhood. Childs Nerv Syst 15:786–788

Finlay J, Boyett J, Yates A et al (1995) Randomized phase III trial in childhood high-grade astrocytomas comparing vincristine, lomustine and prednisone with eight-drug-in-one-day regimen. J Clin Oncol 13:112–123

Finlay JL, Goldman S, Wong MD et al (1996) Pilot study of high-dose thiotepa and etoposide with autologous bone marrow rescue in children and young adults with recurrent CNS tumors. The Children's Cancer Group. J Clin Oncol 14:2495–2503

Gajjar A, Heideman RL, Kovnar EH et al (1993) Response of pediatric low grade gliomas to chemotherapy. Pediatr Neurosurg 19:113–121

Gajjar A, Bhargava R, Jenkins JJ et al (1995) Low grade astrocytoma with neuraxis dissemination at diagnosis. J Neurosurg 83:67–71

Garvey G, Packer RJ (1996) An integrated approach to the treatment of chiasmatic-hypothalamic gliomas. J Neuro Oncol 28:167–183

Giannini C, Scheithauer BW, Burger PC et al (1999) Cellular proliferation in pilocytic and diffuse astrocytomas. J Neuropathol Exp Neurol 58:46–53

Glass J, Hochberg FH, Gruber ML et al (1992) The treatment of oligodendrogliomas and mixed oligodendroglioma-astrocytomas with PCV chemotherapy. J Neurosurg 76:741–745

Grovas AC, Boyett JM, Lindsley K et al (1999) Regimen-related toxicity of myeloablative chemotherapy with BCNU, thiotepa, and etoposide followed by autologous stem cell rescue for children with newly diagnosed glioblastoma multiforme: report from the Children's Cancer Group. Med Pediatr Oncol 33:83–87

Gururangan S, Cavazos CM, Ashley D et al (2002) Phase II study of carboplatin in children with low-grade gliomas. J Clin Oncol 20:2951–2958

Haglund MM, Berger MS, Kunkel DD et al (1992) Changes in gamma-aminobutyric acid and somatostatin in epileptic cortex associated with low-grade gliomas. J Neurosurg 77:209–216

Heideman RL, Douglass EC, Krance RA et al (1993) High-dose chemotherapy followed by autologous bone marrow rescue followed by interstitial and external-beam radiotherapy in newly diagnosed pediatric malignant gliomas. J Clin Oncol 11:1458–1465

Hirsch JF, Sainte Rose C, Pierre-Khan A et al (1989) Benign astrocytic and oligodendrocytic tumors of the cerebral hemispheres in children. J Neurosurg 70:568–572

Hoffman HJ, Rutka JT (1999) Optic pathway gliomas in children. In: Albright L, Pollack I, Adelson D (eds) Principles and practice of pediatric neurosurgery. Thieme Medical Publishers, New York, pp 535–543

Housepian EM (1977) Management and results in 114 cases of optic glioma. Neurosurgery 1:67–68

Housepian EM (1993) Complications of transcranial orbital surgery. In: Post KD, Friedman ED, McCormick P (eds) Postoperative complications in intracranial neurosurgery. Thieme, New York, pp 87–90

Imes RK, Hoyt WF (1986) Childhood chiasmal gliomas. Update on the fate of patients in the 1969 San Francisco study. Br J Ophthalmol 70:179–182

Ito S, Hashino T, Shibuya M, Prados MD, Edwards MSB, Davis RL (1992) Proliferative characteristics of juvenile pilocytic astrocytomas determined by bromodeoxyuridine labeling. Neurosurgery 31:413–419

Janss AJ, Grundy R, Cnaan A et al (1995) Optic pathway and hypothalamic / chiasmatic gliomas in children younger than age 5 years with a 6-year follow-up. Cancer 75:1051–1059

Keles GE, Berger MS (2000) Seizures associated with brain tumors. In Bernstein M, Berger MS (eds) Neuro-oncology essentials. Thieme Medical Publishers, New York, pp 473–477

Keles GE, Lamborn KR, Berger MS (2001) Low-grade hemispheric gliomas in adults: a critical review of extent of resection as a factor influencing outcome. J Neurosurg 95:735–745

Kepes JJ, Kepes M, Slowik F (1973) Fibrous xanthomas and xanthosarcomas of the meninges and the brain. Acta Neuropathol 23:187–199

Kleihues P, Cavenee WK (2000) Pathology and genetics of Tumors of the nervous system. IARC Press, Lyon

Kleihues P, Schauble B, zur Hausen A et al (1997) Tumors associated with p53 germline mutations: a synopsis of 91 families. Am J Pathol 150:1–13

Kovalic JJ, Grigsby PW, Shepard MJ, Fineberg BB, Thomas PR (1990) Radiation therapy for gliomas of the optic nerve and chiasm. Int J Radiat Oncol Biol Phys 18:927–932

Lashford LS, Thiesse P, Jouvet A (2002) United Kingdom Children's Cancer Study Group and French Society for Pediatric Oncology Intergroup Study: Temozolomide in malignant gliomas of childhood. J Clin Oncol 20:4684-4691

Lewis RA, Riccardi VM, Gerson LP, Whitford R, Axelson KA (1984) Von Recklinghausen neurofibromatosis. II. Incidence of optic nerve gliomata. Ophthalmology 91:929–935

Lindboe CF, Cappelen J, Kepes JJ (1992) Pleiomorphic xanthoastrocytoma as a component of a cerebellar ganglioglioma: case report. Neurosurgery 31:353–355

Lindegaard KF, Mork SJ, Eide GE et al (1987) Statistical analysis of clinicopathological features, radiotherapy, and survival in 170 cases of oligodendroglioma. J Neurosurg 67:224–230

Listernick R, Charrow J, Gutmann DH (1999) Intracranial gliomas in neurofibromatosis type 1. Am J Med Genet 89:38–44

Litofsky NS, Hinton D, Raffel C (1994) The lack of a role for p53 in astrocytomas in pediatric patients. Neurosurgery 34:967–72

Longee DC, Friedman HS, Albright RE et al (1990) Treatment of patients with recurrent gliomas with cyclophoshamide and vincristine. J Neurosurg 72:583–588

Lote K, Egeland T, Hager B, Skullerud K, Hirschberg H (1998) Prognostic significance of CT contrast enhancement within histological subgroups of intracranial glioma. J Neurooncol 40:161–170

Mamelak AN, Prados MD, Obana WG, Cogen PH, Edwards MSB (1994) Treatment options and prognosis for multicentric juvenile pilocytic astrocytoma. J Neurosurg 81:24–30

Maroon JC, Kennerdell JS (1976) Lateral microsurgical approach to intraorbital tumors. J Neurosurg 44:556–561

Mason WP, Grovas A, Halpern S et al (1998) Intensive chemotherapy and bone marrow rescue for young children with newly diagnosed malignant brain tumors. J Clin Oncol 29:563–567

Mork SJ, Lindegaard KF, Halvorsen TB et al (1985) Oligodendroglioma: incidence and biological behavior in a defined population. J Neurosurg 63:881–889

Neumann E, Kalousek DK, Norman MG, Steinbok P, Cochrane DD, Goddard K (1993) Cytogenetic analysis of 109 pediatric central nervous system tumors. Cancer Genet Cytogenet 71:40–49

Oakes WJ (1990) Recent experience with the resection of pilocytic astrocytomas of the hypothalamus. In: Marlin A (ed) Concepts in pediatric neurosurgery, vol 10. Karger, Basel, p 108

Oxenhandler DC, Sayers MP (1978) The dilemma of childhood optic gliomas. J Neurosurg 48:34–41

Packer RJ, Sutton LN, Bilaniuk LT et al (1988) Treatment of chiasmatic/hypothalamic gliomas of childhood with chemotherapy: an update. Ann Neurol 23:79–85

Packer RJ, Ater J, Allen J et al (1997) Carboplatin and vincristine chemotherapy for children with newly diagnosed progressive low-grade gliomas. J Neurosurg 86:747–754

Packer RJ, Vezina G, Nicholson HS, Chadduck WM (1999) Childhood and adolescent gliomas. In: Albright L, Pollack I, Adelson D (eds) Principles and practice of pediatric neurosurgery. Thieme Medical Publishers, New York, pp 689–701

Paleologos NA, Macdonald DR, Vick NA et al (1999) Neoadjuvant procarbazine, CCNU, and vincristine for anaplastic and aggressive oligodendroglioma. Neurology 53:1141–1143

Phuphanich S, Edwards MS, Levin VA et al (1984) Supratentorial malignant gliomas of childhood. Results of treatment with radiation therapy and chemotherapy. J Neurosurg 60:495–499

Pollack IF, Claassen D, al-Shboul Q et al (1995) Low-grade gliomas of the cerebral hemispheres in children: an analysis of 71 cases. J Neurosurg 82:536–547

Pollack IF, Finkelstein SD, Woods J (2002) Children's Cancer Group: Expression of p53 and prognosis in children with malignant gliomas. N Engl J Med 346:420–427

Powell SZ, Yachnis AT, Rorke LB et al (1996) Divergent differentiation in pleomorphic xanthoastrocytoma: evidence for a neuronal element and possible relation to ganglion cell tumors. Am J Surg Pathol 20:80–85

Prados MD, Edwards MSB, Rabbitt J et al (1997) Treatment of pediatric low-grade gliomas with nitrosourea based multiagent chemotherapy regimen. J Neuro Oncol 32:235–241

Razak N, Baumgartner J, Bruner J (1998) Pediatric oligodendrogliomas. Pediatr Neurosurg 28:121–129

Recht LD, Lew R, Smith TW (1992) Suspected low-grade glioma: is deferring therapy safe? Ann Neurol 31:431–436

Reifenberger J, Reifenberger G, Liu L et al (1994) Molecular genetic analysis of oligodendroglial tumors shows preferential allelic deletions on 19q and 1p. Am J Pathol 145:1175–1190

Roberts HC, Roberts TP, Brasch RC, Dillon WP (2000) Quantitative measurement of microvascular permeability in human brain tumors achieved using dynamic contrast-enhanced MR imaging: correlation with histologic grade. AJNR 21:1570–1571

Roberts P, Chumas PD, Picton S, Bridges L, Livingstone JH, Sheridan E (2001) A review of the cytogenetics of 58 pediatric brain tumors. Cancer Genet Cytogenet 131:1–12

Ron E, Modan B, Boice JD et al (1988) Tumors of the brain and nervous system after radiotherapy in childhood. N Engl J Med 319:1033–1039

Rubinstein LJ (1972) Oligodendrogliomas. Tumors of the central nervous system. Armed Forces Institute of Pathology, Washington DC, pp 85–104

Ruggieri M (1999) The different forms of neurofibromatosis. Childs Nerv Syst 15:295–308

Rush JA, Younge BR, Campbell RJ, MacCarty CS (1982) Optic glioma: long-term follow-up of 85 histopathologically verified cases. Ophthalmology 89:1213–1219

Scott JN, Brasher PM, Sevick RJ, Rewcastle NB, Forsyth PA (2002) How often are nonenhancing supratentorial gliomas malignant? A population study. Neurology 59:947–949

Shafqat S, Hedley-White ET, Henson JW (1999) Age-dependent rate of anaplastic transformation in low-grade astrocytoma. Neurology 52:867–869

Smith JS, Perry A, Borell TJ et al (2000) Alterations of chromosome arms 1p and 19q as predictors of survival in oligodendrogliomas, astrocytomas, and mixed oligoastrocytomas. J Clin Oncol 187:636–645

Sposto R, Ertel IM, Jenkin RDT et al (1989) The effectiveness of chemotherapy for treatment of high-grade astrocytoma in children: results of a randomized trial. J Neurooncol 7:165–171

Stern J, Jakobiec FA, Housepian EM (1980) The architecture of optic nerve gliomas with and without neurofibromatosis. Arch Ophthalmol 98:505–511

Streffer J, Schabet M, Bamberg M et al (2000) A role for preirradiation PCV chemotherapy for oligodendroglial brain tumors. J Neurol 247:297–302

Stupp R, Dietrich PY, Ostermann Kraljevic S et al (2002) Promising survival for patients with newly diagnosed glioblastoma multiforme treated with concomitant radiation plus temozolomide followed by adjuvant temozolomide. J Clin Oncol 20:1375–1382.

Sun ZM, Genka S, Shitara N et al (1988) Factors possibly influencing the prognosis of oligodendroglioma. Neurosurgery 22:886–891

Tao ML, Barnes PD, Billett AL et al (1997) Childhood optic chiasm gliomas: radiographic response following radiotherapy and long-term clinical outcome. Int J Radiat Oncol Biol Phys 39:579–587

Taratuto AL, Monges J, Lylyk P et al (1984) Superficial cerebral astrocytoma attached to dura: report of six cases in infants. Cancer 54:2505–2512

Turner CD, Gururangan S, Eastwood J et al (2002) Phase II study of irinotecan (CPT-11) in children with high-risk malignant brain tumors: the Duke experience. Neuro-oncol 4:102–108

Varley JM, Evans DG, Birch JM (1997) Li-Fraumeni syndrome – a molecular and clinical review. Br J Cancer 76:1–14

Walker MD, Alexander E, Hunt WE et al (1978) Evaluation of BCNU and/or radiotherapy in the treatment of anaplastic gliomas. A cooperative clinical trial. J Neurosurg 49:333–343

Wisoff JH, Abbott R, Epstein F (1990) Surgical management of exophytic chiasmatic-hypothalamic tumors of childhood. J Neurosurg 73:661–667

Wisoff JH, Boyett JM, Berger MS et al (1998) Current neurosurgical management and the impact of the extent of resection in the treatment of malignant gliomas of childhood: a report of the Children's Cancer Group trial no CCG-945. J Neurosurg 89:52–59

Wolff JEA, Gnekow AK, Kortmann RD et al (2002) Preradiation chemotherapy for pediatric patients with high-grade glioma. Cancer 94:264–271

Wong JY, Uhl V, Wara WM, Sheline GE (1987) Optic gliomas: a reanalysis of the UCSF experience. Cancer 60:1847–1855

Zulch KJ (1986) Brain tumors: their biology and pathology, 3rd edn. Springer, Berlin Heidelberg New York, pp 210–213

Cerebellar Astrocytomas

J. H. Chi · N. Gupta

Contents

2.1 Introduction

Although astrocytomas as a group are the most common tumor of the central nervous system (CNS) in childhood, cerebellar astrocytomas account for only 10 to 17 % of all pediatric brain tumors (Reddy and Timothy 2000; Smoots et al. 1998) and 20 to 35 % of all posterior fossa tumors in children (Morreale et al. 1990; Reddy and Timothy 2000; Steinbok and Mutat 1999; Viano et al. 2001). Long-term survival after surgical resection is common and is dependent on histologic type, extent of invasion, and completeness of tumor removal.

Although the term "cerebellar astrocytoma" has become synonymous with a benign tumor, a variety of histological grades are encountered. The majority (80 %) of cerebellar astrocytomas in children are pilocytic (WHO grade I; see Sect. 2.3.2 for WHO grading) and demonstrate a benign histology (Morreale et al. 1990). Higher grade tumors, fibrillary astrocytomas (WHO grade II), account for 15 % of the total, while anaplastic astrocytomas (WHO grade III) and glioblastoma multiforme (GBM; WHO grade IV) are each less than 5 % of the total (Steinbok and Mutat 1999). The treatment of choice, originally reported by Cushing in 1931, is surgical gross total resection (GTR). Survival after GTR of grade I lesions is greater than 90 % at 5-years and 70 to 80 % at 10-years. Unfortunately, grade II lesions are estimated to have a 5-year survival of only 50 %, and the prognosis for higher-grade tumors remains very poor (Morreale et al. 1990).

Recent laboratory investigations have attempted to define the molecular genetic features of different grades of cerebellar astrocytoma. Clinical studies have focused on approaches to the treatment of residual/recurrent tumor, the role of adjuvant therapy, functional outcomes after treatment, and the management of complications, such as pseudomeningocele, hydrocephalus, and cerebellar mutism.

2.2 Epidemiology

2.2.1 Spontaneous Cerebellar Astrocytoma

Cerebellar astrocytomas account for 5 to 8% of all gliomas and 3.5% of all primary intracranial neoplasms in the general population (Morreale et al. 1990). In the pediatric population (<17-years of age), astrocytomas account for approximately 50% of all primary CNS tumors (Rickert et al. 1997). They can arise within the optic pathway (5%), hypothalamus (10%), cerebellum (15 to 25%), cerebral hemisphere (12%), spine (10 to 12%), and brain stem (12%) (Pollack 1999). Infratentorial tumors account for 50 to 60% of all intracranial tumors in childhood and include cerebellar astrocytomas (20 to 35%), medulloblastoma/PNET (30 to 35%), brain stem glioma (25%), ependymoma (10%), and other miscellaneous types (5%) (Pollack 1999).

The incidence of cerebellar astrocytoma is difficult to determine accurately, but is estimated to be 0.2 to 0.33 cases per 100,000 children per year (Berger 1996; Gjerris et al. 1998; Rosenfeld 2000). The incidence peaks between ages 4 and 10-years with a median age at diagnosis of 6-years (Steinbok and Mutat 1999). Twenty percent of these tumors occur in children less than 3-years of age (Rickert 1998). Gender does not play a role in prognosis or survival, and several case series show only slight male or female predominance (Rickert and Paulus 2001; Viano et al. 2001). International studies do not demonstrate a geographical or ethnic propensity for the occurrence of cerebellar astrocytomas, unlike craniopharyngiomas and germ cell tumors (Gjerris et al. 1998; Rickert 1998; Rickert and Paulus 2001).

The incidence of pediatric brain tumors was recently believed to be rising, based on studies from the US and Europe (Gjerris et al. 1998; Gurney et al. 1996). This trend has been refuted and is now attributed to increased surveillance and reporting (detec-

tion bias) during the preceding two decades and in the initial recruitment phase of large population-based studies (Rickert and Paulus 2001; Smith et al. 1998). Environmental factors such as parental smoking and residential proximity to electromagnetic field sources have not been linked to pediatric brain tumors, though parental occupation in the chemical/electrical industry might be associated with an increased risk of astroglial tumors in offspring (Gold et al. 1993). Conversely, prenatal vitamin supplementation in mothers may confer a slight protective effect (Preston-Martin et al. 1998). Prior cranial radiation therapy is a risk factor for developing malignant cerebellar astrocytomas as those children become older (Steinbok and Mutat 1999).

2.2.2 Neurofibromatosis Type I

Neurofibromatosis type 1 (NF1) is associated with an increased risk of intracranial tumors, with approximately 15 to 20% of patients presenting with low grade intracranial tumors. Pilocytic astrocytomas arise in a variety of locations in NF1, but most commonly in the optic nerve, hypothalamus, and cerebellum. The growth of intracranial tumors is the main cause of death amongst NF1 patients. Five percent of NF1 patients will develop pilocytic cerebellar astrocytomas (Li et al. 2001).

The *NF1* gene is located on chromosome 17q and encodes a GTPase activating protein (GAP), termed neurofibromin, involved in regulating the ras-p21 signaling pathway. Mutations in the *NF1* gene lead to the manifestations of the disease. The exact reason why loss of neurofibromin expression or expression of defective neurofibromin leads to the formation of astrocytomas is unknown. NF1 may arise from sporadic mutations in the *NF1* gene, or through germline transmission of an established mutation (Gutmann et al. 2000). NF1-associated CNS tumors, such as spontaneous pilocytic astrocytomas, rarely demonstrate alterations in other known oncogenic genes such as *p53*, *EGFR*, *PDGF* and *p21* (Gutmann et al. 2000). In general, NF1-associated cerebellar astrocytomas resemble spontaneous pilocytic astrocytomas and are benign (Vinchon et al. 2000).

Figure 2.1 a,b

Histopathological features of pilocytic astrocytoma. a Field of tumor cells demonstrating increased cellularity, mild nuclear atypia, and lack of mitoses. b Tumor edge with gliotic border (*left of image*) and neovascularization.

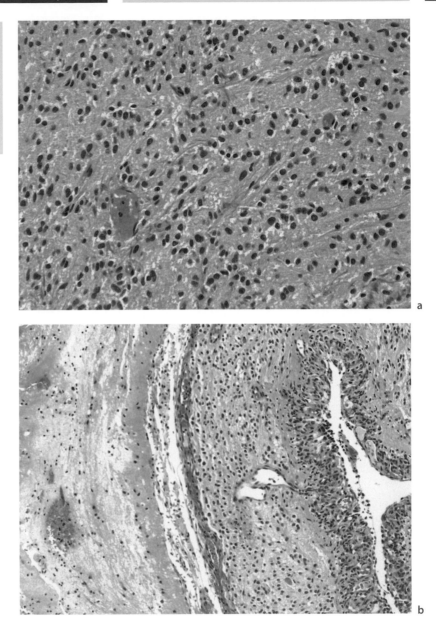

a

b

2.3 Pathology

2.3.1 Histopathology and Genetics

Cerebellar astrocytomas are divided into two distinct histologic groups: pilocytic and diffuse. Pilocytic astrocytomas are divided exhibit a biphasic pattern of compact, bipolar, highly fibrillated astrocytes accompanied by Rosenthal fibers alternating with loose-textured microcystic regions of eosinophilic granular astrocytes (Fig. 2.1). Pleomorphism, mitotic figures, hypercellularity, endothelial proliferation, and necrosis may be present and do not indicate malignancy or, unlike such findings in malignant astrocytomas, poor prognosis (Steinbok and Mutat 1999). Local lep-

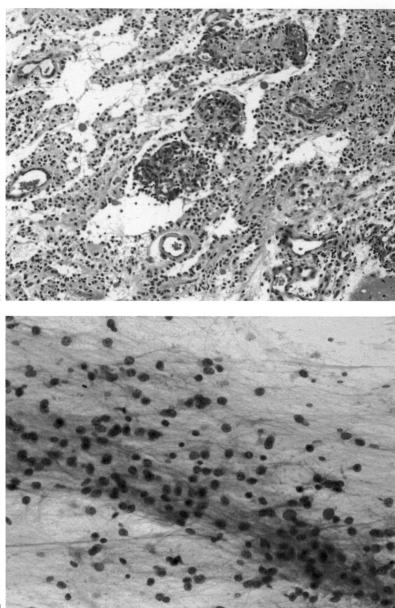

Figure 2.1 c,d

c Biphasic pattern of compact, fibrillated astrocytes and loosely textured microcysts with a focus of endothelial proliferation. d Squash preparations demonstrating thin glial processes ("pili") extending from bipolar tumor cells

tomeningeal invasion is apparent in half of all cases and has no prognostic significance (Burger et al. 2000). Because pilocytic astrocytomas are most common in the first two decades of life, they are often termed *juvenile* pilocytic astrocytomas (JPA). Pilocytic astrocytomas can be found throughout the neuraxis (optic pathway, hypothalamus, cerebral hemisphere), although 80% are found in the cerebellum (Dirven et al. 1997). Cytogenetic abnormalities include gains on chromosomes 1, 7, and 8 and loss of 17p and 17q (Wernicke et al. 1997; White et al. 1995; Zattara-Cannoni et al. 1998). The majority of pilocytic astrocytomas, however, demonstrate normal cytogenetic findings (Bigner et al. 1997; Griffin et al. 1988; Karnes et al. 1992). Mutations of *p53* are extremely rare, even in cases that undergo malignant transformation (Ishii et al. 1998).

Diffuse cerebellar astrocytomas belong to one of three histologic subtypes. Fibrillary astrocytoma is the most common subtype and demonstrates a uniform, compact arrangement of fibrillary astrocytes with varying degrees of cellular atypia on a background of loosely structured tumor matrix (Steinbok and Mutat 1999). Protoplasmic astrocytomas demonstrate low cellularity and extensive mucoid degeneration with numerous, occasionally confluent microcysts (Kaye and Walker 2000). Gemistocytic astrocytomas contain tumor cells with large, slightly eosinophilic cytoplasm with nuclei displaced to the periphery (Kaye and Walker 2000). Diffuse astrocytomas resemble low-grade astrocytomas of the cerebral hemispheres with poorly circumscribed borders and invasion of the surrounding parenchyma. These tumors generally occur in older children and young adults and can undergo malignant transformation (Burger et al. 2000). Mutations of *p53* are commonly reported (up to 80% in gemistocytic variants) and probably represent an early event in malignant progression (Kosel et al. 2001; Watanabe et al. 1998). Other aberra-

tions include allelic losses on chromosomes 10p, 19, and 22q (Bello et al. 1994; von Deimling et al. 1994). Recent experimental studies indicate that grade II tumors have higher mitotic indices, higher percentages of cells in S phase, and more VEGF expression than grade I tumors (Reddy and Timothy 2000).

2.3.2 WHO Classification

In the recent World Health Organization (WHO) classification of central nervous system tumors, cerebellar astrocytomas were organized into four grades (Table 2.1). WHO grade I corresponds to pilocytic cerebellar astrocytoma and accounts for approximately 70 to 80% of pediatric cases (Steinbok and Mutat 1999). Diffuse cerebellar astrocytomas are considered WHO grade II and represent 15% of childhood cases (Steinbok and Mutat 1999) (see 2.2.1). Experimental evidence suggests that grade I and II cerebellar astrocytomas develop from different precursor cells (Li et al. 2001). PEN5, a recently identified oligodendroglial antibody epitope, is positive in grade I tumors but not in grade II tumors. Also, NF1 related cerebellar astrocytomas demonstrate PEN5 immunoreactivity, indicating that both spontaneous grade I and NF1 related grade I cerebellar as-

Table 2.1. Comparison of cerebellar astrocytoma sub-types

WHO grade	Name	Histology	Genetics	Average survival
I	Pilocytic	Low cellularity Biphasic: compact bipolar cells and loose multipolar cells with microcysts and granular bodies Rosenthal fibers Rare mitoses	Nothing consistently reported	>10 years
II	Diffuse	Well-differentiated fibrillary astrocytes Loose tumor matrix Moderate cellularity, nuclear atypia and few mitoses Microcysts may or may not be present	p53 mutations (~60%) Allelic losses on chromosomes 10 and 19 PDGF amplification?	6–8 years

trocytomas come from the same precursor cells, which are different from those preceding grade II tumors.

Cerebellar grade III and IV tumors (anaplastic astrocytoma and glioblastoma multiforme) are rarely encountered in childhood and are identical to their adult counterparts in histology and prognosis. Grade III/IV tumors frequently show gains of chromosomes 7 and 10, structural changes of chromosomes 1, 9, 17, and 22, and loss of alleles on chromosome 17 (Biegel 1997). Mutation and over-expression of *p53* is common in both grade III and VI tumors. *EGFR* gene amplification, observed in approximately 30% of adult tumors, seems to be rarer in pediatric high grade astrocytomas (Sung et al. 2000). *PTEN* mutations were found in 20 to 30% of grade IV tumors, 5.9% of grade III tumors, and 0% of grade II tumors (Raffel et al. 1999).

2.3.3 Gross Pathology

Grossly, cerebellar astrocytomas can be cystic, solid, or have a mixed character. Pilocytic astrocytomas (WHO grade I) are typically described as cystic tumors containing yellow-brown fluid and a neoplastic mural nodule. The cyst wall may contain either neoplastic cells or a pseudocapsule of non-neoplastic glial tissue (Steinbok and Mutat 1999). This classic appearance occurs in less then 50% of cases. Diffuse subtypes are almost always solid tumors composed of somewhat circumscribed neoplastic cells without evidence of cysts. Very commonly, however, cerebellar astrocytomas demonstrate mixed appearance and consist of both cystic and solid portions of tumor. Cystic lesions tend to occur in the cerebellar hemispheres while solid tumors often arise in the midline near the vermis and potentially extend to the brain stem (Abdollahzadeh et al. 1994).

2.3.4 Miscellaneous Grading Scales

Several other histopathologic classifications for cerebellar astrocytomas have been published. Winston and Gilles identified three clusters of histologic fea-

tures that correlated with prognosis (Conway et al. 1991; Steinbok and Mutat 1999). "Glioma A" tumors have microcysts, leptomeningeal deposits, Rosenthal fibers, or foci of oligodendroglioma. "Glioma B" tumors have a combination of perivascular pseudorosettes, hypercellularity, mitosis, necrosis, and/or calcification in the absence of any glioma A features. "Glioma C" tumors are the remaining tumors that do not match either of these categories. Five year survival for groups A and B were 100% and 41% respectively, while 10-year survival was 94% for glioma A, 29% for glioma B and 69% for glioma C (Campbell and Pollack 1996). However, this schema has been criticized for including a heterogeneous group of tumors encompassing features such as mitosis/necrosis and pseudorosettes that indicate higher grade glioma and ependymoma, respectively, in the "Glioma B" category, which may contribute to its association with a poorer prognosis (Campbell and Pollack 1996).

The Kernohan and St. Anne-Mayo classification systems, which are used to describe astrocytomas in any location, are rarely used to describe pediatric cerebellar astrocytomas.

2.4 Clinical Features: Signs and Symptoms

The mean age at diagnosis for cerebellar astrocytomas in children is 6.8-years of age (range 6 months to 17-years) and the average duration of symptoms is approximately 3 to 5 months (with a range of 3 days to 3-years) (Reddy and Timothy 2000; Steinbok and Mutat 1999). The slow growing, indolent characteristics of these tumors allows functional compensation of adjacent brain tissue, and most cerebellar astrocytomas tend to be large at time of diagnosis. With greater availability of high resolution neuroimaging, detection of these lesions is occurring earlier than in the past. Attempts to correlate age at diagnosis and prognosis have been inconclusive, and though patients diagnosed at younger ages tend to have better outcomes, more of these tumors tend to have a benign pathology (Morreale et al. 1997). However, a very short duration of symptoms may be associated with higher malignancy (grade III/VI) and poorer prognosis.

Table 2.2. Signs and symptoms of cerebellar astrocytoma (Abdollahzadeh et al. 1994; McCowage et al. 1996; Rickert 1998; Sgouros et al. 1995)

Presenting symptoms	Percent
Headache	82–87
Vomiting	65–85
Gait disturbance	12–79
Visual disturbance	12–17
Diplopia	10–31
Decreased level of consciousness	9–21
Vertigo	1.5–9
Head tilt	3–18
Behavior changes	2–7
Neck pain/stiffness	2–23
Seizures	2

Signs	Percent
Cerebellar signs/ataxia	74–89
Papilledema	69–88
CN palsy	15–40
Dysmetria	23–39
Nystagmus	10–40
Pyramidal signs	4–13
Increased head circumference	1–16
Hydrocephalus	85
Parinaud's	29
Hemiparesis	1.8–3

Initial signs and symptoms (Table 2.2) are usually mild and nonspecific and are caused by increased intracranial pressure (ICP). Headache is the most common presenting complaint (75 to 97%) (Abdollahzadeh et al. 1994; Berger 1996; Steinbok and Mutat 1999; Viano et al. 2001) and frequently occurs with recumbency. Decreased venous return and hypoventilation during sleep and recumbency exacerbates raised intracranial pressure (Steinbok and Mutat 1999). Headaches begin frontally and may migrate to the occiput.

Constant occipital headache and neck pain with hyperextension is an ominous sign of tonsillar herniation into the foramen magnum. Respiratory depression, preceded by cluster or ataxic breathing, may follow shortly (Rosenfeld 2000). Vomiting, found in 64 to 84% of patients, is the second most frequent presenting symptom and is also caused by hydrocephalus and raised ICP (Steinbok and Mutat 1999; Viano et al. 2001). In the absence of tumor infiltration of the area postrema, vomiting is usually not accompanied by nausea, unlike ependymomas and other lesions arising from the fourth ventricle itself.

Signs of cerebellar dysfunction include ataxia (88%), gait disturbance (56%), appendicular dysmetria (59%), and wide-based gait (27%) (Abdollahzadeh et al. 1994; Pencalet et al. 1999; Steinbok and Mutat 1999; Viano et al. 2001). Lesions of a cerebellar hemisphere produce ataxia and dysmetria in the ipsilateral limbs, while midline lesions produce truncal and gait ataxia (Berger 1996). Other clinical features include behavioral changes (32%), neck pain (20%), and papilledema (55 to 75%) (Abdollahzadeh et al. 1994; Steinbok and Mutat 1999). Some degree of hydrocephalus occurs in 92% of cases, while seizures are extremely rare (2 to 5%) (Abdollahzadeh et al. 1994). Cranial nerves and descending motor tracts are usually not affected, unless there is significant tumor extension, and involvement indicates probable brain stem infiltration. The only clinical feature related to poor prognosis is the presence of brain stem dysfunction (level of consciousness, motor tract signs) regardless of histology (Sgouros et al. 1995).

2.5 Natural History

Cerebellar astrocytomas were once considered generic brain tumors, probably congenital, localized to the posterior fossa, and requiring treatment only when symptomatic. Patients would typically report longstanding headaches and emesis since childhood, with occasional periods of relief. Patients with long standing cerebellar symptoms often developed symptoms of syringomyelia, indicating unrelieved hydrocephalus. It was commonly believed that the cyst wall and cyst fluid were the pathological culprits.

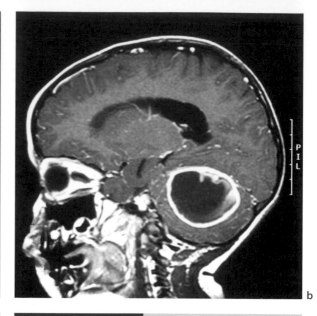

a

b

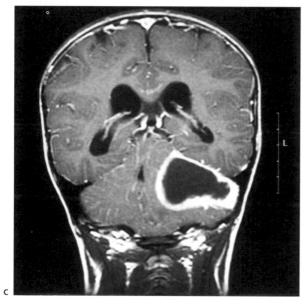

c

Figure 2.2 a–c

MRI images of a typical pilocytic cerebellar astrocytoma. a Axial, b sagittal, c coronal T1-weighted MRI with gadolinium contrast demonstrating cystic hemispheric lesion with mural nodule. In this case the cyst wall enhances brightly following gadolinium and does represent tumor

the true pathology lay in the mural nodule and that removal of the mural tumor may result in cure (Cushing 1931). If left untreated, the patient would experience increasing bouts of cerebellar fits, become blind, and ultimately become comatose and succumb.

2.6 Diagnosis and Neuroimaging

2.6.1 Computed Tomography and Magnetic Resonance Imaging

Thus, early treatment consisted of cyst fluid decompression and cyst wall removal. Symptoms were relieved temporarily, but patients often returned within months to years with cyst recurrence and sometimes tumors with malignant progression. Not until Cushing reported his surgical experience with 76 cerebellar astrocytomas in 1931 did it become clear that

Computed tomography (CT) and magnetic resonance imaging (MRI) are the preferred techniques used to diagnose cerebellar astrocytomas. CT is faster and less costly than MRI, but bone artifact limits visualization of the posterior fossa. MRI is preferred preoperatively because of its accurate anatomic localization, superior resolution (no bone artifact and increased tissue distinction), and multiplanar capability. The disadvantages of MRI include increased study time and the requirement of general anesthesia in younger children and infants. Both CT and MRI allow for contrast injection and adequately demonstrate the degree of hydrocephalus present.

The classic radiological appearance of a pilocytic cerebellar astrocytoma, observed in 30 to 60% of cases, is a large cyst with a solid mural nodule (found in 90% of these lesions; Fig. 2.2) localized to one of the cerebellar hemispheres (Reddy and Timothy 2000; Steinbok et al. 1996). On CT the cyst is hypodense to brain and hyperdense to CSF due to its high protein content, while on MRI the cyst appears hypointense to brain on T1 weighted images (T1-WI) and hyperintense on T2 weighted images (T2-WI). The mural nodule is hypo- to isodense to brain on CT and hyperintense to brain on T1-WI. The mural nodule enhances uniformly following contrast administration on both CT and MRI, while the cyst is not affected by contrast. The cyst wall, however, may demonstrate contrast enhancement if neoplastic cells are present. Most surgeons regard a contrast-enhancing cyst wall as neoplastic tissue and attempt to resect the entire cyst wall. In certain cases, the compressed glial reactive tissue surrounding a cyst may also show limited enhancement (Fig. 2.3). Other variations include multiple mural nodules, a single large nodule filling in a portion of the cyst, and/or an irregular cyst contour.

Cerebellar astrocytomas can also appear as solid lesions in 17 to 56% of cases, with 90% arising from or involving the vermis (Pencalet et al. 1999; Reddy and Timothy 2000). CT shows a lesion hypo- to isodense to brain and MRI demonstrates a solid mass hyperintense to brain. The solid tumor enhances uniformly following contrast administration in the majority of cases, but variations include regions of non-enhancement and small intratumoral cysts in up to 30% of solid tumors (Campbell and Pollack 1996). Quite often, cerebellar astrocytomas will appear with both cystic and solid features and may have a rind-like enhancement pattern with varying degrees of cyst formation. Brain stem involvement is seen in 8 to 30% of cases (Reddy and Timothy 2000; Steinbok and Mutat 1999; Viano et al. 2001), while the cerebel-

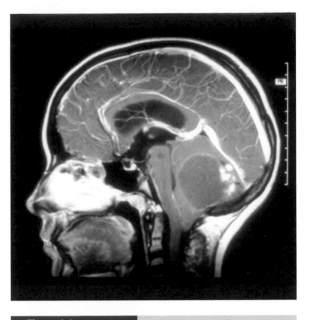

Figure 2.3

Sagittal MRI of a cerebellar astrocytoma showing an irregular, enhancing nodule located posterior to a large cyst. The cyst wall appears to enhance slightly but this represents gliotic brain tissue

lar peduncles are affected in 34% (Hayostek et al. 1993; Pencalet et al. 1999). Calcifications are present in 10 to 17% of tumors and hemorrhage in only 4.5% (Berger 1996). Edema may be evident in some cases but does not indicate malignancy or poor prognosis.

2.6.2 Magnetic Resonance Spectroscopy

Unfortunately, neither classic tumor appearance nor location on neuroimaging can confidently distinguish cerebellar astrocytoma from PNET and ependymoma. Biopsy with histological examination is necessary to establish a definitive diagnosis. Recently, magnetic resonance spectroscopy (MRS) has been used to distinguish various pediatric cerebellar tumors based on differential levels of tumor metabolites and macromolecules. Pilocytic astrocytomas demonstrate increased choline/N-acetyl-aspartate (CHO:NAA) ratios and elevated lactate levels when compared to normal brain, similar to many other tumor types (Hwang et al. 1998; Wang et al. 1995; Warren et al. 2000). In one study, low grade astrocytomas had higher NAA:CHO ratios than PNET, but lower ratios than ependymoma, while creatine:CHO ratios were highest for ependymoma and lowest for PNET (Hwang et al. 1998; Wang et al. 1995). MRS may be useful for distinguishing posterior fossa tumors in children after initial CT/MRI scanning. Other metabolites differentially detected in PNET and astrocytoma in vitro include glutamate, glycine, taurine, and myoinositol. One study examined subtotally resected low-grade astrocytomas and reported that higher normalized CHO levels significantly related to tumor progression for 2-years following resection (Lazareff et al. 1998). Alternatively, high levels of lactate in pilocytic astrocytoma carries no indication of malignancy and may reflect aberrant glucose utilization in these tumors (Wang et al. 1995).

2.7 Treatment

2.7.1 Preoperative Management

Preoperative management is dependent on the clinical presentation of the patient. An asymptomatic, incidentally discovered lesion can be observed with surgery planned electively. More commonly, however, patients present with signs of increased intracranial pressure and cerebellar dysfunction, warranting urgent medical intervention. High dose dexamethasone can relieve headache, nausea, and vomiting within 12 to 24 hours and allow for several days of relief prior to a surgical procedure. An initial loading dose of 0.5 to 1.0 mg/kg IV followed by 0.25 to 0.5 mg/kg/day divided every 6 hours is the typical regimen (Rosenfeld 2000). In a patient who is stuporous and lethargic, with cardiorespiratory instability, relief of elevated ICP is of utmost importance and should be performed immediately. This is done by placing an external ventricular drain (EVD). In less urgent situations, an endoscopic third ventriculocisternostomy (ETV) can also be considered (Sainte-Rose et al.

2001). This procedure consists of placing a fenestration in the floor of the third ventricle to allow CSF to bypass an obstructive lesion in the posterior fossa. ETV, although not always successful, can avoid permanent shunt placement. Currently, most surgeons will promptly proceed with tumor resection in the hope that relief of the obstructing mass will also treat the associated hydrocephalus.

Ventriculoperitoneal (VP) shunting has been shown to improve survival after surgical resection of posterior fossa tumors. This procedure carries the risk of upward herniation and subdural hematoma from overshunting, and also renders the patient dependent for life on the shunt, with all of its associated complications. The risk of upward herniation is estimated at 3% and presents with lethargy and obtundation around 12 to 24 hours after shunt placement with the potential for compression of the posterior cerebral artery at the tentorial hiatus, causing occipital lobe ischemia/stroke (Steinbok and Mutat 1999). Postoperative CSF diversion (with VP shunting) following complete tumor removal and unblockage of the aqueduct and fourth ventricle is required in 10 to 40% of cases (Imielinski et al. 1998).

2.7.2 Operative Treatment

2.7.2.1 Gross Total Resection

Gross total resection (GTR) is the preferred treatment goal and is achieved in 60 to 80% of operative cases (Campbell and Pollack 1996; Gajjar et al. 1997). GTR is defined as the removal of all identifiable tumor during surgery, and is accomplished only when both the surgeon's report and postoperative neuroimaging are concordant. MRI with gadolinium is recommended within 24 to 48 hours after resection. Postoperative changes, including swelling, edema, and gliosis appear by 3 to 5 days following surgery and may interfere with the identification of residual tumor (Berger 1996). Residual tumor after GTR is detected by imaging in 15% of cases, while postoperative imaging fails to demonstrate known residual tumor as reported by the surgeon in 10% of cases (Dirven et al. 1997). The clear presence of residual tumor is managed by reoperation to achieve complete resection.

Classic cystic tumors with a mural nodule may only require removal of the nodule to achieve complete resection, but the management of cyst wall is more controversial. Contrast enhancement of cyst wall on post-contrast MRI scans is believed to represent neoplastic tissue, and complete removal of all enhancing portions is considered essential to prevent recurrence. Non-enhancing areas do not require resection, though recent studies have shown that enhancement of the cyst wall does not always indicate tumor and may only represent vascularized reactive gliosis (Burger et al. 2000; Steinbok and Mutat 1999). There is also some evidence to suggest that patients who undergo complete cyst-wall removal may have a poorer prognosis at 5-years than those with cyst walls left intact (Sgouros et al. 1995). Some support biopsy of the cyst wall during resection for frozen section, but pathological assessment is usually indeterminate and the sampling error is high, making biopsy of little value. Surgeons may choose conservative management of enhancing cyst wall, especially if such enhancement is thin (indicating gliosis rather than tumor), biopsy samples unremarkable for clear pathology, and gross appearance benign (Steinbok and Mutat 1999).

2.7.2.2 Subtotal Resection

Subtotal resection (STR) is recommended when GTR would result in unacceptable morbidity and neurologic dysfunction, usually in the setting of brain stem invasion, involvement of the floor of the fourth ventricle, leptomeningeal spread, and metastasis. Involvement of the cerebellar peduncles was once thought to preclude GTR, but several authorities contend that GTR can be achieved in this circumstance (Berger 1996; Steinbok and Mutat 1999), as postoperative deficits from resection involving the cerebellar peduncles tend to be transient. Management of incompletely resected tumors remains controversial and depends on clinical circumstances.

2.7.3 Follow-up Neuroimaging

Postoperative surveillance imaging in children with benign cerebellar astrocytomas depends on the extent of initial resection and the histology of tumor. While no standard schedule for surveillance imaging exists, large centers tend to obtain MRI scans at 3 and 6 months, then annually for 3 to 4 years. Routine imaging after confirmed GTR for a typical JPA can be stopped 3 to 5 years following resection if there is no evidence of recurrence. However, due to the well-documented late-recurrence behavior of a small percentage of benign cerebellar astrocytomas, sometimes decades after GTR, clinical changes should warrant re-imaging. STR requires closer serial neuroimaging due to higher rates of tumor recurrence. Diffuse/fibrillary histology (grade II) is associated with STR; however, GTR of this histologic subtype seems to demonstrate prognosis and recurrence rates rivaling those of juvenile pilocytic cerebellar tumors (grade I). Nevertheless, most practitioners tend to follow grade II lesions more closely with serial exams and neuroimaging.

2.7.4 Management of Recurrence

Management of recurrence remains the most challenging aspect of treating cerebellar astrocytomas. Treatment options include a combination of reoperation, radiation therapy, and chemotherapy (Fig. 2.4). Recurrence following GTR is rare and can occur several years to decades from the initial operation. Fortunately, the majority of these patients do well after reoperation and rarely require further treatment. Reoperation with the goal of GTR is the recommended treatment for recurrence following STR, although this is usually not possible because the primary reason for incomplete resection is usually involvement of vital structures such as the brain stem (Aguiar et al. 1995). At reoperation, only 30% of recurrences result in GTR, while 70% continue to have residual tumor (Dirven et al. 1997). An interesting biologic feature of low-grade astrocytomas is spontaneous regression or involution of residual tumors (see Sect. 2.8.2). For this reason many authors advocate a

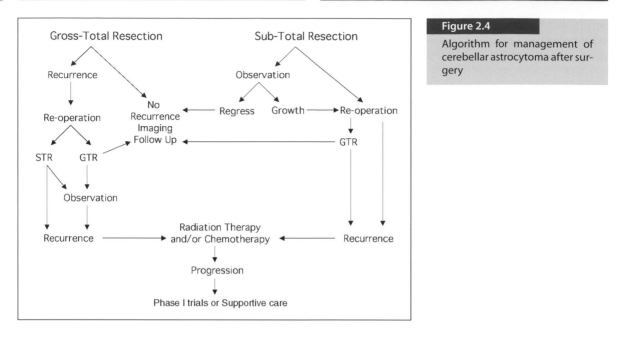

period of observation for residual disease prior to re-operation. This approach is favored at our institution particularly since a second procedure is associated with increased morbidity afterward (Dirven et al. 1997).

Eighty-eight percent of all patients who recurred had undergone STR, while 20 to 50 % had brain stem invasion (Pencalet et al. 1999). Following STR, 30 to 40 % of patients recur within 3 years (mean 54 months), while more than 60 % recur by 5 to 6 years (Dirven et al. 1997). Diffuse/fibrillary histology is more prone to recurrence, but this association is not reported consistently in all series. Of all recurrent tumors, 65 % are pilocytic and 31 % are diffuse/fibrillary (Gjerris et al. 1998; Sgouros et al. 1995). Recurrences are more often found in the midline or vermis. Smoot et al. (1998), using multivariate analysis, noted that the only factor that predicted disease progression was volume of residual disease. This study also showed that only fibrillary histology, and not brain stem invasion or postoperative radiation therapy, significantly affects postoperative tumor volume. Unfortunately, the relationship between STR, brain stem invasion, residual tumor volume, and

histology confound each other in almost all other series.

2.7.5 Adjuvant Therapy for Recurrence

Radiation therapy after resection plays an important role in the control of PNET and ependymoma, but its utility in cerebellar astrocytoma is incompletely understood. Postoperative irradiation in subtotally resected tumors of any grade improves local control and recurrence rates, but survival rates seem to be unaffected (Garcia et al. 1990; Herfarth et al. 2001). One retrospective, nonrandomized study comparing patients with recurrent grade I and II cerebellar astrocytoma found no significant difference in survival at both 5 and 9 years follow-up (Akyol et al. 1992). Radiation doses range from 30 to 54 Gy over 3 to 6 weeks, and some evidence suggests that doses greater than 53 Gy are necessary to see beneficial effects (Herfarth et al. 2001; Tamura et al. 1998). However, the detrimental effects on the developing nervous system precludes its use in infants less than 3 years of age and current trends favor delaying radiation therapy as long as possible to maximize cognitive development prior to radiation therapy. The risks of radiation therapy include decreased cognitive function (Chadderton et al. 1995) and increased risk of malignant transformation (Herfarth et al. 2001).

Currently, there is no consensus on the use of radiation therapy for the treatment of benign recurrent cerebellar astrocytoma, though some authors suggest its use if the recurrent tumor displays more aggressive growth features (Akyol et al. 1992; Garcia et al. 1990). Experience with Gamma Knife (Elekta AB, Stockholm) radiosurgery for the treatment of small-volume residual or recurrent tumors is still too limited at this time for adequate assessment; it may have a role for the treatment of very limited disease (Campbell and Pollack 1996; Somaza et al. 1996).

Chemotherapy has an insignificant role in the treatment of benign cerebellar astrocytoma, but has been used in rare instances of multifocal disease, leptomeningeal spread, and malignant transformation (Castello et al. 1998; Tamura et al. 1998). Combination chemotherapy has been used in adjuvant management of inoperable low-grade astrocytomas. The most widely used regimens are carboplatin/vincristine (Packer et al. 1993) and 6-thioguanine/procarbazine/CCNU/vincristine (Prados et al. 1997). Both regimens have been associated with complete and partial responses in subgroups of tumors. Chronic etoposide treatment showed stable tumor lesions at 7 months in patients with recurrent nonresectable cerebellar astrocytomas in one study (Chamberlain 1997). Cyclophosphamide has been applied in the treatment of cerebellar astrocytoma with leptomeningeal spread (McCowage et al. 1996). To date, no study has shown clear benefits in recurrence or survival with chemotherapy for residual or recurrent cerebellar astrocytomas.

2.8 Outcome

2.8.1 Prognostic Factors

2.8.1.1 Brain Stem Invasion

Brain stem invasion carries a poor prognosis with only 40% of patients alive at 5-years after diagnosis (Sgouros et al. 1995). Conversely, 84% of patients with no evidence of brain stem involvement are alive at 5-years (Sgouros et al. 1995). Brain stem invasion significantly impacts survival irrespective of histology, as noted in several large series (Campbell and Pollack 1996). Smoots et al. (1998) also contend that residual tumor volume within the brain stem is the only prognostic factor for disease progression after multivariate analysis.

2.8.1.2 Tumor Grade

The impact of histology on outcome and progression-free survival (PFS) has been controversial (Pencalet et al. 1999). Hayostek et al. (1993) showed that pilocytic cerebellar astrocytoma has 5, 10, and 20-year survival rates of 85%, 81%, and 79%, respectively, while diffuse subtypes have dramatically reduced survival rates of 7% at each of the 5, 10, and 20-year timepoints. Unfortunately, the mean age of patients in both groups differed greatly (14-years for pilocytic, 51-years for diffuse) making any meaningful comparison difficult. Also, diffuse tumors in this study had more malignant histology (mitosis, necrosis, etc.), which suggests that higher-grade lesions might have been included inappropriately. More recent series have reported 78% survival with 89% PFS for pilocytic histology and 44% survival with 52% PFS for diffuse subtypes at 5-years (Sgouros et al. 1995). Diffuse/fibrillary histology is reported as the single most important determinant for residual tumor volume, which according to one study is the only predictor of tumor recurrence at any site after multivariate analysis (Smoots et al. 1998). Comparing GTR and STR between grade I and grade II tumors has been difficult because grade II lesions are more often subtotally resected due to tumor location and invasion. Two authors, after multivariate analyses, suggest that only extent of resection contributes to outcome in children with grade I and grade II cerebellar astrocytoma (Sgouros et al. 1995; Smoots et al. 1998).

2.8.1.3 Tumor Appearance

Older reports state that tumors with cystic morphology have a greater 5-year PFS than do solid tumors. More recent studies have now shown that cystic tumors are more often completely resectable than are solid tumors, which often invade surrounding parenchyma, making their complete removal difficult. After controlling for extent of tumor removal, most series do not demonstrate a survival advantage based on tumor morphology (Sgouros et al. 1995; Smoots et al. 1998). Also, tumor location (hemispheric vs. vermian/midline) does not appear to affect prognosis (Smoots et al. 1998). Complete resection is more often achieved with a hemispheric location than in the midline, probably due to the ability to perform a more aggressive resection.

2.8.1.4 Clinical Features

Few clinical characteristics at time of presentation contribute to overall outcome. Gender and age at diagnosis do not correlate to survival (Campbell and Pollack 1996; Gilles et al. 1995; Smoots et al. 1998), though earlier age at presentation might indicate earlier progression of disease in those with recurrences (Gajjar et al. 1997). A short duration of symptoms at time of presentation is generally associated with a more rapidly growing tumor, and therefore one more likely to be of higher grade. Longer preoperative symptomatology may indicate progressed disease and larger tumor volume (Pencalet et al. 1999). Patients with neurofibromatosis sometimes present with malignant histology, but the majority of NF patients with cerebellar astrocytomas appear to have a quiescent course (Freeman et al. 1998; Smoots et al. 1998), though absolute numbers are small. The only clinical feature related to poorer prognosis and survival is evidence of brain stem dysfunction. Long tract signs, nystagmus, apnea, and decreased consciousness indicate brain stem invasion by tumor, but also can result from raised ICP and mass effect.

2.8.2 Gross Total and Subtotal Resection

The prognosis for patients with grade I tumors and GTR is excellent with 5 and 10-year progression-free survival of 80 to 100% in nearly all studies. Also, 30-year PFS is not uncommon with long term follow-up in these patients. Patients with grade II tumors have 5-year survival rates of 50 to 80% after GTR. As expected, grade III and IV lesions continue to have poor survival at 2-years despite GTR. GTR is more commonly reported in tumors of pilocytic histology with cystic morphology and peripheral/hemispheric location. Recurrence after confirmed GTR grade I tumors is rare and occurs in less than 5% of cases, though recurrences have been reported as late as 45-years after initial resection (Boch et al. 2000). GTR is reported in 53% of patients with pilocytic cerebellar astrocytomas operated upon, while only 19% of non-pilocytic cerebellar tumors achieve GTR (Campbell and Pollack 1996).

In general, STR is associated with future tumor recurrence and poorer outcome (Pencalet et al. 1999). Approximately 75% of patients with STR will recur during follow-up. The 5-year survival rate ranges from 29 to 80%, and 10-year survival ranges from 0 to 70% (Campbell and Pollack 1996; Sgouros et al. 1995). These variations in survival are explained by inconsistent study design. STR is more commonly reported with solid, midline tumors that are usually grade II or higher. A number of reports demonstrate that patients with STR remain stable, both clinically and on serial imaging, without any evidence of progression for several years (Krieger et al. 1997). In one prospective study, only 50% of patients with STR and no brain stem involvement demonstrated progression of disease at 8-years follow-up (Sutton et al. 1996). In the same study, 1.5% of documented residual tumors spontaneously regressed without further treatment. Smoot et al. observed that 4 of 17 patients with residual tumors had complete disappearance of tumor without additional intervention (Smoots et al. 1998; Steinbok and Mutat 1999). Unfortunately, the number of reported involuted tumors was too small to allow for any meaningful sub-analysis. Pilocytic astrocytoma of the optic pathways or hypothalamic region is known to resolve without any treatment, and most of the spontaneously regressing tumors were of this type (Berger 1996; Freeman et al. 1998). The biologic reason behind tumor quiescence or regression is unknown.

2.8.3 Malignant Transformation

Malignant transformation of pilocytic astrocytomas is an exceedingly rare event (Berger 1996; Mamelak et al. 1994). Several case reports describe malignant degeneration in pilocytic cerebellar astrocytomas at recurrence several years from initial resection. Standard indices of aggressive histology such as necrosis, vascular proliferation, and mitoses do not indicate malignancy in pilocytic astrocytomas, though increased perivascular cellularity may serve as a marker of future anaplastic change (Krieger et al. 1997).

2.8.4 Metastasis

Leptomeningeal dissemination (LMD) of low-grade astrocytomas occurs rarely and is associated mainly with hypothalamic tumor location (Morikawa et al. 1997; Pollack et al. 1994; Tamuar et al. 1998). Spinal metastases are the most common and were found in 3 of 72 patients in one series (Pollack et al. 1994) and in 7% of diffuse cerebellar astrocytoma patients at the time of diagnosis in one other study (Hayostek et al. 1993). Long-term outcome is not known, but there is anecdotal evidence that LMD indicates impending malignant degeneration (Krieger et al. 1997). Aggressive resection of isolated metastasis combined with aggressive chemotherapy and additional radiation therapy may result in progression-free survival (Berger 1996; Pollack et al. 1994; Tamura et al. 1998). CSF sampling offers no aid in detecting early LMD (Pollack et al. 1994).

2.8.5 Survival

Progression-free survival and overall outcome is dependent upon several factors including extent of resection, brain stem involvement, and histologic subtype (Table 2.3). Patients with complete tumor removal enjoy 5 and 10-year PFS in greater than 90% of cases (Gajjar et al. 1997; Steinbok and Mutat 1999). Incomplete tumor resection results in approximately 50% 5-year survival in most series, but with reoperation to remove residual tumor, outcome may improve to 80% PFS at 5-years, 74% at 10-years, and 40% at 20-years (Gajjar et al. 1997). STR with recurrence carries a 25% PFS at 5-years from the time of recurrence; reoperation tends to lower subsequent recurrence rates, but does not affect overall survival (Sgouros et al. 1995). Radiation therapy in the setting of

Table 2.3. Survival outcomes for cerebellar astrocytoma (Campbell and Pollack 1996; Li et al. 2001; Raffel et al. 1999)

Factor		5-year (%)	10-year (%)	20-year (%)
Degree of resection	Gross total	80–100	90	90
	Subtotal	30–80	0–79	42
Brain stem involvement	Yes	40	N/A	N/A
	No	83	N/A	N/A
Tumor appearance	Cystic	88	N/A	N/A
	Solid	52	N/A	N/A
At recurrence		29	N/A	N/A

N/A = not reported

STR or recurrence has not been shown to confer any benefit on overall survival in nearly all studies, but some do report a trend towards lowering the rate of local progression.

2.9 Complications

Surgical resection of cerebellar astrocytomas may lead to both non-neurological and neurological complications (Table 2.4). Fortunately, the majority of these adverse effects are either transient or treatable, making the overall morbidity for surgical treatment of cerebellar astrocytomas quite low.

2.9.1 Neurological Complications

2.9.1.1 Cerebellar Dysfunction

Worsening of cerebellar function, limb/truncal ataxia and cranial nerve (CN) palsy (usually of CN VI) following surgery is not uncommon (Cochrane et al. 1994). Increased ataxia and dysmetria are usually due to retraction injury or cerebellar swelling and improve after several weeks to months. Restiform body injury may result in permanent ipsilateral limb ataxia (Rosenfeld 2000). Significant injury to the vermis can cause severe disabling truncal ataxia, which may resolve only after a prolonged period of time. New neurological deficits are found in 30% of postoperative patients and include CN VI and VII dysfunction, nystagmus, bulbar signs, pseudobulbar syndrome, long tract motor signs, and transient mutism (Cochrane et al. 1994). Impaired initiation of chewing, voiding, and eye opening may present after injury to areas of the cerebellum responsible for repetitive motor movement memory.

Patients with these deficits commonly have tumor involving the floor of the fourth ventricle, brain stem, and cerebellar peduncles. Sometimes, removal of a hemispheric tumor creates enough intracranial shift to affect CN VI and cause transient diplopia. Approximately one half of those with new deficits experience complete recovery of function (Ersahin et al. 1996; Pollack et al. 1995; Steinbok and Mutat 1999).

Table 2.4. Complications following surgery for cerebellar astrocytoma (Abdollahzadeh et al. 1994; Raffel et al. 1999; Rickert 1998)

Complication	Percent
Pseudomeningocele	12–24
Wound infection	2–5
Aseptic meningitis	4.5
Septic meningitis	6
Persistent HCP	10
Hematoma	
Epidural	3
Subdural	3
Operative site	1.5
Transient CN palsy	4.5
Hemiplegia	1.5
Transient mutism	1.5
Permanent neurological deficit	15

2.9.1.2 Cerebellar Mutism

Cerebellar mutism is a well-recognized complication of surgical removal of large midline posterior fossa tumors in children. Patients demonstrate transient mutism with unimpaired consciousness, intact comprehension, and no detectable cranial nerve or motor deficits. The majority of cases will awake from surgery with intact speech function, but then develop mutism within 24 to 94 hours (Pollack et al. 1995). In the largest series to date, the incidence was 8.5% for all posterior fossa tumors and 12% for vermian tumors, but did vary with histology (Catsman-Berrevoets et al. 1999). Patients with malignant tumors commonly involving the brain stem, fourth ventricle, and vermis experienced mutism more often (20%) than those with less invasive tumors (1%) (Doxey et al. 1999; Ersahin et al. 1996).

Clinical improvement begins as profoundly dysarthric and abnormal speech, usually with isolated words and phrases, and progressively improves to full sentences. Recovery can begin as early as 2 weeks after onset of symptoms or as late as 2 months after onset. Most patients recover fluent speech within 4 months of surgery with an average duration of mutism lasting 6 weeks (Aguiar et al. 1995; Ersahin et al. 1996; Pollack et al. 1995). Twenty percent of patients may have permanent dysarthria following recovery from mutism. There are no identifiable clinical predictors of cerebellar mutism, and all cases report normal preoperative speech (Pollack et al. 1995). A small case-controlled radiological review identified bilateral edema in the brachium pontis as the only factor significantly associated with mutism (Pollack et al. 1995).

2.9.1.3 Neuropsychological Consequences

Surgery of the cerebellum also leads to alterations in higher cognitive function, an effect usually attributed to damage to the cerebral hemispheres. One study of children following surgery of the posterior fossa for tumor demonstrated neuropsychological changes at 2-year follow-up, which included visual-spatial dysfunction in 37%, expressive language problems in 37 %, verbal memory decline in 33%, and difficulty with affect control in 15 to 56% (Levisohn et al. 2000). Irritability, impulsiveness, and disinhibition were the most common changes in affect and increased in parallel with greater involvement of the vermis. These neuropsychological consequences seem to also be temporary, but long term studies are not available.

School performance and IQ are also affected by cerebellar surgery, but current studies are confounded by the inability to separate the emotional and psychological effects of childhood illness and stress from cerebellar surgery itself. Strong evidence is lacking for cerebellar astrocytomas, but estimates indicate that greater than 60% of these patients will have an IQ greater than 90 after surgery, equivalent to patients with ependymoma and far better than patients with PNETs (only 10% will have an IQ greater than 90 after treatment for PNET) (Hoppe-Hirsch et al. 1995). Postoperative radiation therapy is strongly associated with lower IQ during childhood, and affects younger children more than older ones (Grill et al. 1999).

2.9.2 Non-neurological Complications

2.9.2.1 Pseudomeningocele

Pseudomeningocele, the formation of a CSF collection outside the confines of the subarachnoid space, is reported in 12 to 24% of patients postoperatively (Abdollahzadeh et al. 1994). It occurs 1 to 2 weeks after the initial surgery and presents as a fluctuant, occasionally tense mass under the incision. A pseudomeningocele predisposes surgical incisions to infection and dehiscence, which can then lead to more serious complications including meningitis. The formation of a pseudomeningocele may indicate the presence of untreated hydrocephalus, a CSF fistula, or a wound infection. Most pseudomeningoceles resolve within days to weeks without intervention. Wound breakdown and hydrocephalus are indications for CSF diversion/shunting and antibiotic treatment if meningitis or other infection is suspected. Percutaneous aspiration for cell count and culture is not recommended as risk of infection rises with skin puncture, although it may provide temporary relief of pain from skin tension, or prevention of complete wound dehiscence.

2.9.2.2 Hydrocephalus

Hydrocephalus (HCP) can develop from obstruction anywhere along the CSF pathway from blood clot, swelling, or inflammation. Persistent hydrocephalus is reported in 10% of postoperative patients. Asymptomatic HCP requires no immediate intervention and the patient can be followed for 6 to 8 weeks before permanent shunt placement is considered. Acute hydrocephalus warrants immediate CSF diversion and may also occur in the setting of hemorrhage within the resection cavity, necessitating urgent evacuation. Ventriculoperitoneal shunting is indicated with raised ICP, persistent pseudomeningocele, and CSF leak, and is required in 10 to 26% of patients following posterior fossa surgery (Imielinski et al. 1998; Rosenfeld 2000; Steinbok and Mutat 1999). The risk of extra-neural metastasis from shunting in children with cerebellar astrocytomas is virtually nonexistent (Berger et al. 1991).

2.9.2.3 Other

Wound infection and breakdown are rare (2 to 5%). Risk factors include poor nutritional state, formation of a CSF pseudomeningocele, poor surgical closure, wound hematoma, and premature removal of sutures. Meningitis occurs in 3 to 8% of patients (Abdollahzadeh et al. 1994). Aseptic meningitis is a well-described postoperative finding after posterior fossa surgery in children. Patients complain of increasing headache 4 to 7 days following surgery, accompanied by fever, nuchal rigidity, and CSF pleocytosis (Rosenfeld 2000). CSF culture and gram stain are negative. No treatment is necessary, though bacterial meningitis must be excluded. The risk of bacterial meningitis is higher in patients with pseudomeningocele and shunts. Cervical spine instability requiring structural support is exceedingly rare, but can occur when a laminectomy extends below C1. Radiation treatment and infection are additional risk factors.

2.10 Conclusion

Among pediatric brain tumors, cerebellar astrocytomas have among the most favorable prognosis. The great majority of cerebellar astrocytomas are low-grade neoplasms (juvenile pilocytic/grade I tumors) with excellent cure rates and long-term survival following surgery. Only a small minority have dismal outcomes (grade III and IV tumors). Tumor recurrence, when it does occur, is a challenging management problem and is most often seen with grade II tumors, subtotal resection, or brain stem invasion. There is no consensus among authorities regarding the optimal method in treating recurrence, though reoperation is advocated for first time recurrence, and for subsequent recurrence many endorse following the repeat surgery with radiation therapy. Chemotherapy is reserved for rare cases of leptomeningeal spread and those tumors that do not respond to radiation, although its use may also be considered prior to radiation in young children with inoperable tumors. Other management considerations encountered with cerebellar astrocytomas include pre- or postoperative CSF diversion to control hydrocephalus and perioperative steroid administration. Surgical removal of cerebellar astrocytomas may be complicated by cerebellar dysfunction, cranial nerve palsies, and mutism. These risks need to be discussed preoperatively with the patient and parents. Fortunately, the majority of patients recovers completely from adverse postperative events.

References

Abdollahzadeh M, Hoffman HJ, Blazer SI, Becker LE, Humphreys RP, Drake JM, Rutka JT (1994) Benign cerebellar astrocytoma in childhood: experience at the Hospital for Sick Children 1980–1992. Childs Nerv Syst 10:380–383

Aguiar PH, Plese JP, Ciquini O, Marino R (1995) Transient mutism following a posterior fossa approach to cerebellar tumors in children: a critical review of the literature. Childs Nerv Syst 11:306–310

Akyol FH, Atahan IL, Zorlu F, Gurkaynak M, Alanyali H, Ozyar E (1992) Results of post-operative or exclusive radiotherapy in grade I and grade II cerebellar astrocytoma patients. Radiother Oncol 23:245–248

Bello MJ, de Campos JM, Kusak ME, Vaquero J, Sarasa JL, Pestana A, Rey JA (1994) Molecular analysis of genomic abnormalities in human gliomas. Cancer Genet Cytogenet 73:122–129

Berger MS (1996) Cerebellar astrocytoma, chap 119. In: Becker DP, Dunsker SB, Friedman WA, Hoffman HJ, Smith RR, Wilson CB (eds) Tumors. Saunders, Philadelphia, pp 2593–2602

Berger MS, Baumeister B, Geyer JR, Milstein J, Kanev PM, LeRoux PD (1991) The risks of metastases from shunting in children with primary central nervous system tumors. J Neurosurg 74:872–877

Biegel JA (1997) Genetics of pediatric central nervous system tumors. J Pediatr Hematol Oncol 19:492–501

Bigner SH, McLendon RE, Fuchs H, McKeever PE, Friedman HS (1997) Chromosomal characteristics of childhood brain tumors. Cancer Genet Cytogenet 97:125–134

Boch AL, Cacciola F, Mokhtari K, Kujas M, Philippon J (2000) Benign recurrence of a cerebellar pilocytic astrocytoma 45-years after gross total resection. Acta Neurochir (Wien) 142:341–346

Burger PC, Scheitauer BW, Paulus W, Szymas J, Gianni C, Kleihues P (2000) Pilocytic Astrocytoma, chap 1. In: Kleihues P and Cavenee WK (eds) Pathology and genetics. Tumors of the nervous system: IARC Press, Lyon

Campbell JW, Pollack IF (1996) Cerebellar astrocytomas in children. J Neurooncol 28:223–231

Castello MA, Schiavetti A, Varrasso G, Clerico A, Cappelli C (1998) Chemotherapy in low-grade astrocytoma management. Childs Nerv Syst 14:6–9

Catsman-Berrevoets CE, Van Dongen HR, Mulder PG, Paz y Geuze D, Paquier PF, Lequin MH (1999) Tumour type and size are high risk factors for the syndrome of "cerebellar" mutism and subsequent dysarthria. J Neurol Neurosurg Psychiatry 67:755–757

Chadderton RD, West CG, Schuller S, Quirke DC, Gattamaneni R, Taylor R, Schulz S (1995) Radiotherapy in the treatment of low-grade astrocytomas. II. The physical and cognitive sequelae. Childs Nerv Syst 11:443–448

Chamberlain MC (1997) Recurrent cerebellar gliomas: salvage therapy with oral etoposide. J Child Neurol 12:200–204

Cochrane DD, Gustavsson B, Poskitt KP, Steinbok P, Kestle JR (1994) The surgical and natural morbidity of aggressive resection for posterior fossa tumors in childhood. Pediatr Neurosurg 20:19–29

Conway PD, Oechler HW, Kun LE, Murray KJ (1991) Importance of histologic condition and treatment of pediatric cerebellar astrocytoma. Cancer 67:2772–2775

Cushing H (1931) Experiences with the cerebellar astrocytomas: a evitical review of seventy-sy cases. Surg Gynecd Obstet 52:120–128

Dirven CM, Mooij JJ, Molenaar WM (1997) Cerebellar pilocytic astrocytoma: a treatment protocol based upon analysis of 73 cases and a review of the literature. Childs Nerv Syst 13:17–23

Doxey D, Bruce D, Sklar F, Swift D, Shapiro K (1999) Posterior fossa syndrome: identifiable risk factors and irreversible complications. Pediatr Neurosurg 31:131–136

Ersahin Y, Mutluer S, Cagli S, Duman Y (1996) Cerebellar mutism: report of seven cases and review of the literature. Neurosurgery 38:60–65

Freeman CR, Farmer JP, Montes J (1998) Low-grade astrocytomas in children: evolving management strategies. Int J Radiat Oncol Biol Phys 41:979–987

Gajjar A, Sanford RA, Heideman R, Jenkins JJ, Walter A, Li Y, Langston JW, Muhlbauer M, Boyett JM, Kun LE (1997) Low-grade astrocytoma: a decade of experience at St Jude Children's Research Hospital. J Clin Oncol 15:2792–2799

Garcia DM, Marks JE, Latifi HR, Kliefoth AB (1990) Childhood cerebellar astrocytomas: is there a role for postoperative irradiation? Int J Radiat Oncol Biol Phys 18:815–818

Gilles FH, Sobel EL, Tavare CJ, Leviton A, Hedley-Whyte ET (1995) Age-related changes in diagnoses, histological features, and survival in children with brain tumors: 1930–1979. The Childhood Brain Tumor Consortium. Neurosurgery 37:1056–1068

Gjerris F, Agerlin N, Borgesen SE, Buhl L, Haase J, Klinken L, Mortensen AC, Olsen JH, Ovesen N, Reske-Nielsen E, Schmidt K (1998) Epidemiology and prognosis in children treated for intracranial tumours in Denmark 1960–1984. Childs Nerv Syst 14:302–311

Gold EB, Leviton A, Lopez R, Gilles FH, Hedley-Whyte ET, Kolonel LN, Lyon JL, Swanson GM, Weiss NS, West D et al (1993) Parental smoking and risk of childhood brain tumors. Am J Epidemiol 137:620–628

Griffin CA, Hawkins AL, Packer RJ, Rorke LB, Emanuel BS (1988) Chromosome abnormalities in pediatric brain tumors. Cancer Res 48:175–180

Grill J, Renaux VK, Bulteau C, Viguier D, Levy-Piebois C, Sainte-Rose C, Dellatolas G, Raquin MA, Jambaque I, Kalifa C (1999) Long-term intellectual outcome in children with posterior fossa tumors according to radiation doses and volumes. Int J Radiat Oncol Biol Phys 45:137–145

Gurney JG, Davis S, Severson RK, Fang JY, Ross JA, Robison LL: 1996. Trends in cancer incidence among children in the U.S. Cancer 78:532–541,

Gutmann DH, Donahoe J, Brown T, James CD, Perry A (2000) Loss of neurofibromatosis 1 (*NF1*) gene expression in *NF1*-associated pilocytic astrocytomas. Neuropathol Appl Neurobiol 26:361–367

Hayostek CJ, Shaw EG, Scheithauer B, O'Fallon JR, Weiland TL, Schomberg PJ, Kelly PJ, Hu TC (1993) Astrocytomas of the cerebellum. A comparative clinicopathologic study of pilocytic and diffuse astrocytomas. Cancer 72:856–869

Herfarth KK, Gutwein S, Debus J (2001) Postoperative radiotherapy of astrocytomas. Semin Surg Oncol 20:13–23

Hoppe-Hirsch E, Brunet L, Laroussinie F, Cinalli G, Pierre-Kahn A, Renier D, Sainte-Rose C, Hirsch JF (1995) Intellectual outcome in children with malignant tumors of the posterior fossa: influence of the field of irradiation and quality of surgery. Childs Nerv Syst 11:340–345

Hwang JH, Egnaczyk GF, Ballard E, Dunn RS, Holland SK, Ball WS Jr (1998) Proton MR spectroscopic characteristics of pediatric pilocytic astrocytomas. AJNR Am J Neuroradiol 19:535–540

Imielinski BL, Kloc W, Wasilewski W, Liczbik W, Puzyrewski R, Karwacki Z (1998) Posterior fossa tumors in children – indications for ventricular drainage and for V-P shunting. Childs Nerv Syst 14:227–229

Ishii N, Sawamura Y, Tada M, Daub DM, Janzer RC, Meagher-Villemure M, de Tribolet N, van Meir EG (1998) Absence of *p53* gene mutations in a tumor panel representative of pilocytic astrocytoma diversity using a *p53* functional assay. Int J Cancer 76:797–800

Karnes PS, Tran TN, Cui MY, Raffel C, Gilles FH, Barranger JA, Ying KL (1992) Cytogenetic analysis of 39 pediatric central nervous system tumors. Cancer Genet Cytogenet 59:12–19

Kaye AH, Walker DG (2000) Low grade astrocytomas: controversies in management. J Clin Neurosci 7:475–483

Kosel S, Scheithauer BW, Graeber MB (2001) Genotype-phenotype correlation in gemistocytic astrocytomas. Neurosurgery 48:187–193

Krieger MD, Gonzalez-Gomez I, Levy ML, McComb JG (1997) Recurrence patterns and anaplastic change in a long-term study of pilocytic astrocytomas. Pediatr Neurosurg 27:1–11

Lazareff JA, Bockhorst KH, Curran J, Olmstead C, Alger JR (1998) Pediatric low-grade gliomas: prognosis with proton magnetic resonance spectroscopic imaging. Neurosurgery 43:809–817

Levisohn L, Cronin-Golomb A, Schmahmann JD (2000) Neuropsychological consequences of cerebellar tumour resection in children: cerebellar cognitive affective syndrome in a paediatric population. Brain 123:1041–1050

Li J, Perry A, James CD, Gutmann DH (2001) Cancer-related gene expression profiles in NF1-associated pilocytic astrocytomas. Neurology 56:885–890

Mamelak AN, Prados MD, Obana WG, Cogen PH, Edwards MS (1994) Treatment options and prognosis for multicentric juvenile pilocytic astrocytoma. J Neurosurg 81:24–30

McCowage G, Tien R, McLendon R, Felsberg G, Fuchs H, Graham ML, Kurtzberg J, Moghrabi A, Ferrell L, Kerby T, Duncan-Brown M, Stewart E, Robertson PL, Colvin OM, Golembe B, Bigner DD, Friedman HS (1996) Successful treatment of childhood pilocytic astrocytomas metastatic to the leptomeninges with high-dose cyclophosphamide. Med Pediatr Oncol 27:32–39

Morikawa M, Tamaki N, Kokunai T, Nagashima T, Kurata H, Yamamoto K, Imai Y, Itoh H (1997) Cerebellar pilocytic astrocytoma with leptomeningeal dissemination: case report. Surg Neurol 48:49–51

Morreale VM, Ebersold MJ, Quast LM, Parisi JE (1997) Cerebellar astrocytoma: experience with 54 cases surgically treated at the Mayo Clinic, Rochester, Minnesota, from 1978 to 1990. J Neurosurg 87:257–261

Packer RJ, Lange B, Ater J, Nicholson HS, Allen J, Walker R, Prados M, Jakacki R, Reaman G, Needles MN et al (1993) Carboplatin and vincristine for recurrent and newly diagnosed low-grade gliomas of childhood. J Clin Oncol 11:850–856

Pencalet P, Maixner W, Sainte-Rose C, Lellouch-Tubiana A, Cinalli G, Zerah M, Pierre-Kahn A, Hoppe-Hirsch E, Bourgeois M, Renier D (1999) Benign cerebellar astrocytomas in children. J Neurosurg 90:265–273

Pollack IF (1999) Pediatric brain tumors. Semin Surg Oncol 16:73–90

Pollack IF, Hurtt M, Pang D, Albright AL (1994) Dissemination of low grade intracranial astrocytomas in children. Cancer 73:2869–2878

Pollack IF, Polinko P, Albright AL, Towbin R, Fitz C (1995) Mutism and pseudobulbar symptoms after resection of posterior fossa tumors in children: incidence and pathophysiology. Neurosurgery 37:885–893

Prados MD, Edwards MS, Rabbitt J, Lamborn K, Davis RL, Levin VA (1997) Treatment of pediatric low-grade gliomas with a nitrosourea-based multiagent chemotherapy regimen. J Neurooncol 32:235–241

Preston-Martin S, Pogoda JM, Mueller BA, Lubin F, Modan B, Holly EA, Filippini G, Cordier S, Peris-Bonet R, Choi W, Little J, Arslan A (1998) Prenatal vitamin supplementation and pediatric brain tumors: huge international variation in use and possible reduction in risk. Childs Nerv Syst 14:551–557

Raffel C, Frederick L, O'Fallon JR, Atherton-Skaff P, Perry A, Jenkins RB, James CD (1999) Analysis of oncogene and tumor suppressor gene alterations in pediatric malignant astrocytomas reveals reduced survival for patients with PTEN mutations. Clin Cancer Res 5:4085–4090

Reddy ATM, Timothy B (2000) Cerebellar astrocytoma, chap 74. In: McLone DG (ed) Pediatric neurosurgery: surgery of the developing nervous system. Saunders, New York, pp 835–843

Rickert CH (1998) Epidemiological features of brain tumors in the first 3-years of life. Childs Nerv Syst 14:547–550

Rickert CH, Paulus W (2001) Epidemiology of central nervous system tumors in childhood and adolescence based on the new WHO classification. Childs Nerv Syst 17:503–511

Rickert CH, Probst-Cousin S, Gullotta F (1997) Primary intracranial neoplasms of infancy and early childhood. Childs Nerv Syst 13:507–513

Rosenfeld JV (2000) Cerebellar astrocytoma in children, chap 37. In: Kaye AH, Black PM (eds) Operative neurosurgery. Churchill Livingstone, New York, pp 447–463

Sainte-Rose C, Cinalli G, Roux FE, Maixner R, Chumas PD, Mansour M, Carpentier A, Bourgeois M, Zerah M, Pierre-Kahn A, Renier D (2001) Management of hydrocephalus in pediatric patients with posterior fossa tumors: the role of endoscopic third ventriculostomy. J Neurosurg 95:791–797

Sgouros S, Fineron PW, Hockley AD (1995) Cerebellar astrocytoma of childhood: long-term follow-up. Childs Nerv Syst 11:89–96

Smith MA, Freidlin B, Ries LA, Simon R (1998) Trends in reported incidence of primary malignant brain tumors in children in the United States. J Natl Cancer Inst 90:1269–1277

Smoots DW, Geyer JR, Lieberman DM, Berger MS (1998) Predicting disease progression in childhood cerebellar astrocytoma. Childs Nerv Syst 14:636–648

Somaza SC, Kondziolka D, Lunsford LD, Flickinger JC, Bissonette DJ, Albright AL (1996) Early outcomes after stereotactic radiosurgery for growing pilocytic astrocytomas in children. Pediatr Neurosurg 25:109–115

Steinbok P, Hentschel S, Cochrane DD, Kestle JR (1996) Value of postoperative surveillance imaging in the management of children with some common brain tumors. J Neurosurg 84:726–732

Steinbok P, Mutat A (1999) Cerebellar astrocytoma, chap 35. In: Albright AL, Pollack IF, Adelson PD (eds) Principles and practice of pediatric neurosurgery. Thieme, New York, pp 641–662

Sung T, Miller DC, Hayes RL, Alonso M, Yee H, Newcomb EW (2000) Preferential inactivation of the p53 tumor suppressor pathway and lack of EGFR amplification distinguish de novo high grade pediatric astrocytomas from de novo adult astrocytomas. Brain Pathol 10:249–259

Sutton LN, Cnaan A, Klatt L, Zhao H, Zimmerman R, Needle M, Molloy P, Phillips P (1996) Postoperative surveillance imaging in children with cerebellar astrocytomas. J Neurosurg 84:721–725

Tamura M, Zama A, Kurihara H, Fujimaki H, Imai H, Kano T, Saitoh F (1998) Management of recurrent pilocytic astrocytoma with leptomeningeal dissemination in childhood. Childs Nerv Syst 14:617–622

Viano JC, Herrera EJ, Suarez JC (2001) Cerebellar astrocytomas: a 24-year experience. Childs Nerv Syst 17:607–610

Vinchon M, Soto-Ares G, Ruchoux MM, Dhellemmes P (2000) Cerebellar gliomas in children with NF1: pathology and surgery. Childs Nerv Syst 16:417–420

Von Deimling A, Nagel J, Bender B, Lenartz D, Schramm J, Louis DN, Wiestler OD (1994) Deletion mapping of chromosome 19 in human gliomas. Int J Cancer 57:676–680

Wang Z, Sutton LN, Cnaan A, Haselgrove JC, Rorke LB, Zhao H, Bilaniuk LT, Zimmerman RA (1995) Proton MR spectroscopy of pediatric cerebellar tumors. AJNR Am J Neuroradiol 16:1821–1833

Warren KE, Frank JA, Black JL, Hill RS, Duyn JH, Aikin AA, Lewis BK, Adamson PC, Balis FM (2000) Proton magnetic resonance spectroscopic imaging in children with recurrent primary brain tumors. J Clin Oncol 18:1020–1026

Watanabe K, Peraud A, Gratas C, Wakai S, Kleihues P, Ohgaki H (1998) *p53* and *PTEN* gene mutations in gemistocytic astrocytomas. Acta Neuropathol (Berl) 95:559–564

Wernicke C, Thiel G, Lozanova T, Vogel S, Witkowski R (1997) Numerical aberrations of chromosomes 1, 2, and 7 in astrocytomas studied by interphase cytogenetics. Genes Chromosomes Cancer 19:6–13

White FV, Anthony DC, Yunis EJ, Tarbell NJ, Scott RM, Schofield DE (1995) Nonrandom chromosomal gains in pilocytic astrocytomas of childhood. Hum Pathol 26:979–986

Zattara-Cannoni H, Gambarelli D, Lena G, Dufour H, Choux M, Grisoli F, Vagner-Capodano AM (1998) Are juvenile pilocytic astrocytomas benign tumors? A cytogenetic study in 24 cases. Cancer Genet Cytogenet 104:157–160

Brainstem Gliomas

E. Pan · M. Prados

Contents

3.1 Introduction

Historically, brainstem gliomas (BSGs) were regarded as a homogeneous category of central nervous system neoplasms with a uniformly poor prognosis. With the advent of magnetic resonance imaging (MRI), BSGs are now recognized as a heterogeneous group of neoplasms with distinct subtypes that vary widely with respect to prognosis and growth patterns. They can be classified broadly into two categories: the diffuse intrinsic gliomas and the nondiffuse brainstem tumors (Table 3.1). The diffuse intrinsic gliomas, which constitute the majority of brainstem tumors and conform to the stereotype of BSGs, occur most often in the pons, infiltrate throughout the brainstem, and have a uniformly poor prognosis. The nondiffuse brainstem tumors include focal midbrain, dorsally exophytic, and cervicomedullary tumors. Almost all of these tumors are slow-growing, low-grade neoplasms that have a more favorable prognosis and response to treatment (specifically surgery) than the diffuse intrinsic gliomas. The management plan for these tumors is individualized to each distinct brainstem tumor type and is based strongly upon their MRI characteristics and clinical presentations. It should be appreciated that other tumors and non-tumor conditions such as brain abscess, neuroepithelial cyst, and inflammatory conditions can also present with lesions in the brainstem, but these entities are exceptionally rare and will not be discussed further.

Table 3.1. Overview of the brainstem glioma subtypes[a]

Tumor type	Approximate frequency (%)	Clinical presentation	Imaging characteristics	Predominant pathology
Diffuse intrinsic	75–85	Multiple bilateral CN deficits	Diffuse pontine enlargement	Fibrillary astrocytoma (Grades II-IV)
		LTS	T1 hypointensity	
		Ataxia	T2 hyperintensity	
		Short clinical history	Little contrast enhancement	
Focal midbrain	5–10[b]	Signs and symptoms of raised ICP	Small, well-circumscribed	Low-grade astrocytoma (Grades I and II)
		Isolated CN deficit	No edema	Ganglioglioma
		Ataxia	T1 hypointensity	
		Hemiparesis (rarer)	T2 hyperintensity	
		Torticollis	Variable enhancement	
			Ventriculomegaly	
Dorsally exophytic	10–20	Signs and symptoms of raised ICP	Arise from floor of 4th ventricle	Pilocytic astrocytoma (Grade I)
		CN dysfunction	T1 hypointensity	Grade II astrocytoma
		Prominent nystagmus	T2 hyperintensity	
		Torticollis	Bright enhancement	
		FTT (infants)		
		LTS typically absent		
Cervicomedullary	5–10	Lower CN dysfunction	Arise from lower medulla/upper cervical cord	Low-grade astrocytoma
		LTS		
		Apnea	Bulges dorsally toward 4th ventricle	Ganglioglioma
		Sensory loss	T1 hypointensity	
		Torticollis	T2 hyperintensity	
		Hydrocephalus (rarer)	Commonly enhances	

[a] Adapted from Freeman and Farmer (1998)
[b] Frequency reflects incidence of focal tumors of the midbrain and medulla
CN, cranial nerve; ICP, increased intracranial pressure; LTS, long tract signs; FTT, failure to thrive

3.2 Epidemiology

Brainstem tumors account for approximately 10 to 20 % of all intracranial tumors in children (Panitch and Berg 1970; Farwell et al. 1977; Albright et al. 1983); 90 % are glial in origin (Pierre-Kahn et al. 1993). Seventy-five percent of BSGs occur in patients before age 10 (Panitch and Berg 1970; Farwell et al. 1977). Historically, the prognosis for children with BSGs (particularly diffuse intrinsic gliomas) has been exceedingly poor, with median survival ranging from 4 to 15 months (Fulton et al. 1981). The median time to disease progression of diffuse intrinsic gliomas is only 5 to 6 months, and only 6 to 10 % of these patients survive beyond 2 years after treatment (Freeman and Perilongo 1999). The overall 5-year survival rates are in the range 20 to 30 % for all brainstem tumors (Freeman and Farmer 1998).

Diffuse pontine gliomas represent 80 % of all pediatric BSG subtypes (Freeman and Farmer 1998). The nondiffuse brainstem tumors, including focal midbrain, dorsally exophytic, and cervicomedullary tumors, occur less frequently but have much better prognoses. One study noted a 4-year progression-free survival rate (PFS) of 94 % and a total 4-year survival rate of 100 % in 17 patients with focal midbrain tumors, which included tectal gliomas (Robertson et al. 1995). Pollack et al. (1993) noted that 17 of 18 patients (94 %) with dorsally exophytic brainstem tumors were alive at the conclusion of their study; follow-up periods ranged from 33 to 212 months. Patients with cervicomedullary tumors have been noted to have a 5-year PFS rate of 60 % and an overall 5-year survival rate of 89 % after initial resection (Weiner et al. 1997). Thus, the incidence and prognosis of BSG vary depending on the specific tumor subtype and location.

3.3 Pathology

Brainstem gliomas are not designated as a specific pathological category in the World Health Organization (WHO) classification of central nervous system tumors. Rather, BSGs are classified by location rather than histology. For this reason, BSGs comprise tumors of varying behavior and grade. Benign and low-malignancy brainstem tumors tend to occur in the midbrain and medulla, while higher-grade gliomas occur more frequently in the pons. The major utility of examining BSGs as a separate group from other posterior fossa tumors is that distinct therapeutic and prognostic concerns are related to neoplasms in this location.

3.3.1 Histopathology

3.3.1.1 Diffuse Pontine Glioma

Similar to astrocytomas elsewhere in the CNS, most diffuse pontine gliomas are fibrillary astrocytomas and are characterized by the presence of nuclear atypia, scant cytoplasm, and microcysts. Increased mitotic activity and nuclear pleomorphism are features of grade III (anaplastic) astrocytoma, while microvascular proliferation and necrosis are required for a diagnosis of grade IV astrocytoma (glioblastoma multiforme). Fibrillary astrocytomas also exhibit immunohistochemical reactivity to glial fibrillary acidic protein (GFAP) and vimentin. It is difficult to accurately determine the frequency of low- versus high-grade tumors with diffuse intrinsic gliomas, since biopsies are performed in only one-fourth to one-third of all cases. An additional complicating factor is the unavoidability of sampling error when a stereotactic biopsy is performed (Freeman and Farmer 1998). At autopsy, most pontine tumors are high-grade gliomas with extensive brainstem involvement, a finding that is most consistent with the poor outcome associated with these tumors (Mantravadi et al. 1982).

3.3.1.2 Nondiffuse Brainstem Glioma

The overwhelming majority of focal midbrain tumors, either tectal or tegmental, are grade I (pilocytic) or grade II astrocytomas (Hoffman et al. 1980; Robertson et al. 1995). Anaplastic astrocytomas have been reported to occur in this region; however, they are recognized to have a more benign course than similar tumors in the cerebral hemispheres (Raffel et al. 1988). Most cervicomedullary tumors are low-grade astrocytomas. Both gangliogliomas, which contain both neoplastic glial cells and dysplastic neurons, and ependymomas, which arise from ependymal cells that line the ventricles, have also been reported in this region (Epstein and Farmer 1993; Weiner et al. 1997). Anaplastic astrocytomas were noted in 4 of 39 patients (10 %; Weiner et al. 1997) and 4 of 44 patients (9 %) with cervicomedullary tumors (Epstein and Farmer 1993). Thus, approximately 90 % of cervicomedullary tumors are believed to be low-grade in nature.

Dorsally exophytic tumors are largely low-grade astrocytomas. Khatib et al. reported in their series that 11 of 12 patients (92 %) with dorsally exophytic tumors had classic grade I pilocytic astrocytomas (Khatib et al. 1994). Histologically, these tumors are characterized by a biphasic pattern of compacted bipolar cells with loose-textured multipolar cells, low cellularity, and Rosenthal fibers, which are eosinophilic, hyaline, corkscrew-shaped intracytoplasmic masses. Mitoses are rare in these tumors. Gangliogliomas (Hoffman et al. 1980) and anaplastic astrocytomas (Pollack et al. 1993) have also been reported, although these tumors rarely occur as dorsally exophytic tumors.

3.3.2 Molecular Biology

The molecular characterization of BSG, particularly of diffuse intrinsic pontine gliomas, is only at the beginning stages. Sawyer et al. reported an extra copy of the long arm of chromosome 1 (trisomy 1q) that was translocated onto the distal end of one copy of chromosome 7 as the sole chromosomal abnormality in a patient with a high-grade pontine astrocytoma (Sawyer et al. 1990). Analysis of 13 pontine gliomas of juvenile onset revealed a high incidence of multiple or tandem mutations of probable somatic (not germline) origin in the *p53* gene. These mutations appear to be characteristic for pontine gliomas, as cerebral gliomas do not usually have multiple mutations (Zhang et al. 1993). Louis et al. (1993) also reported allelic losses of chromosomes 17p (including the *p53*

gene) and 10 in pediatric brainstem glioblastoma multiforme (GBM) patients, with no epidermal growth factor receptor (*EGFR*) gene amplifications noted. This pattern of genetic alterations (i.e., *p53* mutations without *EGFR* amplification) is similar to that of secondary GBMs in young adults, which are believed to arise from lower-grade astrocytomas (Watanabe et al. 1996). The significance of such findings remains unclear. An important challenge in understanding the biology of these tumors is the relative paucity of human tissue available for molecular analysis, as few diffuse pontine gliomas undergo biopsy.

3.4 Clinical Features

The array of clinical signs and symptoms caused by BSGs is dependent upon their exact location and the affected anatomic structures. For example, focal midbrain tectal gliomas typically cause extraocular motor palsies and hydrocephalus, while hemiparesis is much less common. Dorsally exophytic tumors arise primarily within the medulla and extend posteriorly into the fourth ventricle. They often present with signs and symptoms of raised intracranial pressure, including headache, nausea, vomiting, papilledema, gait ataxia, and stupor. In infants, such tumors often present insidiously with failure to thrive. Other signs include torticollis, prominent nystagmus, and cranial nerve dysfunction (Pollack et al. 1993). Long tract signs such as paresis, hyperreflexia, spasticity, and the Babinski reflex are typically absent in patients with these tumors. Cervicomedullary tumors originate in the lower medulla and upper cervical spinal cord, which contain the lower cranial nerve nuclei (IX to XII), medullary respiratory center, descending motor corticospinal tracts, and ascending sensory tracts. Thus, presenting signs and symptoms of cervicomedullary tumors typically include dysphagia, dysarthria, nausea, vomiting, apnea, failure to thrive in infants, upper motor neuron dysfunction, sensory loss, and torticollis. Unlike in patients with dorsally exophytic tumors, hydrocephalus is unusual and long tract signs are common in patients with cervicomedullary tumors.

The pons is the largest of the three brainstem components and primarily contains motor tracts destined for the spinal cord and cerebellum. Diffuse intrinsic pontine gliomas may present with a "triad" of clinical signs: cranial nerve dysfunction (particularly CN VI and VII), long tract signs, and ataxia. While these three signs present simultaneously in only about 35 % of diffuse pontine glioma patients (Farmer et al. 2001), the majority of patients present with at least one of these cardinal signs. These tumors typically have a short duration of symptoms prior to diagnosis (median of 1 month), and only about 10 % of patients present with hydrocephalus at diagnosis (Freeman and Farmer 1998).

3.4.1 Growth Pattern

Many of the BSGs, when subclassified correctly according to clinical presentation and location, have stereotypical growth patterns. The growth and shape of these tumors, especially the benign, slow-growing neoplasms, are strongly influenced by existing anatomical structures. This was observed by Scherer (1938), who stated that fiber tracts and pial borders direct the growth of low-grade lesions. Focal midbrain tumors often remain circumscribed within the dorsal area of the midbrain (tegmentum and tectal plate) (Rubin et al. 1998). Diffuse pontine gliomas,

in comparison, grow unhindered along the medullary axis both rostrally and caudally, without involving the fourth ventricle (Epstein and Farmer 1993). Unlike low-grade tumors, the expansion of a high-grade tumor is not contained or controlled by the surrounding tissue matrix (Scherer 1938).

Dorsally exophytic tumors originate within the substance of the medulla. Initially, the lesion causes focal swelling of the medulla and displaces the axially-oriented fiber tracts. Because of rostral and caudal anatomic barriers, the tumor grows toward the avenue of least resistance, which in this region is the floor of the fourth ventricle, thus becoming dorsally exophytic (Fig. 3.1a–c) (Epstein and Farmer 1993).

Cervicomedullary tumors originate within the upper cervical cord below the cervicomedullary barrier. Caudal growth is limited by the circumferential pia of the upper cord and follows a cylindrical shape, similar to spinal cord tumors. Rostral growth is limited by the crossing fibers of the low medulla, and thus directs the growth toward the least resistant area, the obex, which is the midline point of the dorsal medulla that marks the caudal angle of the fourth ventricle (Fig. 3.2 a,b) (Epstein and Farmer 1993). From there the tumor may rupture through the obex into the fourth ventricle and cause obstructive hydrocephalus.

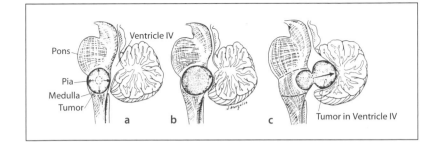

Figure 3.1 a–c

Illustrations of growth patterns of benign medullary tumors. a Focal medullary tumor displaces axially oriented fibers as it grows (*arrows*). b Larger focal medullary tumor tends to grow subependymally (*arrowhead*) since its axial growth is limited by barriers. c Subependymal lesion becomes dorsally exophytic (*arrow*) because of the limited resistance to growth offered by the ependyma. (Reprinted with permission from Epstein and Farmer 1993)

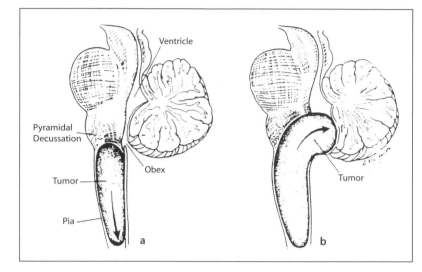

Ventricle

Pyramidal
Decussation

Obep

Tumor

Pia

a

Tumor

b

Figure 3.2 a,b

Illustrations of growth patterns of cervicomedullary lesions. a Caudal growth is cylindrical, as for spinal cord tumors (*arrow*). b Rostral growth is directed toward the obex (*arrow*) as a result of hindrance from pial elements and decussating fibers. Note the rostral displacement of the barrier. (Reprinted with permission from Epstein and Farmer 1993)

3.4.2 Prognostic Factors

A number of studies have addressed the question of which factors are predictive for prognosis. Albright et al. (1986) found that early presentation of cranial nerve palsies and presence of mitoses on histologic examination were statistically significant negative prognostic factors, whereas calcification or Rosenthal fibers in the tumor histology were significant favorable prognostic factors. Other studies have also found a significant correlation of early cranial nerve involvement with poor outcome. Other features associated with poor outcome include presence of long tract signs (Freeman et al. 1993), young age (less than 2 years), and short duration of signs and symptoms prior to diagnosis (Panitch and Berg 1970). Favorable outcome is associated with older age, absence of cranial nerve and long tract signs at presentation, longer duration of signs and symptoms, and neurofibromatosis type 1 (NF1) (Kaplan et al. 1996). It is not clear why cranial nerve and long tract signs portend poor outcomes, but they may reflect the aggressive behavior of high-grade gliomas.

3.5 Diagnosis and Imaging

3.5.1 Computed Tomography and Magnetic Resonance Imaging

High-quality neuroimaging, specifically MRI, is the diagnostic tool of choice for BSGs. On CT, diffuse intrinsic tumors are iso- or hypodense, and enhance poorly after contrast administration. If a posterior fossa lesion is suspected, an MRI scan is mandatory; for most cases of diffuse intrinsic pontine glioma, diagnosis and prognosis is determined from MRI appearance alone. On MRI, diffuse pontine gliomas are usually hypointense on T1-weighted and hyperintense on T2-weighted images (Fig. 3.3a–f). Most do not enhance significantly with gadolinium, although some may exhibit heterogeneous enhancement. The differential diagnosis of diffuse intrinsic pontine mass on MRI includes malignant nonglial tumors (e.g., ependymomas or primitive neuroectodermal tumors), nonmalignant tumors (e.g., gangliogliomas, hamartomas), infarction, infection, and demyelination.

Focal midbrain tumors are also iso- or hypointense on T1-weighted images and hyperintense on T2-weighted images (Fig. 3.4a–f). Lesions that exclusively involve the midbrain tectum rarely enhance with gadolinium (Robertson et al. 1995; Bowers et al.

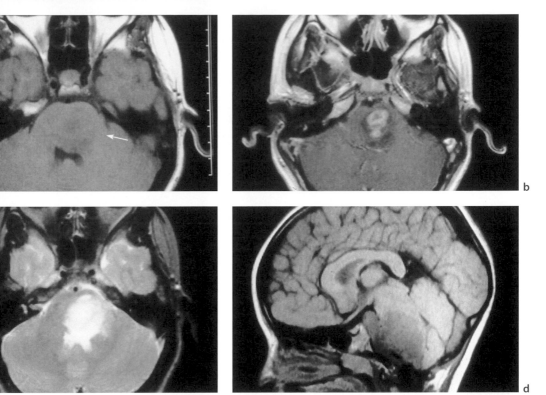

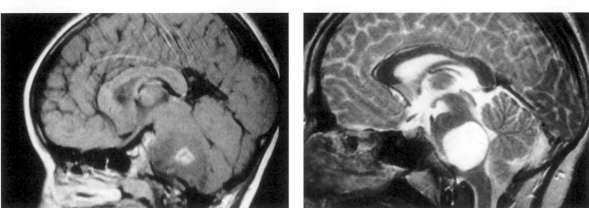

Figure 3.3 a–f

MRI images of diffuse pontine gliomas. **a** Axial T1-weighted image without contrast. The lesion is slightly hypointense compared to the normal pons. **b** Axial T1-weighted image following gadolinium administration. An irregular area of enhancement is seen with a hypointense center. **c** Axial T2-weighted image. The lesion is hyperintense demonstrating the large area of involvement. **d** Sagittal T1-weighted image without contrast. The lesion is hypointense and expands the pons. **e** The same image following contrast. There is a small central area which enhances brightly with gadolinium. **f** Sagittal T2-weighted MRI image. Note the striking hyperintensity of the lesion and the expansion of the pons

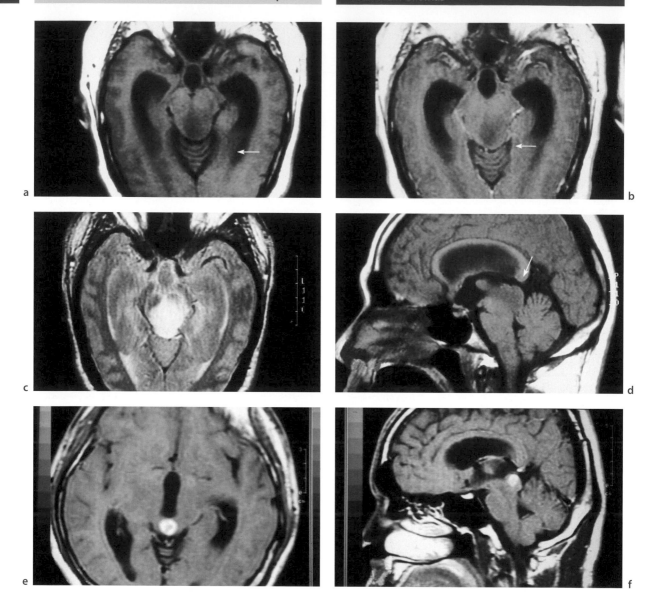

Figure 3.4 a–f

MRI images of tectal gliomas. **a** Axial T1-weighted image without contrast. The lesion is small, well-circumscribed, and produces no edema. **b** Axial T1-weighted image following contrast. Note the lack of enhancement. **c** Axial proton density image. The lesion is notably hyperintense, which contrasts with the hypointense signal of the lesion on T1-weighted pre-contrast images. **d** Sagittal T1-weighted image without contrast. The lesion is hypointense and does not produce significant edema. **e** Axial T1-weighted image following contrast. This tectal glioma exhibits obvious contrast enhancement, illustrating the enhancement variability of tectal gliomas. **f** Sagittal T1-weighted image following contrast. The lesion is well-circumscribed and enhances brightly, which contrasts with the lesion noted in image **b**

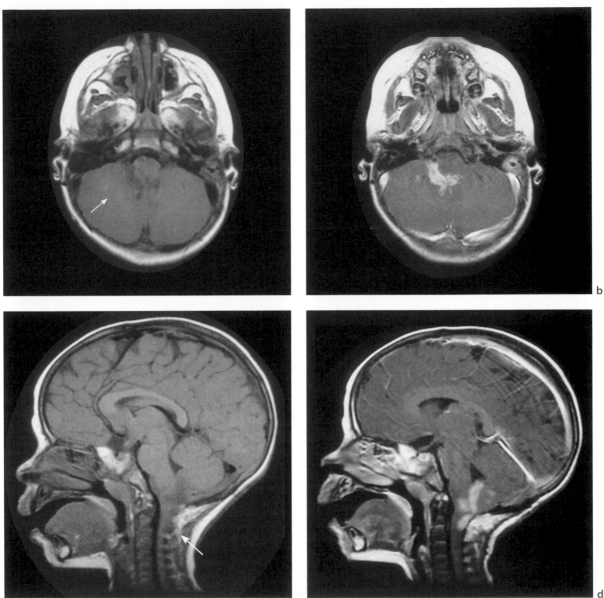

a

b

c

d

Figure 3.5 a–d

MRI images of dorsally exophytic tumors. a Axial T1-weighted image without contrast. The lesion arises from the medulla and is hypointense on T1-weighted images. b Axial T1-weighted image with contrast. The lesion enhances brightly with contrast, which is a typical characteristic for dorsally exophytic tumors. c Sagittal T1-weighted without contrast. The lesion does not invade the intrinsic tissue of the lower brainstem. d Sagittal T1-weighted with contrast. The enhancing lesion extrinsically involves the posterior upper cervical cord, medulla, and fourth ventricle. This patient has recently undergone a craniotomy

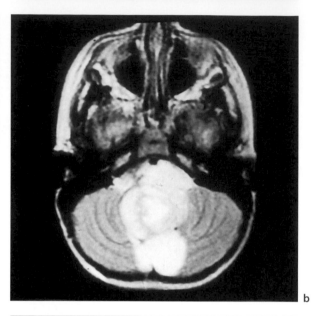

a

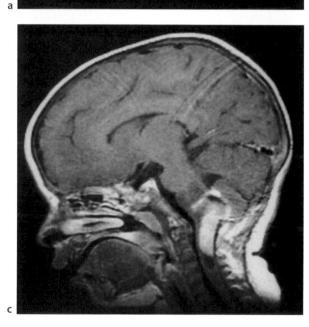

c

Figure 3.6 a–c

MRI images of cervicomedullary tumors. a Axial T1-weighted image with contrast. The lesion enhances heterogeneously and arises from the upper cervical cord. b Axial proton density image. The lesion is hyperintense on T1-weighted image. c Sagittal T1-weighted image following contrast. The lesion bulges dorsally into the fourth ventricle

2000), whereas peritectal and tegmental tumors more frequently demonstrate enhancement (Robertson et al. 1995). Ventriculomegaly secondary to obstructive hydrocephalus can also be readily discerned on MRI.

Dorsally exophytic tumors appear as sharply demarcated hypointense lesions on T1-weighted images and are hyperintense on T2-weighted images (Fig. 3.5a–d). Unlike the other BSGs, bright uniform enhancement and hydrocephalus are commonly noted findings (Khatib et al. 1994). Cervicomedullary tumors appear as solid masses within the lower medulla and upper cervical cord that frequently extend into the fourth ventricle. Like the other BSGs, they are hypointense on T1-weighted and hyperintense on T2-weighted images. They often enhance homogeneously with gadolinium (Fig. 3.6a–c).

With the development of MR imaging, BSG subtypes could be classified by various imaging criteria. Barkovich et al. (1990) retrospectively reviewed 87 pediatric patients with BSG and noted several statistically significant prognostic factors for poor outcome, including location primarily in the pons (as opposed to the midbrain or medulla), moderate to severe brainstem enlargement, and diffuse infiltration. Focal lesions and tumors with identifiable cysts had favorable outcomes; tumor necrosis and hydrocephalus had no prognostic significance (Barkovich et al. 1990). In their review, Moghrabi et al. (1995) found that the presence of MRI enhancement of BSG gave no statistically significant prognostic information. The value of contrast enhancement lies in the follow-up of BSG patients, as new-onset or significantly increased contrast enhancement may indicate tumor progression, particularly if noted prior to radiotherapy.

3.5.2 Role of Diagnostic Biopsy for Diffuse Pontine Glioma

The issue of whether or not to biopsy a diffuse brainstem lesion has been a subject of controversy. Prior to the general availability of MRI, brainstem biopsies were performed to confirm the diagnosis of a neoplasm and identify the histologic grade, thereby contributing to prognosis and formulation of a treatment plan. Currently, most evidence argues against routine biopsies of diffuse brainstem lesions. When the MRI scans and clinical features are consistent with diffuse brainstem glioma, the diagnostic information obtained from biopsy often has little impact on prognosis (Albright et al. 1993). Additionally, other lesions in the differential diagnosis, such as demyelination or encephalitis, have markedly different clinical and radiographic features than those of diffuse brainstem gliomas, and thus often do not require biopsies to distinguish them from BSG. Finally, biopsy of brainstem lesions is subject to sampling error. Cases have been documented where the biopsy revealed a low-grade glioma, yet 1 year later on autopsy the brainstem lesion was noted to be a GBM (Albright et al. 1986).

Although the stereotactic brain biopsy procedure itself is relatively safe (mortality rate is less than 05 % and morbidity is approximately 6 %), risks still exist, such as plegia, hemorrhage, cranial nerve deficits, and the possibility of the biopsy being nondiagnostic (Albright 1996). The potential benefit from a biopsy often does not clearly outweigh the potential risks of such a procedure. Currently, a surgical stereotactic biopsy is indicated only in situations where the clinical and radiographic features are not consistent with diffuse intrinsic pontine glioma. The role of biopsy may become more important with the advent of molecular typing and biologically directed therapies.

3.6 Treatment

3.6.1 Radiotherapy

The conventional treatment for BSGs remains fractionated external beam radiotherapy. The standard radiation dose is 54 to 60 Gray (Gy), or 5400 to 6000 rads, delivered conformally in single daily fractions of 1.8 to 2.0 Gy per day over approximatily 6 weeks. Hyperfractionated external beam radiotherapy (HFRT) is a regimen in which total doses of 64 Gy or more are delivered in twice-daily, smaller-dose fractions (e.g., 1 Gy) over 6 weeks (Jennings et al. 1996). HFRT was originally proposed for the treatment of patients with diffuse intrinsic gliomas. However, Mandell et al. (1999) conducted a phase III randomized study demonstrating that there were no statistically significant differences in PFS or overall survival between diffuse pontine glioma patients treated with standard radiation versus HFRT; median time to death was 8.5 months for patients treated with the standard radiation dose and 8 months for those who received HFRT to 70.2 Gy (Mandell et al. 1999). Furthermore, HFRT was reported to cause significant adverse treatment-related effects in long-term survivors (Freeman et al. 1996). Median survival in untreated diffuse intrinsic glioma patients is approximately 20 weeks (Langmoen et al. 1991).

3.6.2 Chemotherapy
for Diffuse Pontine Glioma

The role of chemotherapy in the management of diffuse intrinsic gliomas is not clear. Numerous chemotherapy regimens have been used to treat recurrent BSG and have not demonstrated significant efficacy. These include PCNU (Allen et al. 1987), cisplatin (Sexauer et al. 1985), topotecan (Blaney et al. 1996), and ifosfamide (Heideman et al. 1995). Chamberlain reported one patient with a complete response, three patients with partial responses, and two patients with stable disease in twelve patients with recurrent BSG treated with oral VP-16 (etoposide); however, two of the partial responders were over age 28 (Chamberlain 1993). Trials involving multiagent chemotherapy regimens for recurrent BSG have not fared better (Pendergrass et al. 1987; Rodriguez et al. 1988; van Eys et al. 1988).

Results from studies of regimens for newly-diagnosed BSG patients that involve combining radiotherapy and chemotherapy, either concurrently or sequentially, have been quite disappointing. Such regimens include radiation with high-dose tamoxifen (Broniscer et al. 2000), HFRT with carboplatin and etoposide concurrently (Walter et al. 1998), and radiation followed by high-dose busulfan and thiotepa (Bouffet et al. 2000). The only phase III trial evaluating chemotherapy in diffuse intrinsic glioma patients involved the randomization of patients to one of two arms: radiotherapy alone versus radiotherapy with a concurrent chemotherapy regimen of vincristine, CCNU, and prednisone. Overall 5-year survival rate was 17% for patients who received radiotherapy alone and 23% for those who received radiotherapy and chemotherapy. These results were not statistically different, and the median survival was 9 months in both trial arms (Jenkin et al. 1987). Chemotherapy administered concurrently with radiation as a radiosensitizing agent also has not demonstrated benefit – in fact, patients who received cisplatin with HFRT had worse outcomes compared with those who received HFRT alone (Freeman et al. 2000).

Another approach to treating diffuse intrinsic gliomas involves immunotherapy, in which the goal is to heighten the patient's anti-tumor immune response. The interferons, a widely used class of immunotherapy agents, are glycoproteins that induce the synthesis of specific proteins, regulate immune effector cells, and inhibit mitotic activity (Packer 1996). However, results of clinical trials involving interferons are conflicting. Wakabayashi et al. (1992) reported 3 patients with complete responses and 9 patients with partial responses in a group of 16 diffuse intrinsic glioma patients treated with interferon-alpha, ACNU, and radiation therapy. Median survival was 15.7 months, which was notably higher than previously reported survival rates for BSG patients (Wakabayashi et al. 1992). However, in a phase I/II study by Packer et al., 30 of 32 diffuse intrinsic glioma patients treated with escalating doses of interferon-alpha and HFRT to 72 Gy developed progressive disease at a median of 5 months. Median survival was only approximately 9 months (Packer et al. 1996).

Currently, there is little evidence to suggest that any standard chemotherapy agent or multiagent regimen has a significant impact on the outcome of pediatric patients with diffuse intrinsic gliomas. Thus, the standard of care for newly diagnosed diffuse intrinsic gliomas is conventional radiotherapy. Chemotherapy should be reserved for cases involving tumor progression. Whenever possible, patients should be given the option for enrollment into clinical research trials. Given the dismal prognosis, any treatment developed in the future that exhibits a modestly significant benefit will have a tremendous impact on the outcome of this patient group.

3.6.3 Surgery and Adjunctive Treatment for Nondiffuse Tumors

Focal midbrain tumors often have an indolent course reflective of their benign pathology and favorable prognosis (Robertson et al. 1995; Bowers et al. 2000). Small tectal tumors can be followed by serial MRI scans, while hydrocephalus can be alleviated with CSF diversion by a shunt or third ventriculostomy. Often, these tectal gliomas will remain unchanged for many years. With tumor progression, surgery is indicated to obtain tissue for diagnosis and potentially achieve a gross total resection. If a tumor happens to be surgically accessible, then gross total resection may be attempted although the difficult location of these tumors usually precludes complete excision. Tegmental and other non-tectal midbrain tumors tend to be larger and more frequently cause signs and symptoms of brainstem involvement (Robertson et al. 1995). Surgery is indicated for these midbrain tumors, and debulking or resection often leads to neurological improvement (Pendl et al. 1990; Vandertop et al. 1992). The role of radiotherapy has not been definitively outlined, but is often used for progressive tumors not amenable to resection. No chemotherapy regimen has been shown to have any meaningful impact on survival in this patient subgroup.

Surgery is also the treatment of choice for dorsally exophytic tumors. Despite the fact that an optimal resection may still leave a thin layer of tumor on the floor of the fourth ventricle, several series have noted excellent results for most of these patients (Pollack et al. 1993; Khatib et al. 1994). Although routine postoperative adjuvant treatment is not indicated, the minority of patients whose tumors recurred after initial resection were noted to have their tumors controlled with repeat resections and radiotherapy (Pollack et al. 1993). Radiation should be considered for patients with high-grade tumors or for those whose tumors progress within 9 months postoperatively (Freeman and Farmer 1998). An increasing number of pediatric patients are being treated with chemotherapy for symptomatic and recurrent low-grade tumors. Regimens include carboplatin plus vincristine, and nitrosourea-containing multiagent chemotherapy drugs.

Like other nondiffuse BSGs, cervicomedullary tumors are mostly of low-grade histology and associated with a favorable prognosis (Epstein and Wisoff 1987; Weiner et al. 1997). Conceptually, they should be regarded as intramedullary spinal cord tumors (Robertson et al. 1994). Thus, surgery is the mainstay of treatment when symptoms of progression arise, and if possible should be performed prior to the occurrence of significant neurologic disability. Most of these tumors have long antecedent presentations (18 to 24 months) and have very slow-developing symptomatic progression (Jennings et al. 1996). Initially, asymptomatic or stable patients may be followed clinically and radiographically. If residual disease is present within the medulla or upper cervical spinal cord, careful observation is probably warranted. Routine adjuvant chemotherapy or radiotherapy is not indicated. However, these treatment modalities may be used to manage the small proportion of high-grade cervicomedullary tumors, which should be treated as if they were diffuse intrinsic gliomas.

3.7 Conclusion

Brainstem gliomas are a heterogeneous group of neoplasms with dissimilar natural histories and prognoses. Distinct tumor subtypes and growth patterns exist that are classified according to location within the brainstem, clinical presentation, and radiographic appearance. They are subdivided into diffuse intrinsic gliomas, which originate primarily in the pons and have a dismal prognosis, and the nondiffuse BSG, of which the overwhelming majority are low-grade in histology and have a very favorable outcome. The diagnosis and treatment approach are made based on noninvasive methods: careful clinical history, physical examination, and MRI characteristics. In the setting of classic neuroradiological and clinical findings, routine biopsy for diagnosis is typically not indicated. Developing effective treatments for diffuse intrinsic gliomas has been especially frustrating, as their infiltrative nature and brainstem location precludes surgical debulking, and chemotherapeutic agents have not demonstrated significant efficacy against them. Conventional conformal radiotherapy is the mainstay of treatment for diffuse intrinsic gliomas, while surgical resection is the treatment of choice for symptomatic or recurrent nondiffuse BSG. Radiotherapy and chemotherapy for nondiffuse BSG are reserved for recurrent or high-grade neoplasms.

Acknowledgements. The authors wish to thank Nancy Fischbein, MD, for the MRI figures and Agnes Ritter for her assistance with slide preparations. This chapter was supported in part by NIH training grants T32 CA09291 and CA 13525.

References

Albright AL (1996) Diffuse brainstem tumors: when is a biopsy necessary? Pediatr Neurosurg 24:252–255

Albright AL, Price RA, Guthkelch AN et al (1983) Brain stem gliomas of children. A clinicopathological study. Cancer 52:2313–2319

Albright AL, Guthkelch AN, Packer RJ et al (1986) Prognostic factors in pediatric brain-stem gliomas. J Neurosurg 65:751–755

Albright AL, Packer RJ, Zimmerman R et al (1993) Magnetic resonance scans should replace biopsies for the diagnosis of diffuse brain stem gliomas: a report from the Children's Cancer Group. Neurosurgery 33:1026–1029

Allen JC, Hancock C, Walker R et al (1987) PCNU and recurrent childhood brain tumors. J Neurooncol 5:241–244

Barkovich AJ, Krischer J, Kun LE et al (1990) Brain stem gliomas: a classification system based on magnetic resonance imaging. Pediatr Neurosurg 16:73–83

Blaney SM, Phillips PC, Packer RJ et al (1996) Phase II evaluation of topotecan for pediatric central nervous system tumors. Cancer 78:527–531

Bouffet E, Raquin M, Doz F et al (2000) Radiotherapy followed by high dose busulfan and thiotepa: a prospective assessment of high dose chemotherapy in children with diffuse pontine gliomas. Cancer 88:685–692

Bowers DC, Georgiades C, Aronson LJ et al (2000) Tectal gliomas: natural history of an indolent lesion in pediatric patients. Pediatr Neurosurg 32:24–29

Broniscer A, Leite CC, Lanchote VL et al (2000) Radiation therapy and high-dose tamoxifen in the treatment of patients with diffuse brainstem gliomas: results of a Brazilian cooperative study. Brainstem Glioma Cooperative Group. J Clin Oncol 18:1246–1253

Chamberlain MC (1993) Recurrent brainstem gliomas treated with oral VP-16. J Neurooncol 15:133–139

Epstein F, Wisoff J (1987) Intra-axial tumors of the cervicomedullary junction. J Neurosurg 67:483–487

Epstein FJ, Farmer JP (1993) Brain-stem glioma growth patterns. J Neurosurg 78:408–412

Farmer JP, Montes JL, Freeman CR et al (2001) Brainstem Gliomas. A 10-year institutional review. Pediatr Neurosurg 34:206–214

Farwell JR, Dohrmann GJ et al (1977) Central nervous system tumors in children. Cancer 40:3123–3132

Freeman CR, Farmer JP (1998) Pediatric brain stem gliomas: a review. Int J Radiat Oncol Biol Phys 40:265–271

Freeman CR, Perilongo G (1999) Chemotherapy for brain stem gliomas. Childs Nerv Syst 15:545–553

Freeman CR, Krischer JP, Flannery JT et al (1993) Final results of a study of escalating doses of hyperfractionated radiotherapy in brain stem tumors in children: a Pediatric Oncology Group study. Int J Radiat Oncol Biol Phys 27:197–206

Freeman CR, Bourgouin PM, Sanford RA et al (1996) Long term survivors of childhood brain stem gliomas treated with hyperfractionated radiotherapy. Clinical characteristics and treatment related toxicities. The Pediatric Oncology Group. Cancer 77:555–562

Freeman CR, Kepner J, Kun LE et al (2000) A detrimental effect of a combined chemotherapy-radiotherapy approach in children with diffuse intrinsic brain stem gliomas? Int J Radiat Oncol Biol Phys 47:561–564

Fulton DS, Levin VA, Wara WM et al (1981) Chemotherapy of pediatric brain-stem tumors. J Neurosurg 54:721–725

Heideman RL, Douglass EC, Langston JA et al (1995) A phase II study of every other day high-dose ifosfamide in pediatric brain tumors: a Pediatric Oncology Group Study. J Neurooncol 25:77–84

Hoffman HJ, Becker L, Craven MA et al (1980) A clinically and pathologically distinct group of benign brain stem gliomas. Neurosurgery 7:243–248

Jenkin RD, Boesel C, Ertel I et al (1987) Brain-stem tumors in childhood: a prospective randomized trial of irradiation with and without adjuvant CCNU, VCR, and prednisone. A report of the Children's Cancer Study Group. J Neurosurg 66:227–233

Jennings MT, Freeman ML, Murray MJ et al (1996) Strategies in the treatment of diffuse pontine gliomas: the therapeutic role of hyperfractionated radiotherapy and chemotherapy. J Neurooncol 28:207–222

Kaplan AM, Albright AL, Zimmerman RA et al (1996) Brainstem gliomas in children. A Children's Cancer Group review of 119 cases. Pediatr Neurosurg 24:185–192

Khatib ZA, Heideman RL, Kovnar EH et al (1994) Predominance of pilocytic histology in dorsally exophytic brain stem tumors. Pediatr Neurosurg 20:2–10

Langmoen IA, Lundar T, Storm-Mathisen I et al (1991) Management of pediatric pontine gliomas. Childs Nerv Syst 7:13–15

Louis DN, Rubio MP, Correa KM et al (1993) Molecular genetics of pediatric brain stem gliomas. Application of PCR techniques to small and archival brain tumor specimens. J Neuropathol Exp Neurol 52:507–515

Mandell LR, Kadota R, Freeman C et al (1999) There is no role for hyperfractionated radiotherapy in the management of children with newly diagnosed diffuse intrinsic brainstem tumors: results of a Pediatric Oncology Group phase III trial comparing conventional vs. hyperfractionated radiotherapy. Int J Radiat Oncol Biol Phys 43:959–964

Mantravadi RV, Phatak R, Bellur S et al (1982) Brain stem gliomas: an autopsy study of 25 cases. Cancer 49:1294–1296

Moghrabi A, Kerby T, Tien RD et al (1995) Prognostic value of contrast-enhanced magnetic resonance imaging in brainstem gliomas. Pediatr Neurosurg 23:293–298

Packer RJ (1996) Brain stem gliomas: therapeutic options at time of recurrence. Pediatr Neurosurg 24:211–216

Packer RJ, Prados M, Phillips P et al (1996) Treatment of children with newly diagnosed brain stem gliomas with intravenous recombinant beta-interferon and hyperfractionated radiation therapy: a Children's Cancer Group phase I/II study. Cancer 77:2150–2156

Panitch HS, Berg BO (1970) Brain stem tumors of childhood and adolescence. Am J Dis Child 119:465–472

Pendergrass TW, Milstein JM, Geyer JR et al (1987) Eight drugs in one day chemotherapy for brain tumors: experience in 107 children and rationale for preradiation chemotherapy. J Clin Oncol 5:1221–1231

Pendl G, Vorkapic P, Koniyama M (1990) Microsurgery of midbrain lesions. Neurosurgery 26:641–648

Pierre-Kahn A, Hirsch JF, Vinchon M et al (1993) Surgical management of brain-stem tumors in children: results and statistical analysis of 75 cases. J Neurosurg 79:845–852

Pollack IF, Hoffman HJ, Humphreys RP et al (1993) The long-term outcome after surgical treatment of dorsally exophytic brain-stem gliomas. J Neurosurg 78:859–863

Raffel C, Hudgins R, Edwards MS et al (1988) Symptomatic hydrocephalus: initial findings in brainstem gliomas not detected on computed tomographic scans. Pediatrics 82:733–737

Robertson PL, Allen JC, Abbott IR et al (1994) Cervicomedullary tumors in children: a distinct subset of brainstem gliomas. Neurology 44:1798–1803

Robertson PL, Muraszko KM, Brunberg JA et al (1995) Pediatric midbrain tumors: a benign subgroup of brainstem gliomas. Pediatr Neurosurg 22:65–73

Rodriguez LA, Prados M, Fulton D et al (1988) Treatment of recurrent brain stem gliomas and other central nervous system tumors with 5-fluorouracil, CCNU, hydroxyurea, and 6-mercaptopurine. Neurosurgery 22:691–693

Rubin G, Michowitz S, Horev G et al (1998) Pediatric brain stem gliomas: an update. Childs Nerv Syst 14:167–173

Sawyer JR, Roloson GJ, Hobson EA et al (1990) Trisomy for chromosome 1q in a pontine astrocytoma. Cancer Genet Cytogenet 47:101–106

Scherer H (1938) Structural development in gliomas. Am J Cancer 34:333–351

Sexauer CL, Khan A, Burger PC et al (1985) Cisplatin in recurrent pediatric brain tumors. A POG Phase II study. A Pediatric Oncology Group Study. Cancer 56:1497–1501

Van Eys J, Baram TZ, Cangir A et al (1988) Salvage chemotherapy for recurrent primary brain tumors in children. J Pediatr 113:601–606

Vandertop WP, Hoffman HJ, Drake JM et al (1992) Focal midbrain tumors in children. Neurosurgery 31:186–194

Wakabayashi T, Yoshida J, Mizuno M et al (1992) Effectiveness of interferon-beta, ACNU, and radiation therapy in pediatric patients with brainstem glioma. Neurol Med Chir (Tokyo) 32:942–946

Walter AW, Gajjar A, Ochs JS et al (1998) Carboplatin and etoposide with hyperfractionated radiotherapy in children with newly diagnosed diffuse pontine gliomas: a phase I/II study. Med Pediatr Oncol 30:28–33

Watanabe K, Tachibana O, Sata K et al (1996) Overexpression of the EGF receptor and p53 mutations are mutually exclusive in the evolution of primary and secondary glioblastomas. Brain Pathol 6:217–223

Weiner HL, Freed D, Woo HH et al (1997) Intra-axial tumors of the cervicomedullary junction: surgical results and long-term outcome. Pediatr Neurosurg 27:12–18

Zhang S, Feng X, Koga H et al (1993) p53 gene mutations in pontine gliomas of juvenile onset. Biochem Biophys Res Commun 196:851–857

Ependymoma

B. N. Horn · M. Smyth

Contents

4.1 Epidemiology

4.1.1 Incidence

Ependymomas are relatively rare gliomas arising from the differentiated ependymal cell layer lining the ventricular system and central canal of the spinal cord. Intracranial ependymomas account for approximately 9% of all brain tumors in the population under 20 years of age, and are the third most common primary brain tumor in children (following astrocytomas and primitive neuroectodermal tumors). According to SEER (Surveillance, Epidemiology and End Results) data from 1975 until 1998, the annual incidence of ependymoma is 2.6 per million for the 0 to 14 age group, and 2.2 per million for the 0 to 20 age group (Ries et al. 1999). Population-based measurements of the incidence of spinal cord ependymoma in children are available from the Connecticut Tumor Registry. Between 1935 and 1973, 5 spinal cord ependymomas and 44 intracranial ependymomas were identified in the Connecticut population under 20 years of age; suggesting that spinal cord ependymoma represents approximately 10% of all ependymal tumors in children and young adults (Dohrmann et al. 1976). Another large institutional series confirmed that spinal cord ependymomas are rare in children under 10 years of age, accounting for less than 1% of all spinal tumors. After age 10, the incidence of spinal cord ependymoma increases, and it represents the majority of intramedullary tumors in patients older than 20 years (Constantini et al. 1997).

4.1.2 Age and Sex Distribution

The incidence of intracranial ependymoma peaks in the 0 to 4 age group (5.2 cases per million) and decreases thereafter to 1.5 per million in the 5 to 14 age group, and 0.9 per million in the 15 to 19 age group. Ependymomas are twice as common in males than in females. The average annual incidence is 3 per million in males, and 1.5 per million in females (Ries et al. 1999).

4.1.3 Etiology – Environmental and Viral Causes

The etiology of ependymomas remains obscure. In most epidemiologic studies ependymomas are grouped with other brain tumors, making definitive identification of specific risk factors impossible. One agent that recently received attention and has been studied for its role in oncogenesis is a specific polyomavirus, simian virus 40 (SV40). Contamination of pools of poliovirus and adenovirus vaccines from 1955 until 1963 with SV40 has raised concern about possible increases in overall cancer incidence and increases in the incidence of rare tumors such as ependymoma and choroid plexus papilloma (Carbone et al. 1997). SV40 virus is capable of transforming cells from different species, including normal human cells, into cells with a neoplastic phenotype. Furthermore, in an animal model, intracerebral inoculation of rodents with SV40 virus induces ependymoma formation (Kirschstein and Gerger 1962). SV40 oncogenicity and transforming ability are dependent on the expression of the early region gene product, large tumor antigen (Tag), which complexes with tumor suppressor genes such as *p53*, *pRb*, *p107*, *p130*, *p300* and *p400*, resulting in their inactivation (Zhen et al. 1999). The SV40 genome can be detected in the tissue of a majority of ependymomas and choroid plexus carcinomas, and also in astrocytomas, meningiomas, glioblastoma multiforme, and medulloblastoma (Bergsagel et al. 1992; Martini et al. 1996). Normal brain tissue is negative for SV40 large tumor antigen. Although provocative, these data are nonspecific and do not provide a causative link for the formation of human tumors. In addition, large epidemiologic studies that evaluated the incidence of neoplasms in patients inoculated with contaminated vaccines after long follow-up periods ranging from 17 to 30 years did not detect an increased overall incidence of ependymoma or other neoplasms (Strickler et al. 1998).

4.1.4 Genetic Predisposition

Neurofibromatosis type 2 (NF2) is the only known genetic defect with a predisposition for development of ependymoma. Patients with NF2 typically develop intramedullary spinal tumors (Lee et al. 1996). NF2 mutations have been found in 25 to 70% of patients with sporadic intraspinal ependymomas. No NF2 mutations were found in ependymomas arising in other locations (Birch et al. 1996; Lamszus et al. 2001). Familial intracranial ependymoma is very rare; however, in one family with four cousins who developed ependymoma, a suspected tumor-suppressor gene locus was located by a segregation analysis to the 22pter–22q11.2 region (Hulsebos et al. 1999). There is currently no evidence that this gene plays a role in sporadic ependymoma. Although there is a case report of a child with a germ-line mutation in the *p53* gene and intracranial ependymoma, ependymoma is usually not considered to be one of the neoplasms associated with Li-Fraumeni syndrome (Hamilton and Pollack 1997). One large population study indicated that parents of children with ependymoma may be at an increased risk of colon cancer (relative risk 3.7; Hemminki et al. 2000). However, another large study did not identify increased risk of any cancer in families of children with brain tumors (Gold et al. 1994).

4.2 Pathology

4.2.1 Histopathological Characteristics

Ependymomas arise from ependymal epithelium, which lines the ventricles of the brain and central canal of the spinal cord. Therefore, the most common

Figure 4.1

Myxopapillary ependymoma, WHO grade I, demonstrates cuboidal to elongated tumor cells arranged in a perivascular papillary pattern around central cores of mucinous perivascular stroma

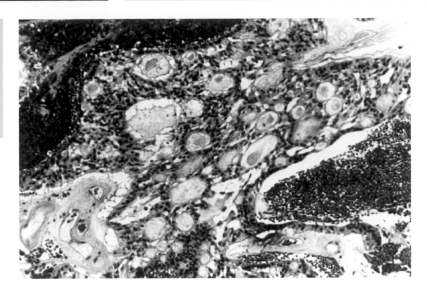

sites for this tumor are the fourth, third, and lateral ventricles, and the lumbosacral spinal cord. Ependymomas are usually well-demarcated tumors that often display areas of calcification, hemorrhage, and cysts. Ependymomas vary from well-differentiated tumors with no anaplasia and little polymorphism to highly cellular lesions with significant anaplasia, mitotic activity, and necrosis that may resemble glioblastoma multiforme. The WHO classification of brain tumors (Kleihues and Cavenee 2000) distinguishes three grades of ependymoma. Two histologic entities are known as grade I (WHO) ependymoma. The first is subependymoma, a rare benign ependymal tumor located in the wall of the ventricular system. Histologically, subependymomas are characterized by clustering of monomorphic cells arranged against a fibrillary background, frequently showing the presence of focal cystic degeneration, vascular hyalinization, hemosiderin deposition, and calcifications. Subependymomas usually show strong immunopositivity for glial fibrillary acidic protein (GFAP) and S-100 antigens. Compared to other ependymal tumors, subependymomas have the lowest rate of cell proliferation, as evidenced by MIB-1 immunostaining (Prayson and Suh 1999). Subependymomas do not show any chromosomal changes and are considered to be hamartomatous lesions

by many authors (Debiec-Rychter et al. 2000). Most subependymomas are incidental tumors discovered at autopsy, but they may grow large enough to be symptomatic. Following surgical resection, these tumors rarely recur and the long-term prognosis is excellent.

Myxopapillary ependymomas, also WHO grade I, are found almost exclusively in the region of the cauda equina, originating from the filum terminale. Myxopapillary ependymomas are slow-growing tumors that may eventually erode into adjacent bone and soft tissues. Grossly, myxopapillary ependymomas are well-circumscribed and separate from the adjacent nerves and spinal cord. The microscopic features are reminiscent of the normal filum terminale (Fig. 4.1). Cuboidal to columnar cells, sometimes with clear cytoplasm, are arranged in a perivascular papillary pattern around a central core whose stroma is composed of connective tissue and blood vessels (Kleihues and Cavene 2000). Although rare, myxopapillary ependymomas can spread along the CNS axis (Woesler et al. 1998) or occur outside the central nervous system in ectopic sites such as the sacrum and presacral tissues, where embryonically derived ependymal rests may be found (Gerston et al. 1985; Ciraldo et al. 1986).

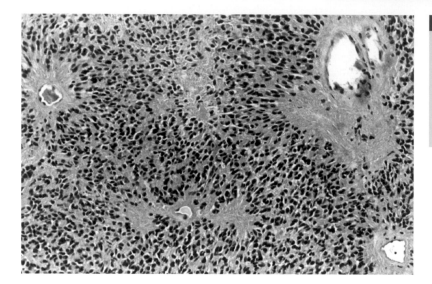

Figure 4.2

Ependymoma, WHO grade II, demonstrates moderate cellularity with low mitotic activity and pseudorosettes (neoplastic cells around a blood vessel with their cytoplasmic processes running between their nuclei and the vessel wall)

WHO grade II ependymomas are usually solid and well demarcated, with limited infiltration of surrounding structures. Histologic features include perivascular pseudorosettes, which consist of neoplastic ependymal cells surrounding a blood vessel with cytoplasmic processes extending from their nuclei to the vessel wall (Fig. 4.2). Less commonly, true ependymal rosettes may form. These are composed of neoplastic cells forming a central space reminiscent of ependymal canals. Grade II ependymomas are moderately cellular with low mitotic activity, but may demonstrate nuclear atypia, occasional mitoses, and foci of necrosis and calcification. Three subtypes of grade II ependymomas are described: cellular ependymoma, which displays conspicuous cellularity but often less prominent pseudorosette or rosette formation; papillary ependymoma, which histologically mimics the pattern of choroid plexus papilloma; and clear-cell ependymoma, which consists of cells with swollen, clear cytoplasm and well-defined plasma membranes (Kleihues Cavenee 2000).

WHO grade III anaplastic (malignant) ependymoma has histologic evidence of anaplasia, including high cellularity, variable nuclear atypia, and hyperchromatism, and marked mitotic activity (Fig. 4.3). Vascular proliferation is often prominent, and necrosis may be widespread (Kleihues et al. 1993). Ependymoblastomas are highly malignant rare tumors of embryonal origin that consist of elements resembling primitive embryonic ependymal cells. Despite their name, these tumors are not ependymal tumors, but highly malignant primitive neuroectodermal tumors (Kleihues and Cavenee 2000; see Chapter 5).

Significant disagreement may exist among neuropathologists over the diagnosis and grading of ependymomas. The rate of misclassification can be as high as 69% (Robertson et al. 1998), and the criteria for distinction between grades II and III are not highly reproducible. Many studies, even with central histology review, could not confirm the correlation between histology and patients' outcomes (Schiffer et al. 1991; Ross and Rubinstein 1989; Perilongo et al. 1997; Robertson et al. 1998).

Immunohistochemistry may be difficult to interpret in ependymomas and does not appear to add useful information to conventional histologic examination. Most ependymomas express GFAP, while the expression of other antigens, such as epithelial membrane antigen (EMA), varies. Vimentin is usually found in perivascular pseudorosette expression. In a study of 22 patients with ependymoma, DNA indices did not correlate with outcomes or histology (Reyes-Mugica et al. 1994).

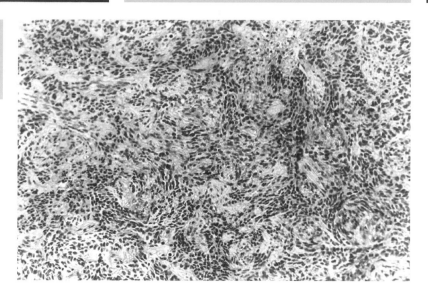

Figure 4.3

Ependymoma, WHO grade 3, demonstrates high cellularity, nuclear atypia, and mitotic activity

Electron microscopy can be useful in establishing the diagnosis of ependymoma when there is atypical appearance under light microscopy. The normal ependymoma cell bears microvilli and cilia on its apical surface (Sara et al. 1994). True rosettes are found in more than 90% of cases by electron microscopy, while they are present in only 30 to 40% of cases by light microscopy (Jinnouchi et al. 1989). However, there are no ultrastructural features that can differentiate low-grade from anaplastic ependymomas.

4.2.2 Cytogenetics

Techniques used for genetic studies of ependymoma include karyotyping, polymerase chain reaction (PCR)-based microsatellite analysis, *NF2* gene sequencing, and comparative genomic hybridization (CGH). Karyotyping depends on successful in vitro culture of tumor tissue, and therefore may not represent the entire tumor cell population. Microsatellite analysis provides limited coverage of the genome. CGH screens the whole genome of all tumor cells and can identify a variety of aberrations, but the sensitivity of CGH and the clinical relevance of aberrations identified remain poorly defined. Recently, several large studies of chromosomal-copy-number aberrations in pediatric intracranial and spinal cord ependymomas have been published, and the summary of their results are presented in Table 4.1.

Between 55% and 100% of intracranial ependymomas and all spinal cord ependymomas demonstrate chromosomal aberrations, usually displaying multiple genomic imbalances. The most common chromosomal losses in pediatric intracranial ependymomas involve chromosome 22 (21/93 patients), 16 (10/93) and 20q (9/93). The most common chromosomal gains involve chromosome 1q (20/93). Higher frequency of imbalanced chromosomal regions, as revealed by CGH, was found in spinal ependymomas and ependymomas of lower histologic grade (Scheil et al. 2001; Hirose et al. 2001). The frequency and variety of chromosomal aberrations identified in combination with the relatively low incidence of ependymoma makes the prognostic utility of these findings unclear. Nevertheless, CGH may prove to be helpful in localizing regions where genes important for development of sporadic ependymoma are located.

Table 4.1. Most frequent genetic aberrations in pediatric ependymoma, using comparative genomic hybridization

Study	Number of samples	Chromosomal losses		Chromosomal gains	
		Chromosome	Frequency	Chromosome	Frequency
Reardon et al. (1999)	22 intracranial ependymomas	X	6/22	1q	4/22
		6q	4/22	9	3/22
		22q	4/22		
Ward et al. (2001)	40 intracranial ependymomas	22	10/40	1q	8/40
		16p	5/40	4q	7/40
		17q	5/40	7q	6/40
		20q	5/40	6q	5/40
				7p	5/40
Hirose et al. (2001)	14 intracranial ependymomas	9	5/14	1q	4/14
		6q	2/14		
		22q	2/14		
	9 spinal cord ependymomas	1, 2, 10	2/9	7	9/9
		22q	2/9	9	8/9
				20	4/9
Scheil et al. (2001)	9 intracranial ependymomas	no pattern identified		1q	4/9
				17	3/9
Zheng et al. (2000)	7 intracranial ependymomas	22q	5/8	13q	3/8
		16	5/8	21q	2/8
		20q	4/8		

4.3 Clinical Features

Intracranial ependymomas predominate in children, representing 90% of all pediatric ependymomas. Only 10% of ependymomas in children are located in the spinal cord (Dohrmann et al. 1976). Supratentorial and infratentrial ependymomas represent approximately one third, and respectively two thirds of intracranial ependymomas. Approximately 35% of tumors are WHO grade III at diagnosis. Seven to fifteen percent of patients with ependymoma have disseminated disease at diagnosis (Robertson et al. 1998; Perilongo et al. 1997). Supratentorial ependymomas present as intracerebral lesions, typically adjacent to the lateral ventricles. Infratentorial ependymomas arise from the fourth ventricle and typically invade adjacent structures or extend into the aqueduct of Sylvius, foramen of Magendie, foramen of Luschka, or to the upper cervical spinal cord. Extraneural ependymomas have been described rarely, usually after progression of intracranial disease. Reported sites of extraneural spread include peritoneum, lymph nodes, lungs, pleura, bone, and liver (Newton et al. 1992).

Table 4.2 illustrates Chang's staging system for posterior fossa tumors. Posterior fossa ependymomas typically present with signs and symptoms of obstructive hydrocephalus including vomiting, headache, and ataxia (Nazar et al. 1990; Ilgren et al. 1984). Infiltration into the brainstem and growth through

Table 4.2. Modified Chang's staging system for posterior fossa tumors

	Definition
Tumor	
T1	Tumor confined to the fourth ventricle
T2	Tumor of the fourth ventricle with contiguous extension inferiorly through the foramen of Magendie and extending to the upper cervical canal
T3	Tumor of the fourth ventricle with lateral extension through the foramen of Luschka into the cerebellomedullary or cerebellopontine cistern
T4	Tumor of the fourth ventricle with invasion of other structures such as the cerebellar peduncle, medulla, pons, midbrain, etc.
Metastases	
M0	No evidence of metastases
M1	Microscopic tumor found in cerebrospinal fluid
M2	Gross nodule seedings in the cerebellar or cerebral subarachnoid space or in the third or lateral ventricles
M3	Gross nodule seedings in the spinal subarachnoid space
M4	Extraneuroaxial metastases

the foramina of Luschka or central canal may result in cranial nerve palsies, torticollis, or meningismus. Children less than 2 years of age tend to present with nonspecific signs such as irritability, vomiting, lethargy, macrocephaly, or gait disturbance (Nazar et al. 1990). The duration of symptoms is usually less than 6 months at the time of diagnosis (Coulon and Till 1977), with 50% of children presenting with duration of symptoms of less than 1 month (Horn et al. 1999). Symptoms of spinal cord ependymoma from an adult series included pain in 75%, sensory changes in 71%, and weakness in 68%. Average duration of symptoms was 13 months prior to diagnosis (Waldron et al. 1993). Ependymomas of the cauda equina present with limited spinal motion in 50% of patients, paravertebral spasm in 32%, and motor deficits and abolition of reflexes in 34% (Wager et al. 2000).

4.4 Natural History and Risk Factors

In a small retrospective series of 11 untreated intracranial ependymomas, all patients died within 3 years of symptom onset (Mork and Loken 1977). In older series, surgery alone was shown to be curative in a small proportion of patients. For example, in one pediatric series between 1935 and 1973, 4/12 patients with intracranial ependymomas, and 3/3 of patients with spinal cord ependymomas were alive 5 years after surgery (Dohrmann et al. 1976). In another series of patients diagnosed between 1953 and 1974, 2/12 patients with intracranial ependymomas treated with surgery alone were alive 5 years after the surgery, and 10/17 patients with intramedullary ependymomas were alive 10 years after the surgery (Mork and Loken 1977). A recent series using better diagnostic imaging studies noted that if gross total resection (GTR) was accomplished, surgery alone may be curative for a subgroup of children with a low grade intracranial ependymoma. In that study, 5/7 patients following GTR without adjunctive therapy remained in remission 24 to 70 months following surgery (Awaad et al. 1996). It should be noted that longer observation of patients is necessary since recurrences continue to occur past 5 years from diagnosis.

While most studies agree that achievement of GTR of intracranial and intramedullary spinal cord ependymoma correlates with superior outcomes, other risk factors including location of tumor, histology, and use of adjuvant chemotherapy, have not been unequivocally confirmed to predict outcome (Perilongo et al. 1977; Rousseau et al. 1994; Robertson et al. 1998; Cervoni et al. 1994). Younger children with ependymoma historically have had worse outcomes. It is not clear if age alone, or a combination of risk factors such as unfavorable location, which may prevent GTR, and withholding radiation therapy may have contributed to poor outcomes in younger age groups. Current studies stratify patients based on age, histology, and location of ependymoma, despite conflicting literature reports on their validity.

4.5 Diagnosis and Neuroimaging

Evaluation of a patient with ependymoma should include a comprehensive history and physical examination, preoperative and postoperative MRI of the brain, MRI of the spine, and CSF sampling. Ideally, the spinal MRI study should be performed prior to surgery, mainly because postoperative changes can be confused with drop metastases or leptomeningeal spread.

Radiographically, supratentorial ependymomas appear as large, heterogeneous, periventricular or, less commonly, intraventricular masses. Calcifications are present in approximately 50% of tumors examined by computerized tomography. Most supratentorial ependymomas have cystic components and enhance after the administration of intravenous contrast (Furie and Provenzale 1995). Infratentorial ependymomas appear as heterogeneous lesions that grow into the fourth ventricle and cause dilation of its upper part. Usually, the tumor is separated from the vermis by a cleavage plane. In most cases, the solid part of the tumor is isointense with gray matter on T1- and T2-weighted MRI images, and enhances with contrast (Tortori-Donati et al. 1995). The pattern of

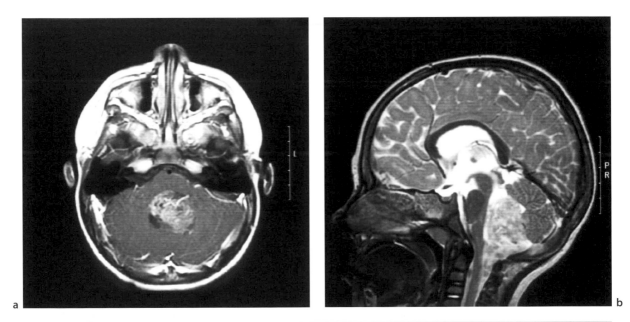

a

b

Figure 4.4 a,b

a Axial T1-weighted image following gadolinium shows a heterogeneous pattern of enhancement with the tumor directly approximated to the floor of the fourth ventricle. b Sagittal T2-weighted image showing a mixed signal mass pushing the cerebellum superiorly and extending inferiorly through the foramen magnum. Note the anterior displacement of the brainstem

enhancement is often heterogeneous (Fig. 4.4a). Often the tumor is noted to extend along CSF spaces, either through the foramen magnum (Fig. 4.4b) or laterally through the foramen of Luschka.

The typical picture of intramedullary spinal cord ependymoma on MRI consists of segmental or diffuse cord expansion with intramedullary intensity abnormalities and prominent nodular gadolinium enhancement (discussed in greater detail in Chap. 10). Intramedullary cysts and hydrosyringomyelia are common, particularly in childhood cases. Gadolinium enhancement usually distinguishes solid tumor from cord edema and from cyst or syrinx (Slasky et al. 1987). Cauda equina ependymomas usually demonstrate homogeneous hypointense signal on T1-weighted MRI sequences, hyperintense signal on T2-weighted sequences, and homogeneous enhancement after gadolinium injection (Wager et al. 2000).

4.6 Treatment

4.6.1 Surgery

The surgical goals are (1) establish a definitive tissue diagnosis, (2) achieve a GTR if possible, and (3) re-establish CSF flow. While the first and last goals are usually always possible, tumor invasion of surrounding tissues and proximity of posterior fossa tumors to the brainstem can preclude complete resection in a substantial proportion of patients. The reason for attempting GTR is based on results from retrospective and prospective studies, where the most important prognostic factor is extent of resection. In a study of 55 patients with anaplastic ependymoma, patients with a GTR followed by other treatments had a 83 % disease-free survival after 3 years of follow-up, compared with 38 % for those without complete resection (Timmermann et al. 2000). In a similar study of 32 children between 2 and 18 years of age with ependymoma, 66 % of patients with complete resection had a 5-year progression-free survival, compared with 11 % of those without complete resection (Robertson et al. 1998).

Some investigators have advocated surgery alone without adjunctive therapy. In one study of ten se-

lected cases with intracranial ependymoma (eight supratentorial and two posterior fossa), seven remained free of disease without any other interventions at a median follow-up of 48 months (Hukin et al. 1998). Investigators at St. Jude Children's Research Hospital have found that 10/16 patients with residual disease after the first surgery achieved GTR after a "second-look" surgery (Osterdock et al. 2000). The role of second-look surgery is debated, and the Children's Oncology Group is developing a study in which second-look surgery will be performed in patients with residual local disease, following adjuvant chemotherapy (see Chapter 13).

Surgical results have been improved by using technical advances such as intraoperative electromyographic monitoring of cranial nerves, computer-assisted navigation, and the operating microscope. Due to the paramount importance of the degree of surgical resection, all children with suspected ependymoma should be referred to a center that can provide the expertise required for optimal management of these tumors.

4.6.2 Radiation Therapy

Radiotherapy is considered the standard adjuvant treatment for intracranial ependymomas in older children, with various definitions of the lower age limit. The approach to radiation therapy of ependymoma, in particular the radiation field, has changed over time. In the 1960s and 1970s, local field radiation was used, as improved outcomes were noted in irradiated patients when compared to historical controls. In 1975, Salazar recommended extending the radiation field to include the whole brain in low-grade ependymomas and the entire craniospinal axis in high-grade ependymomas (Salazar et al. 1975). These recommendations were based on an overestimated risk of dissemination from autopsy findings, and on poor distinction between ependymomas and ependymoblastomas. In the late 1980s and early 1990s, multiple studies questioned the role of craniospinal radiation (Vanuytsel and Brada 1991; Shaw et al. 1987; Goldwein et al. 1991) and reported no difference in failure rates between patients undergoing localized vs. craniospinal radiation. Local relapse was confirmed to be the most significant component of failure, and a local radiation dose of more than 4500 cGy was recommended (Goldwein et al. 1991).

In the late 1980s, cooperative pediatric study groups initiated studies of postoperative chemotherapy in infant brain tumors with the goal of delaying and possibly avoiding radiation in young patients for whom cranial radiation would produce significant morbidity (Duffner et al. 1993; Geyer et al. 1994). Young children with ependymomas were treated in these studies together with patients with primitive neuroectodermal tumors. In the 1990s, attempts were made to replace radiation therapy with high dose chemotherapy consolidation in children less than 6 years of age with malignant brain tumors (Mason et al. 1998a), or to replace radiation with postoperative chemotherapy in children under 5 years of age (Grill et al. 2001). However, radiation was avoided in only 23% of patients in the latter study, and after progression of tumor, only those children who underwent a second complete resection remained in remission following radiation therapy.

The Pediatric Oncology Group conducted a clinical trial of hyperfractionated radiation for localized posterior fossa ependymoma. Forty-six patients older than 3 years of age were enrolled in this study between 1991 and 1994. Hyperfractionated radiation was given using 1.2 Gy in 58 fractions for a total dose of 69.6 Gy. The results of this study are not yet published, but they may answer the question of whether higher doses of radiation will improve disease control in patients with postoperative residual disease, a group that has who historically had a poor outcome despite adjuvant therapy. Other investigators have focused on reducing the radiation field by using conformal techniques. In one such study, 36 children with localized ependymoma underwent conformal radiotherapy with an anatomically defined clinical target volume margin of 10 mm surrounding the postoperative residual tumor and tumor bed. Two failures occurred after a median follow-up period of 15 months. Of note, 30/36 children in this preliminary report had complete surgical resection (Merchant et al. 2000). Radiosurgery has also been used in patients with ependymoma, usually at the time of recurrence, and

can be used safely without significant risk of radionecrosis (Hodgson et al. 2001). In another study, tumor control was achieved in 3/5 patients undergoing radiosurgery for residual localized ependymoma (Aggarwal et al. 1997). It is possible that radiosurgery will have a significant role in local control of ependymoma in the future; however, more studies comparing radiosurgery to standard radiation are necessary.

Current studies have adopted a conformal approach for all patients older than 12 months of age. The American Pediatric Brain Tumor Consortium study for children less than 3 years of age uses intrathecal chemotherapy, systemic chemotherapy, and conformal radiotherapy for patients with higher-risk disease. The Children's Oncology Group proposes the use of conformal radiation therapy in a subgroup of patients older than 1 year of age with higher-risk localized ependymomas. Craniospinal radiation may still be used alone, or in combination with chemotherapy, for an occasional older patient with disseminated ependymoma.

In summary, although the role of radiation therapy has not been confirmed in randomized studies, the high risk of relapse in younger children treated with chemotherapy only, even after gross total resection, warrants its use. Studies are underway to confirm the role of conformal field radiation in local control of ependymoma.

4.6.3 Chemotherapy

Ependymomas are sensitive to chemotherapy. Cisplatin, the most effective single agent, provides a 30% response rate in recurrent tumors (Walker and Allen 1988). A combination of agents, either platinum-based or nitrosourea-based, have resulted in 60% response rates in recurrent adult ependymoma in a small retrospective study (Gornet et al. 1999). In eight children under the age of 4 years with residual ependymoma, an 86% response rate to VETOPEC therapy (vincristine, etoposide, cyclophosphamide, cisplatin, carboplatin) was reported (White et al. 1998). The role of chemotherapy in the treatment of older children with ependymoma has not been established, although some conclusions may be possible when the Children's Cancer Group study (CCG-9942) is published. In that study, investigators used pre-irradiation chemotherapy in children older than 3 years of age with residual disease.

The role of chemotherapy in delaying or avoiding radiation in young children with ependymoma has been well studied. The results of several studies addressing chemotherapy in young children with ependymoma are presented in Table 4.3. The outcomes cannot be directly compared since radiation was planned, although not always given, as a part of earlier studies (Duffner et al. 1993; Geyer et al. 1994). In later studies, radiation was used only after tumor progression, and its use indicated chemotherapy failure (Mason et al. 1998a, b; Grill et al. 2001). Also, 2- or 3-year follow-up is inadequate to accurately assess long-term progression-free survival. While this approach delayed irradiation for a median of 15 months in the most recent study (Grill et al. 2001), progression-free-survival rates are disappointingly low. As a result of the disappointing survival using surgery and chemotherapy, some current ongoing clinical tri-

als for ependymoma are re-incorporating the use of local radiation in all but the youngest patients.

High-dose chemotherapy followed by autologous bone marrow rescue has been used in the setting of recurrent or progressive disease with dismal results. In a study which used a thiotepa, etoposide, and carboplatin conditioning regimen and autologous bone marrow rescue, of 15 children with recurrent ependymoma 5 died of treatment complications and all other patients sustained disease recurrence (Mason et al. 1998a, b). In another study, which used busulfan and thiotepa as a conditioning regimen, of 16 patients one sustained toxic death, and only 3 survived with a follow-up of 15 to 25 months. All three surviving patients received additional radiation (one patient) or surgery and radiation (two patients) after transplant (Grill et al. 1996). Because of the poor outcome in these small studies, high-dose therapy is not recommended in patients with relapsed or progressive disease. Myeloablative therapy is still being studied as an upfront approach for high-risk patients up to 10 years of age in the Headstart protocol.

Table 4.3. Progression-free survival of young children with ependymoma treated with chemotherapy

Study Age groups included	Duffner et al. (1993)[a] <36 months	Geyer et al. (1994) <18 months	Mason et al. (1998) <6 years of age	Grill et al. (2001) <5 years of age
Chemotherapy regimen	7 cycles VCR/CTX alternating with cisplatin/VP-16	8 courses of 8 drugs in 1 day	5 cycles of induction VCR/CTX/cisplatin/VP/16; consolidation with high dose carbo/thiotepa/ VP-16 and stem cell rescue	7-cycles alternating 3 regimens procarbazine/carbo VP-16/cisplatin/ VCR/CTX
Complete resection	19	15 patients total, degree of resection not available	4	46
Incomplete resection	27		6	27
Progression-free survival	42% at 2 years 27% at 5 years	26% at 3 years	30% at 2 years	22% PFS at 4 years

[a] Most patients in this study underwent irradiation following chemotherapy

Currently, chemotherapy is used as an adjuvant treatment in patients with postoperative residual disease. The goal is to achieve a response that would increase the feasibility of second-look surgery and conformal radiation therapy. Chemotherapy may also control microscopic disseminated disease, but it rarely results in complete response of macroscopic disease.

4.6.4 Treatment of Spinal Cord Ependymomas

Spinal cord ependymoma has a more favorable prognosis than its intracranial counterpart. Surgery remains the primary mode of therapy for spinal cord ependymomas, and complete resection is usually curative. Current treatment recommendations are that another resection be attempted if residual tumor is unexpectedly found on the postoperative scan, or in the case of recurrence (Nadkarni and Rekate 1999). Radiation therapy is used when complete resection is not possible. In some studies, excellent control rates of residual tumor were achieved with radiation therapy (80% progression-free survival at 5 years after diagnosis; Waldron et al. 1993; Garrett et al. 1983); while others report higher post-radiation relapse rates (37 to 89%; Whitaker et al. 1991; Cervoni et al. 1994). The management of spinal cord tumors is discussed in greater detail in Chap. 10.

4.6.5 Recurrent Disease

Depending on the completeness of surgical resection and patient age, disease recurs in 25 to 80% of patients. In a retrospective series of 52 relapsed pediatric patients, progression occurred in the majority of cases at the original tumor site (73%), the original and a new site were involved in 16% of cases, and a new site alone in 11% of cases. Thirteen percent of patients with previously localized disease recurred with disseminated disease (Horn et al. 1999). A similar distribution of site of relapse was observed in another retrospective study of 37 relapsed patients (Goldwein et al. 1990). Very similar results were obtained in a prospective study of young children.

Eighty-seven percent of relapses in that study were local and 13% were at a distant site (Grill et al. 2001). A variety of treatments were used after relapse including second surgery, radiation, radiosurgery, chemotherapy, and high dose chemotherapy. Twenty to twenty-eight percent of patients achieved a second complete remission (Goldwein et al. 1990; Grill et al. 2001). Children under 5 years of age who did not receive radiation upfront and who underwent a second complete resection followed by irradiation therapy had the best chance of second complete remission (28%). However, there was no benefit of radiation for recurrent disease if a second complete resection was not achieved (Grill et al. 2001).

Although recurrent ependymoma has poor prognosis, routine neuroimaging surveillance is recommended as patients with asymptomatic recurrences, discovered on routine imaging scans, had longer survival than patients who were symptomatic at the time of tumor recurrence (60% vs. 30% at 2 years post-recurrence; Good et al. 2001).

4.7 Outcome

4.7.1 Neurological Function

With long-term remission rates of at least 50% at 5 years after diagnosis, long-term effects of a tumor and its treatment on neurological functioning have become even more important. Table 4.4 summarizes the results of neurologic exams in children with ependymoma prior to adjuvant treatments and after long-term follow-up. Long-term sequelae most commonly include cranial nerve deficits, abnormal gait, and difficulties with fine motor function. Of note, 30 % of children with supratentorial ependymomas and 50% of those with infratentorial tumors required placement of a ventriculoperitoneal shunt (Horn et al. 1999).

Long-term intellectual outcome has also been studied. Cognitive impairment occurs in most patients with posterior fossa tumors, even after posterior fossa irradiation only. The degree of impairment correlates with the dose of craniospinal irradiation (Grill et al. 1999). The mean full-scale IQ score was

Table 4.4. Results of neurological exam in children with intracranial ependymoma

Neurologic exam	Percent (%) of children with normal findings, 1 month after surgery (n=84)	Percent (%) of surviving children with normal findings, 6 years after diagnosis (n=39)
Consciousness	92	100
Speech	80	82
Memory	98	80
Visual acuity	86	90
Visual fields	80	90
Cranial nerves	49	67
Fine motor function	64	74
Sensory function	97	97
Gait	43	67
Swallowing	84	95
Posterior-fossa mutism[a]	79	93

[a] Only patients with posterior fossa tumors were included

found to be 85 in 12 patients with posterior fossa ependymoma who underwent posterior fossa irradiation as a part of their treatment. This was significantly better than in patients with medulloblastoma who underwent craniospinal irradiation, whose mean full-scale IQ score was 70. Ninety-two percent of children who underwent posterior fossa irradiation alone were able to attend normal schools (Grill et al. 1999).

4.7.2 Progression-Free Survival

Figure 4.5 presents results of overall survival and progression-free survival in a retrospective group of 84 children with ependymoma treated between 1987 and 1991. All age groups and any treatment modality are included. This historic group has close to 50% long-term survival, and somewhat lower progression-free survival. Five-year overall survival rates obtained from SEER registry indicate 56% survival for children with ependymoma treated between 1985 and 1994 (Ries et al. 1999). With current treatment plans, low-risk patients (older patients with complete surgical resection) treated with observation or conformal field radiation can expect 75% progression-free survival. Older patients with postoperative residual disease may achieve 30 to 50% progression free survival when treated with radiation with or without chemotherapy and second-look surgery. Additionally, up to 20% of patients whose disease progresses or recurs may achieve a prolonged second complete remission. Up to 50% of young children treated with upfront surgery and chemotherapy, and rescue surgery and radiation are alive in first or second complete remission at 4 years post diagnosis (Grill et al. 2001). Expectations are that current treatment of infants with chemotherapy and conformal field radiation can sustain similar results.

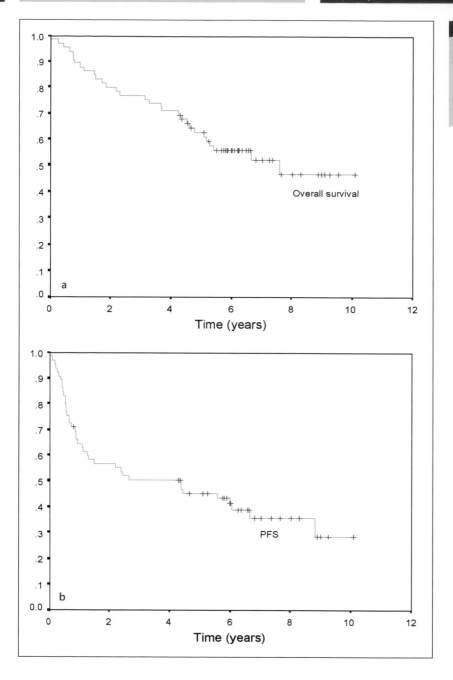

Figure 4.5a,b

Kaplan–Meier curves for 84 children with ependymoma treated between 1987 and 1991: overall survival a and progression-free survival b

4.8 Conclusion

In summary, ependymoma affects 2.6 per million children annually. Children under 4 years of age have the highest incidence of disease. Two-thirds of patients with intracranial ependymomas present with posterior fossa tumors, and more than 85% present with localized disease. Complete surgical resection is the most important predictor of good outcome. Conformal field radiation is recommended as adjuvant therapy in most patients, and chemotherapy is used in control of microscopic dissemination. Currently, overall survival of all children with ependymoma is in the range of 50 to 60%. Most children who underwent posterior fossa irradiation for this tumor are able to pursue normal schooling.

References

Aggarwal R, Yeung D, Kumar P et al (1997) Efficacy and feasibility of stereotactic radiosurgery in the primary management of unfavorable pediatric ependymoma. Radiother Oncol 43:269–273

Awaad Y, Allen J, Miller D et al (1996) Deferring adjuvant therapy for totally resected intracranial ependymoma. Pediatr Neurol 14:216–219

Bergsagel D, Finegold M, Butel J et al (1992) DNA sequences similar to those of Simian virus 40 in ependymomas and choroid plexus tumors of childhood. N Engl J Med 326: 988–993

Birch B, Johnson J, Parsa A et al (1996) Frequent type 2 neurofibromatosis gene transcript mutations in sporadic intramedullary spinal cord ependymomas. Neurosurgery 39:135–140

Carbone M, Rizzo P, Pass H (1997) Simian virus 40, poliovaccines and human tumors: a review of recent developments. Oncogene 15:1877–1888

Cervoni L, Celli P, Fortuna A et al (1994) Recurrence of spinal ependymoma. Risk factors and long-term survival. Spine 19:2838–2841

Ciraldo A, Platt M, Agamanolis D et al (1986) Sacrococcygeal myxopapillary ependymomas and ependymal rests in infants and children. J Pediatr Surg 21:49–52

Constantini S, Allen J, Epstein F (1997) Pediatric and adult primary spinal cord tumors. In: Black P, Loeffler J (eds) Cancer of the nervous system. Blackwell Science, Cambridge, pp 638–639

Coulon R, Till K (1977) Intracranial ependymomas in children. Child's Brain 3:154–168

Debiec-Rychter M, Hagemeijer A, Sciot R (2000) Cytogenetic analysis in three cerebral subependymomas: further evidence for a hamartomatous nature? Cancer Genet Cytogenet 122:63–64

Dohrmann G, Farwell J, Flannery J (1976) Ependymomas and ependymoblastomas in children. J Neurosurg 45:273–281

Duffner P, Horowitz M, Krischer J et al (1993) Postoperative chemotherapy and delayed radiation in children less than three years of age with malignant brain tumors. N Engl J Med 328:1725–1731

Furie D, Provenzale J (1995) Supratentorial ependymomas and subependymomas: CT and MR appearance. J Comput Assist Tomogr 19:518–526

Garrett P, Simpson W (1983) Ependymomas: results of radiation treatment. Int J Radiat Oncol Biol Phys 9:1121–1124

Gerston K, Suprun H, Cohen H et al (1985) Presacral myxopapillary ependymoma presenting as an abdominal mass in a child. J Pediatr Surg 20:276–278

Geyer R, Zeltzer P, Boyett J et al (1994) Survival of infants with primitive neuroectodermal tumors or malignant ependymomas of the CNS treated with eight drugs in 1 day: a report from the Childrens Cancer Group. J Clin Oncol 12:1607–1615

Gold E, Leviton A, Lopez R et al (1994) The role of family history in risk of childhood brain tumors. Cancer 73:1302–1311

Goldwein J, Glauser T, Packer R et al (1990) Recurrent intracranial ependymomas in children. Cancer 66:557–563

Goldwein J, Corn B, Finlay J et al (1991) Is craniospinal irradiation required to cure children with malignant (anaplastic) intracranial ependymomas? Cancer 67:2766–2771

Good C, Wade A, Hayward R et al (2001) Surveillance neuroimaging in childhood intracranial ependymoma: how effective, how often, and for how long? J Neurosurg 94:27–32

Gornet M, Buckner J, Marks R et al (1999) Chemotherapy for advanced CNS ependymoma. J Neurooncol 45:61–67

Grill J, Kalifa C, Doz F et al (1996) A high-dose busulfan-thiotepa combination followed by autologous bone marrow transplantation in childhood recurrent ependymoma. Pediatr Neurosurg 25:7–12

Grill J, Renaux V, Bulteau C et al (1999) Long-term intellectual outcome in children with posterior fossa tumors according to radiation doses and volumes. Int J Radiat Oncol Biol Phys 45:137–145

Grill J, Le Deley M, Gambarelli D et al (2001) Postoperative chemotherapy without irradiation for ependymoma in children under 5 years of age: a multicenter trial of the French Society of Pediatric Oncology. J Clin Oncol 19:1288–1296

Hamilton R, Pollack I (1997) The molecular biology of ependymomas. Brain Pathol 7:807–822

Hemminki K, Li X, Vaittinen P et al (2000) Cancers in the first-degree relatives of children with brain tumours. Br J Cancer 83:407–411

Hirose Y, Aldape K, Bollen A et al (2001) Chromosomal abnormalities subdivide ependymal tumors into clinically relevant groups. Am J Pathol 158:1137–1143

Hodgson D, Goumnerova L, Loeffler J et al (2001) Radiosurgery in the management of pediatric brain tumors. Int J Radiat Oncol Biol Phys 50:929–935

Horn B, Heidman R, Geyer R et al (1999) A multi-institutional retrospective study of intracranial ependymoma in children: identification of risk factors. J Pediatr Hematol Oncol 21:203–211

Hukin J, Epstein F, Fefton D, Allen J (1998) Treatment of intracranial ependymoma by surgery alone. Pediatr Neurosurg 29:40–45

Hulsebos T, Oskam N, Bijleveld E et al (1999) Evidence for an ependymoma tumour suppressor gene in chromosome region 22pter-22q11.2. Br J Cancer 81:1150–1154

Ilgren E, Stiller C, Hughes J et al (1984) Ependymomas: a clinical and pathologic study. I. Biologic features. Clin Neuropathol 3:113–121

Jinnouchi T, Shibata S, Fukushima M et al (1989) Ultrastructure of blood capillary permeability in human brain tumors, part 7. Ependymoma. J Clin Electron Micros 22:57–63

Kirschstein R, Gerger P (1962) Ependymomas produced after intracerebral inoculation of SV40 into newborn hamsters. Nature 195:299–300

Kleihues P, Cavenne WK (2000) Pathology and genetics of the nervous system. IARC Press, Lyon

Lamszus K, Lachenmayer L, Heinemann U (2001) Molecular genetic alterations on chromosomes 11 and 22 in ependymomas. Int J Cancer 91:803–808

Lee M, Rezai A, Freed D et al (1996) Intramedullary spinal cord tumors in neurofibromatosis. Neurosurgery 38:32–37

Martini F, Iaccheri L, Lazzarini L et al (1996) SV40 early region and large T antigen in human brain tumors, peripheral blood cells and sperm fluids from healthy individuals. Cancer Res 56:4820–4825

Mason W, Grovas A, Halpern S et al (1998a) Intensive chemotherapy and bone marrow rescue for young children with newly diagnosed malignant brain tumors. J Clin Oncol 16:210–221

Mason W, Goldman S, Yates A et al (1998b) Survival following intensive chemotherapy with bone marrow reconstitution for children with recurrent intracranial ependymoma. J Neurooncol 37:135–143

Merchant T, Thompson S, Williams T et al (2000) Preliminary results from a phase II trial of conformal radiation therapy for localized pediatric brain tumors. 2000 annual meeting of the American Society of Therapeutic Radiology and Oncology. Boston, MA, 22–26 Oct. Int J Radiol Oncol Biol Phys 48:180–181

Mork S, Loken A (1977) Ependymoma: a follow-up study of 101 cases. Cancer 40:907–915

Nadkarni T, Rekate H (1999) Pediatric intramedullary spinal cord tumors. Child's Nerv Syst 15:17–28

Nazar G, Hoffman H, Becker L et al (1990) Infratentorial ependymomas in childhood: prognostic factors and treatment. J Neurosurg 72:408–417

Newton H, Henson J, Walker R (1992) Extraneural metastases in ependymoma. J Neurooncol 14:135–142

Osterdock R, Sanford R, Merchant T (2000) Pediatric ependymoma (40 in 36 months). 2000 AANS/CNS Section on Pediatric Neurological Surgery Annual Meeting. Coronado, California, 6–9 Dec 2000

Perilongo G, Massimino M, Sotti G et al (1997) Analyses of prognostic factors in a retrospective review of 92 children with ependymoma: Italian Pediatric Neuro-Oncology Group. Med Pediatr Oncol 29:79–85

Prayson R, Suh J (1999) Subependymomas: clinicopathologic study of 14 tumors, including comparative MIB-1 immunohistochemical analysis with other ependymal neoplasms. Arch Pathol Lab Med 123:306–309

Reardon D, Entrekin R, Sublett J et al (1999) Chromosome arm 6q loss is the most common recurrent autosomal alteration detected in primary pediatric ependymoma. Genes Chromosom Cancer 24:230–237

Reyes-Mugica M, Chou PM, Myint MM et al (1994) Ependymomas in children: histologic and DNA-flow cytometric study. Pediatr Pathol 14:453–466

Ries L, Smith M, Gurney J et al (eds) (1999) Cancer incidence and survival among children and adolescents: United States SEER Program 1975–1995, National Cancer Institute, SEER Program. NIH Publ no 99–4649. Bethesda, MD

Robertson P, Zeltzer P, Boyett J et al (1998) Survival and prognostic factors following radiation therapy and chemotherapy for ependymomas in children: a report of the Children's Cancer Group. J Neurosurg 88:695–703

Ross G, Rubinstein L (1989) Lack of histological correlation of malignant ependymomas with postoperative survival. J Neurosurg 70:31–36

Rousseau P, Habrand J, Serrazin D et al (1994) Treatment of intracranial ependymomas of children: review of a 15-year experience. Int J Radiat Oncol Biol Phys 28:381–386

Salazar O, Rubin P, Bassano D et al (1975) Improved survival of patients with intracranial ependymoma by irradiation therapy. Dose escalation and field extension. Cancer 35:1563–1573

Sara A, Bruner J, Mackay B (1994) Ultrastructure of ependymoma. Ultrastruct Pathol 18:33–42

Scheil S, Bruderlein S, Eicker M et al (2001) Low frequency of chromosomal imbalances in anaplastic ependymomas as detected by comparative genomic hybridization. Brain Pathol 11:133–143

Schiffer D, Chio A, Giordana M et al (1991) Histologic prognostic factors in ependymoma. Child's Nerv Syst 7:177–182

Shaw E, Evans R, Scheithauer B et al (1987) Postoperative radiotherapy of intracranial ependymoma in pediatric and adult patients. Int J Radiat Oncol Biol Phys 13:1457–1462

Slasky B, Bydder G, Niendrof H et al (1987) MR imaging with gadolinium-DTPA in the differentiation of tumor, syrinx and cyst of the spinal cord. J Compt Tomogr 11:845–850

Strickler H, Rosenberg P, Devesa S et al (1998) Contamination of poliovirus vaccines with Simian virus 40 (1955–1963) and subsequent cancer rates. JAMA 279:292–295

Timmermann B, Kortmann R, Kuhl J et al (2000) Combined postoperative irradiation and chemotherapy for anaplastic ependymomas in childhood: results of the German prospective trials HIT 88/89 and HIT 91. Int J Radiat Oncol Biol Phys 46:287–295

Tortori-Donati P, Fondelli M, Cama A et al (1995) Ependymomas of the posterior cranial fossa: CT and MRI findings. Neuroradiology 37:238–243

Vanuytsel LJ, Brada M (1991) The role of prophylactic spinal irradiation in localized intracranial ependymoma. Int J. Radiat Oncol Biol Phys 21:825–830

Wager M, Lapierre F, Blanc J et al (2000) Cauda equina tumors: a French multicenter retrospective review of 231 adult cases and review of the literature. Neurosurg Rev 23:119–129

Waldron J, Laperriere N, Jaakkimainen L et al (1993) Spinal cord ependymomas: a retrospective analysis of 59 cases. Int J Radiat Oncol Biol Phys 27:223–229

Walker R, Allen J (1988) Cisplatin in the treatment of recurrent primary brain tumors. J Clin Oncol 6:62–66

Ward S, Harding B, Wilkins P et al (2001) Gain 1q and loss of 22 are the most common changes detected by comparative genomic hybridisation in pediatric ependymoma. Genes Chromosom Cancer 32:59–66

White L, Kellie S, Gray E et al (1998) Postoperative chemotherapy in children less than 4 years of age with malignant brain tumors: promising initial response to a VETOPEC-based regimen. J Pediatr Hematol Oncol 20:125–130

Whitaker S, Bessel E, Ashley S et al (1991) Postoperative radiotherapy in the management of spinal cord ependymoma. J Neurosurg 74:720–728

Woesler B, Moskopp D, Kuchelmeister K et al (1998) Intracranial metastasis of a spinal myxopapillary ependymoma: Case report. Neurosurg Rev 21:62–65

Zhen H, Zhang X, Bu X et al (1999) Expression of the Simian virus 40 large tumor antigen (Tag) and formation of Tag-p53 and Tag-pRb complexes in human brain tumors. Cancer 86:2124–2132

Zheng P, Pang J, Hui A et al (2000) Comparative genomic hybridization detects losses of chromosomes 22 and 16 as the most common recurrent genetic alterations in primary ependymomas. Cancer Genet Cytogenet 122:18–15

Embryonal Tumors

P.G. Fisher

Contents

5.1 Introduction

Embryonal tumors account for a large fraction of pediatric brain tumors. Their cell of origin, histopathological classification, and treatment are all areas of controversy. The prognosis for these tumors was at one time exceedingly poor, but advances in treatment have led to substantial improvement in survival. Intensive treatment strategies often lead to debilitating and severe late effects.

Historically, all embryonal tumors, regardless of their site of origin in the central nervous system (CNS), were grouped under the umbrella term primitive neuroectodermal tumor (PNET) (Rorke 1983). These tumors were distinguished by a homogeneous histologic appearance consisting of poorly cohesive, undifferentiated neuroepithelial cells, often with a high mitotic rate. These small, monomorphic, round cells sometimes demonstrate neuroblastic differentiation. All embryonal tumors were conjectured to arise from a common precursor cell of the subependymal matrix in the CNS. The tendency for these neoplasms to disseminate though cerebrospinal fluid (CSF) pathways was believed to contribute to a poor outcome. The term medulloblastoma is often used interchangeably with infratentorial PNET. Bailey and Cushing believed that the cells of origin were "medulloblasts," one of the primitive cell types of the neural tube. Medulloblasts have never been identified; other cells of origin include cells of the subependymal layer, external granule layer, and internal granule layer.

Growing evidence suggest that rather than being one uniform group of tumors, PNETs are a heterogeneous group of neoplasms. Indeed, gene-expression profiling favors the older concept of a site-specific origin for distinct embryonal tumors (Pomeroy et al. 2002; Gilbertson 2002). Embryonal tumors are better identified by their more classic descriptions, based on tumor location, divergent histopathologic origins, and patterns of differentiation. These embryonal neoplasms include medulloblastoma, atypical teratoid/rhabdoid tumor, pineoblastoma, ependymoblastoma, cerebral neuroblastoma, ganglioneuroblastoma, medulloepithelioma, and supratentorial embryonal tumor. Children with average-risk medulloblastoma have significantly higher survival rates than those with other embryonal neoplasms (McNeil et al. 2002). In this chapter we shall consider and discuss separately the entities of medulloblastoma, atypical teratoid/rhabdoid tumor, pineoblastoma, and other embryonal tumors as recognized by the current World Health Organization (WHO) classification of tumors (Kleihues and Cavenee 2000).

5.2 Medulloblastoma

5.2.1 Epidemiology

The incidence of pediatric CNS neoplasms is approximately 3.5 per 100,000 children per year. Medulloblastoma accounts for about 20 percent of these cases (Gurney et al. 1999). By the 1990s, multimodal therapies were associated with increasing survival from medulloblastoma (McNeil et al. 2002; Gurney et al. 1999), while incidence was considered to be decreasing slightly (Thorne et al. 1994; Morland 1995). A more recent report, however, suggests no change in medulloblastoma occurrence (McNeil et al. 2002). Regardless, medulloblastoma remains the second most common pediatric brain tumor, following pilocytic astrocytoma. Peak occurrence is around 4 years of age (Gurney et al. 1999; Morland 1995). Up to 20% or more of cases occur in patients over 15 years of age (Peterson and Walker 1995; Prados et al. 1995; Roberts et al. 1991). Boys are affected one and a half times more frequently than girls, and females have a better outcome (McNeil et al. 2002; Gurney et al. 1999; Weil et al. 1998).

The etiology for this tumor is unclear, except in a small fraction of children who harbor a germline mutation of a tumor-suppressor gene, such as in Gorlin's syndrome or, even more rarely, Turcot's syndrome (Hamilton et al. 1995), Li-Fraumeni syndrome (Pearson et al. 1982), ataxia telangiectasia (Shuster et al. 1966), or Coffin-Siris syndrome (Rogers et al. 1988). Gorlin's syndrome is identified by nevoid basal cell carcinoma, jaw cysts, palmar and plantar pits, rib anomalies, hyporesponsiveness to parathyroid hormone, and medulloblastoma (Gorlin and Goltz 1960; Gorlin et al. 1965). Environmental exposures such as to JC and SV40 viruses have been described as putative causes for medulloblastoma, but epidemiological studies are inconclusive (Fine 2002). Maternal consumption of cured meats and exposure to N-nitroso compounds have been posited as risk factors for childhood brain tumors, yet evidence is inconsistent (Gurney et al. 1999).

5.2.2 Pathology

5.2.2.1 Grading

Most clinicians and neuropathologists now agree that medulloblastoma is a distinct cerebellar cancer. The WHO classifies medulloblastoma as a malignant neuroepithelial embryonal neoplasm of the cerebellum with predominantly neuronal differentiation, distinct from other embryonal tumors, and with a tendency to metastasize via CSF pathways (Kleihues and Cavenee 2000). All tumors are classified as grade IV because of their highly malignant phenotype. However, some data suggest that this grading system may be an oversimplification. Less differentiation and increasing anaplasia tend to be associated with a significantly worse outcome (Eberhart et al. 2002).

5.2.2.2 Histopathology

Histologically, classic medulloblastoma is a small, round-cell, embryonal tumor composed of tightly packed and poorly differentiated cells with scanty cytoplasm and dense basophilic nuclei, as well as a number of mitotic figures (Fig. 5.1). Glial or neuronal differentiation may be present. Perivascular

Figure 5.1

Hematoxylin and eosin micrograph of classic medulloblastoma. There are dense sheets of small cells with scant cytoplasm. This appearance has been described as typical for "small blue cell tumors"

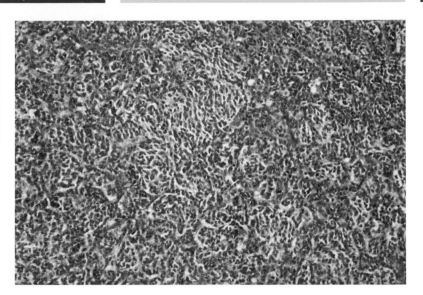

Figure 5.2

Hematoxylin and eosin micrograph of Homer–Wright rosettes in medulloblastoma

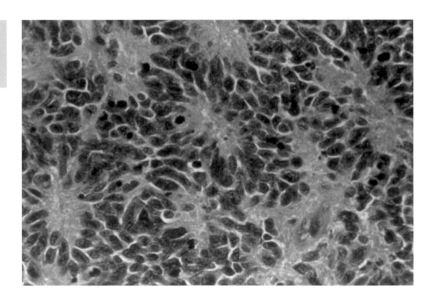

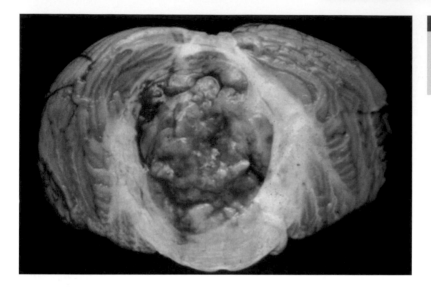

Figure 5.3

Gross specimen of circumscribed medulloblastoma at the level of the cerebellar vermis and fourth ventricle

pseudorosettes or Homer-Wright rosettes (neuroblastic rosettes of nuclei in a circle around tangled cytoplasmic processes) may be present in a minority of cases (Fig. 5.2). Vascular proliferation and hemorrhage are seldom noted. Grossly, the tumor often sits at the cerebellar vermis or within the fourth ventricle as a circumscribed yet friable, tan to pink mass of several centimeters (Fig. 5.3). On MRI the mass demonstrates homogeneous low signal intensity on T1-weighted images, and intermediate- or rarely hyper-intensity on T2-weighted images. Enhancement with gadolinium may be patchy or dense (Fig. 5.4).

A variety of histologic variants of medulloblastoma have been identified to date. While exceedingly rare, medullomyoblastoma, with striated muscle or muscle antigen, and melanotic medulloblastoma, with a minor component of melanin-forming neuroepithelial cells, were described decades ago (Marinesco and Goldstein 1933; Fowler and Simpson 1962). Both of these subtypes may carry a worse prognosis than classic medulloblastoma. More recently, desmoplastic medulloblastoma and large-cell medulloblastoma have been described as distinct subtypes, and the separate entity of an atypical teratoid/rhabdoid tumor has clearly been established (see Section 5.3).

Desmoplastic medulloblastoma is characterized microscopically by an abundant stromal component of dense reticulin surrounding nodular foci of tumor (so-called pale islands) (Fig. 5.5). Macroscopically, this variant appears as a mass at the superficial edge of a cerebellar hemisphere (Fig. 5.6), occurring perhaps most often in adolescents or young adults (Levy et al. 1997). There may be extensive infiltration of the overlying meninges.

Large-cell medulloblastoma is identified histologically by pleomorphic, large, round to irregular nuclei with prominent nucleoli and a more abundant cytoplasm than classic medulloblastoma (Fig. 5.7) (Giangspero et al. 1992). Numerous mitoses and a high apoptotic rate are common. Large-cell tumors stain uniformly for synaptophysin, and may stain for chromogranin. These tumors may constitute up to 4% of medulloblastomas, and are frequently associated with bulky spinal metastases at diagnosis (Fig. 5.8) and an aggressive disease course (Brown et al. 2000). Overall survival at 5 years from diagnosis may be as low as 10%.

Atypical teratoid/rhabdoid tumor (ATRT; see section 5.3) is a newly recognized tumor that despite distinct histologic and biologic features was previously misclassified with medulloblastoma. It is a distinct malignant neoplasm with a very high mortality rate in infants and young children. Since patients with this

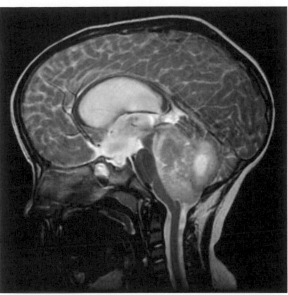

a

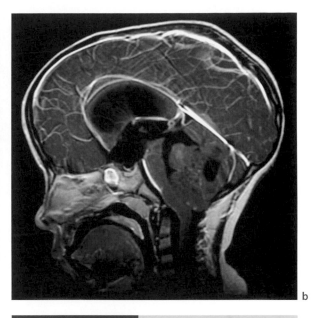

b

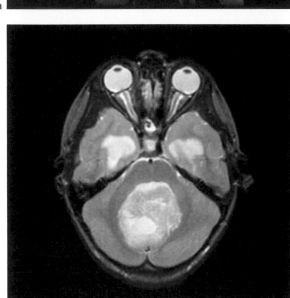

c

Figure 5.4 a–c

MR images of a five year old boy with a typical posterior fossa medulloblastoma. a T2-weighted sagittal image showing a large heterogeneous, partially cystic mass arising within the cerebellar vermis, displacing the brainstem anteriorly, and with associated ventricular enlargement. b T1-weighted image with contrast demonstrates minimal enhancement, which is a common finding. c T2-weighted axial image showing that the tumor extends to the floor of the fourth ventricle but does not invade the brainstem. This tumor was resected completely

highly aggressive tumor were considered years ago to harbor medulloblastoma, they were undoubtedly treated on clinical trials for medulloblastoma. Thus, overall survival rates reported for very young children with "medulloblastoma" might underestimate the true survival to be expected with medulloblastoma.

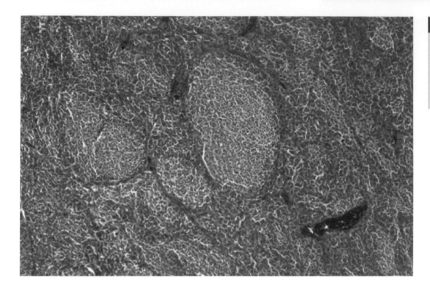

Figure 5.5

Hematoxylin and eosin micrograph of desmoplastic medulloblastoma with pale islands of tumor cells and intervening dense reticulin

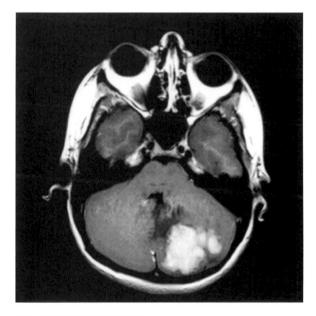

Figure 5.6

Transverse T1-weighted axial MR image following contrast demonstrating a superficial left cerebellar desmoplastic medulloblastoma in a 16-year-old girl

5.2.2.3 Molecular Biology and Cytogenetics

Improved characterization of the histologic variants of medulloblastoma has also led to an improved understanding of the underlying biologic features. Better knowledge of the molecular and cytogenetic changes associated with outcome in medulloblastoma (Table 5.1) will be necessary to refine stratification of disease risk, which at present is based solely on clinical features (see below). In the future, ascertainment of molecular variations may allow for individually tailored therapy using specific or novel targets.

In the 1970s and 1980s, descriptive histopathologic features such as desmoplasia and increased cellular differentiation were correlated with improved survival (Caputy et al. 1987; Chatty and Earle 1971), although one report suggested that patients with differentiating neoplasms fare less well (Packer et al. 1984). More recently, a low proliferative index (as determined by Ki-67 antigen/MIB-1 antibody identification of cycling, non G_0/G_1 phase cells) has been found to predict a better outcome (Grotzer et al. 2001). A high rate of apoptosis also predicts an improved outcome (Haslam et al. 1998).

Figure 5.7

Hematoxylin and eosin micrograph of a large-cell medulloblastoma with cells having abundant cytoplasm, irregular nuclei, and prominent nucleoli

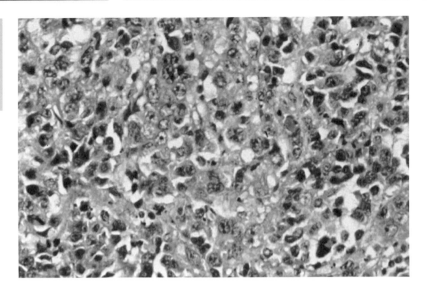

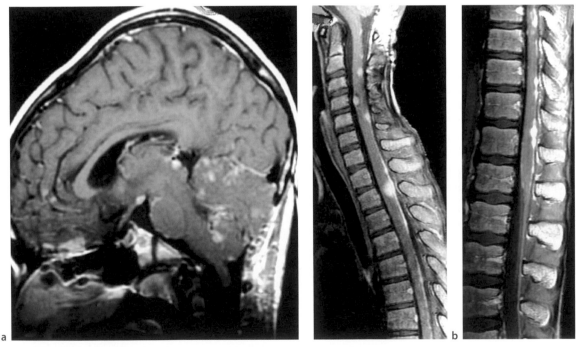

Figure 5.8 a–c

T1-weighted sagittal post-gadolinium images of the brain **a**, thoracic spine **b**, and lumbar spine **c** of a 10-year-old with a widely metastatic large-cell medulloblastoma just after resection of a vermian primary mass. Widespread tumor spread is visualized as "sugar coating" of the surface of the cerebellum and spinal cord

Table 5.1. Cytogenetic and molecular features associated with medulloblastoma outcome

Good prognosis
Hyperdiploidy (Gajjar et al. 1993)
High *trkC* expression (Grotzer et al. 2000; Kim et al. 1999)

Poor prognosis
Isolated 17p loss of heterozygosity (Gilbertson et al. 2001)
Elevated *erbB2* expression (Gilbertson et al. 2001)
Elevated *c-myc* expression (Scheurlein et al. 1998)
Overexpression of calbindin-D_{28k} (Pelc et al. 2002)

Cytogenetic studies over the last ten years have yielded a number of findings. Isochromosome *17q* is seen in about half of cases of medulloblastoma (Bigner et al. 1988), and is associated with large-cell medulloblastoma (Brown et al. 2000). Loss of heterozygosity of 17p may be seen with isochromosome 17q. Isolated 17p loss appears to be associated with poor prognosis (Gilbertson et al. 2001). Chromosome-1 rearrangements and 1q loss have been inconsistently noted in medulloblastoma (Bigner et al. 1988). Hyperdiploidy appears to be associated with a better outcome than diploidy (Gajjar et al. 1993), yet one study found diploidy to be associated with a better outcome than aneuploidy (Zerbini et al. 1993). Comparative genomic hybridization has revealed that high-level chromosomal gain at 8q24 (the locus of *c-myc*, see below) may be associated with large-cell medulloblastoma (Brown et al. 2000).

Molecular markers recently associated with medulloblastoma have thus far included the genetic loci *c-myc*, *trkC* and *erbB2*. In a study of 55 patients, elevated expression of *erbB2*, a gene for class I receptor tyrosine kinases, was associated with reduced patient survival (Gilbertson et al. 2001). High expression of *trkC*, a neurotrophin-receptor gene that promotes apoptosis in medulloblastoma, has consistently predicted a favorable clinical outcome (Grotzer et al. 2000; Kim et al. 1999). Amplification of the c-*myc* proto-oncogene has been linked to a very poor prognosis and was found in 8 of a series of 32 medullo-

blastomas (Scheurlein et al. 1998). The c-myc proto-oncogene has been found to be amplified in large-cell medulloblastomas (Brown et al. 2000). Overexpression of the calcium-binding protein calbindin-D_{28k} is associated with a high risk of medulloblastoma relapse (Pelc et al. 2002). This protein protects cells from calcium overload and may prevent apoptosis.

Recent laboratory reports have implicated a key role for the human homolog of the *Drosophila* gene patched (*PTCH*). Mutations in this gene occur in some medulloblastoma tumors (Pietsch et al. 1997; Raffel et al. 1997; Wolter et al. 1997; Xie et la. 1997). The *PTCH* protein product serves as a transmembrane receptor where the antagonist ligand sonic hedgehog protein (Shh) binds, a key ligand–receptor signal-transduction pathway in cerebellar development (Gilbertson 2002). The mechanism by which *PTCH* signal dysregulation leads to tumorigenesis is unclear, but appears to stem from a principal defect in *PTCH*. Overexpression of *PTCH* and two other Shh downstream target genes – *GLI* and n-*myc* – is highly correlated with desmoplastic medulloblastoma (Pomeroy et al. 2002). Patients with Gorlin's syndrome have germline mutations in the *PTCH* gene at chromosome 9q31, and their medulloblastomas are often desmoplastic (Pietsch et al. 1997). Mutations in other genes in the Shh pathway, such as the human suppressor of fused (*SUFU*), have also been identified as leading to medulloblastoma (Taylor et al. 2002).

Further research is being driven by the use of transgenic mouse models of medulloblastoma. Inactivation of one *PTCH* allele in the mouse leads to a 14% incidence of medulloblastoma (Wetmore et al. 2000). These tumors demonstrate features of both glial and neuronal differentiation, also observed in human tumors. An additional genetic mutation in a critical tumor suppressor gene such as *p53* leads to virtually all mice developing medulloblastoma (Wetmore et al. 2001). Interestingly, transgenic mice deficient for both DNA ligase IV (Lig4; a component of the DNA repair machinery) and *p53* also develop medulloblastoma (Lee et al. 2002). A confounding variable in the interpretation of these results is that *p53* mutations are not commonly observed in human tumors. Nonetheless, these animal studies suggest that alterations in multiple genetic pathways may result in medulloblastoma.

5.2.3 Clinical Features

Since medulloblastoma occurs most often in the midline cerebellum at the level of the fourth ventricle, children present frequently with symptoms and signs of obstructive hydrocephalus and cerebellar dysfunction over a period of 2 to 6 months. Early symptoms may include irritability, behavioral changes, and declining school performance. The child may go on to experience emesis, particularly upon awakening, horizontal diplopia, head tilt, clumsiness, and occipital or frontal headaches. Within 6 months of headache onset, virtually all children will have associated neurologic signs, such as papilledema, strabismus, ataxia, or weakness (Honig and Charney 1982). Infants may display microcephaly, splitting of the cranial sutures, or a bulging anterior fontanelle.

5.2.4 Natural History

Among all childhood brain tumors, medulloblastoma has the greatest tendency for subarachnoid space seeding and extraneural spread. At diagnosis, 14% to 43% of patients are reported to have microscopic or nodular seeding in the subarachnoid space of the spine or brain (Tarbell et al. 1991; Deutsch and Reigel 1980). Spread outside the CNS at any point in the disease course occurs in less than 5% of cases (Kleinman et al. 1981).

More than half of all children with medulloblastoma can now be cured of their disease. Relapse occurs most often at the primary tumor site or elsewhere within the cerebellum, with or without neuraxis spread (Halberg et al. 1991). Median time to recurrence is 14 months from diagnosis, although for infants the time to progression is just 6 months (Minn et al. 2001; Duffner et al. 1993). Subarachnoid tumor spread has been noted in many patients at autopsy. These data on tumor relapse derive from children treated with 36 Gy of craniospinal radiation, or infants treated without radiotherapy. As the dose of prophylactic neuraxis radiation is decreased and systemic and intrathecal chemotherapies added or altered, these patterns of relapse may change.

The relationship of age at diagnosis to natural history has been debated. Children of less than 3 years have significantly worse survival than older children, but there do not appear to be significant differences between age groups 4 to 9, 10 to 14, and 15 to 19 years (McNeil et al. 2002). Thus, the adverse effect of very young age on outcome may be confounded by the absence of irradiation during treatment. Outcome is unaffected by race (McNeil et al. 2002).

5.2.5 Diagnosis, Surgery, and Staging

5.2.5.1 Diagnosis

A child presenting with the clinical features described above should be immediately evaluated by a brain imaging study. Initially, this will be a computed tomography (CT) scan of the head because of its simplicity, speed, and availability in most communities. In addition, sedation can often be avoided with the rapid acquisition of images using newer CT scanners. A high quality CT scan will almost always detect a posterior fossa mass. Nonetheless, anatomic definition and preoperative planning require a high-quality MRI scan. MRI can also add to preoperative treatment planning with the ability to reformat three-dimensional volumetric data for tumor localization. In many centers, full-spine MRI is also obtained simultaneously with the brain MRI to determine if there is leptomeningeal dissemination. A child with a posterior fossa mass might have obstructive hydrocephalus and be at risk for deterioration from transient increases in intracranial pressure while supine or sedated during a prolonged MRI. Dexamethasone 0.1 to 0.3 mg/kg divided twice to four times daily may be initiated for vasogenic edema. At times, a ventriculostomy may be required prior to further imaging to allow CSF drainage and ICP monitoring.

5.2.5.2 Surgery

Virtually all children with a posterior fossa mass will undergo an open craniotomy. The goals of surgery are relief of mass effect, tissue diagnosis, and cytoreduction to facilitate further treatment. In general, there is no indication for stereotactic or open biopsy unless the cerebellar tumor is diffuse or there is extensive leptomeningeal seeding. An effort should be made for a near-total or gross total resection. Children who are left with less than 1.5 cm^2 of residual disease on postoperative imaging have an improved prognosis for long term, relapse-free survival (Zeltzer et al. 1999). Preoperative tumor infiltration of the brainstem does not affect prognosis (Zeltzer et al. 1999). Thus, removal of tiny components of medulloblastoma invading the brainstem or lying at the floor or exit of the fourth ventricle is not warranted and should be avoided in order to minimize neurologic injury. A postoperative brain MRI should be obtained 48 to 72 hours following surgery, before obscuring gliosis and evolving blood products lessen the ability to distinguish residual tumor.

Many children will require a postoperative ventriculostomy (i.e., external drain) for temporary diversion of CSF as obstructive hydrocephalus resolves. Usually, weaning from the ventriculostomy will take place over the first week or ten days either by gradually elevating the external drain, or by clamping the drain with continuous monitoring of the ICP. This is usually done in an intensive-care setting. If ICP rises, or if ventricular enlargement occurs with such weaning, the presence of true hydrocephalus must be presumed and a permanent ventriculoperitoneal shunt should be placed. Shunt placement does not appear to increase the risk of systemic tumor spread (Berger et al. 1991). If the ventriculostomy can be removed successfully, careful observation of ventricular size and clinical symptoms must continue as delayed hydrocephalus can still occur.

5.2.5.3 Staging

Following surgery, the child requires a simple staging protocol for further evidence of tumor spread. If not already done, a full spine MRI with and without gadolinium is mandatory. Spine imaging should be delayed at least for 10 to 14 days following surgery, as blood products in the subarachnoid space can be misinterpreted as metastatic tumor. A lumbar puncture should be obtained in the same time period to assess cytology for microscopic tumor spread. Ventricular sampling of CSF for cytology has inferior sensitivity and should not be used unless a lumbar sample absolutely cannot be obtained (Gajjar et al. 1999). A bone scan is often obtained to search for extraneural spread, but bone marrow biopsy is no longer recommended.

With these findings from staging, children over age 3 years are stratified into two risk groups, based on resection extent and Chang metastasis staging (Tables 5.2 and 5.3) (Chang et al. 1969). "Average risk" includes children with less than 1.5 cm^2 residual and no metastasis. "High risk" is defined by more than 1.5 cm^2 residual or metastatic disease. However, the impact of M1 disease on survival remains debatable. In both trials Children's Cancer Group (CCG) 921 and HIT '91, overall survival was not significantly different in children staged as M1 or M0 (Zeltzer et al. 1999; Kortmann et al. 2000). Histologic variants such as large-cell medulloblastoma or cellular markers may portend a poor outcome, but are not used to establish high risk.

Previously, brainstem invasion (Chang stage T3b) was another indication for stratification as high risk, but such does not appear to affect prognosis (Duffner et al. 1993). The older term "low risk," indicating less than 1.5 cm^2 residual tumor, M0, and no brainstem invasion has been abandoned.

Radiotherapy or chemotherapy does not usually commence until three to four weeks after surgery because of time required for wound healing, neurologic recovery, and staging. Baseline assessment of endocrine and cognitive function should be performed in the postoperative period, as craniospinal irradiation may adversely affect the pituitary and thyroid glands along with the cerebrum.

Table 5.2. Chang metastasis staging system for medulloblastoma (Gajjar et al. 1999)

M0 No evidence of gross subarachnoid or hematogenous metastasis

M1 Microscopic tumor cells found in cerebrospinal fluid

M2 Gross nodular seeding demonstrated in the cerebellar, cerebral subarachnoid space, or in the third or lateral ventricles

M3 Gross nodular seeding in spinal subarachnoid space

M4 Extraneural metastasis

Table 5.3. Risk stratification for medulloblastoma in children ≥3 years

Average risk

<1.5 cm^2 postoperative residual tumor and Stage M0

High risk

>1.5 cm^2 postoperative residual tumor or Stage M1–4

5.2.6 Treatment

Medulloblastoma is radiosensitive, and thus for many years craniospinal irradiation followed by an additional radiation boost to the posterior fossa has been the mainstay of adjuvant therapy for this tumor. Indeed, attempts to omit craniospinal irradiation in children of less than 3 years or to exclude the entire neuraxis from the radiation field resulted in reduced survival (Duffner et al. 1993; Bouffet et al. 1992). The cognitive and endocrinologic sequelae (see below) of craniospinal radiotherapy, along with the poor survival of children with high-risk medulloblastoma, has led to sustained efforts by cooperative groups to introduce chemotherapy in order to reduce radiation dosage, improve survival, or delay irradiation.

In the late 1970s, the International Society of Pediatric Oncology (SIOP I), CCG (CCG 942), and the Pediatric Oncology Group (POG 7909) each performed prospective randomized trials of craniospinal irradiation alone versus post-irradiation chemotherapy, heavily based on alkylators (lomustine or nitrogen mustard/procarbazine) plus vincristine, with or without prednisone (Tait et al. 1990; Evans et al. 1990; Krischer et al. 1991). An improvement in overall survival from chemotherapy was not apparent for all children, but a benefit did appear in those who had bulky residual disease or metastatic disease, i.e., high-risk disease. These experiences and a series of subsequent trials demonstrated that medulloblastoma is one of the most chemotherapy-sensitive of all brain tumors. Alkylators and platinum compounds have remained the foundation of adjuvant chemotherapy, particularly lomustine, cisplatin, and sometimes procarbazine, cyclophosphamide, ifosfamide, or carboplatin. The mitotic inhibitor vincristine is often administered weekly during irradiation and then during adjuvant chemotherapy. In addition, the topoisomerase II inhibitor etoposide has shown promising activity in disseminated medulloblastoma and infant medulloblastoma, and its use is increasing (Duffner et al. 1993; Ashley et al. 1996). The antimetabolite methotrexate has been used in European trials, particularly before irradiation, but there remains concern in the United States about its potential for causing leukoencephalopathy.

In average-risk medulloblastoma, a series of trials from SIOP, the French Society of Pediatric Oncology (SFOP), POG and CCG [now merged into the Children's Oncology Group (COG)], and the German Society of Pediatric Oncology (GPO and the HIT trials) have attempted to reduce craniospinal irradiation, with the addition of either pre-irradiation "neoadjuvant" chemotherapy or, more commonly, post-irradiation chemotherapy (Table 5.4) (Kortmann et al. 2000; Bailey et al. 1995; Gentet et al. 1995; Thomas et al. 2000; Kühl et al. 1998; Packer et al. 1999; Taylor et al. 2001). The study POG 8631/CCG 923 compared directly 23.4 Gy versus 36 Gy craniospinal irradiation, without any chemotherapy in either group. This study was suspended in 1990 when an interim statistical analysis revealed an increased rate of relapse in the reduced-dosage radiotherapy group (Thomas et al. 2000). Regardless, follow-up of this cohort over time has provided very important data. First, the children receiving 36 Gy experienced an event-free survival (EFS) of 67% at 5 years and 60% at 8 years. These results serve as a benchmark for average-risk

Table 5.4. Cooperative group studies for average-risk medulloblastoma, age ≥3 years

Study	Years of accrual	Number of eligible patients	Pre-irradiation chemotherapy x cycles	Craniospinal radiotherapy[a] (Gy)	Post-irradiation chemotherapy x cycles	Percent event-free survival at 5 years	Comments
SIOP II[b,c] (Bailey et al. 1995)	1984–1989	40 36 38 36	none none PCZ/VCR/MTX x 1 PCZ/VCR/MTX x 1	35 25 35 25	none none none none	60±8 69±8 75±7 42±8	No significant benefit from "sandwich" chemotherapy, but negative interaction between "sandwich" chemotherapy and reduced irradiation
SFOP M7[b,d] (Gentet et al. 1995)	1985–1988	31	"8-in-1"[e] x 2, HD MTX x 2	30–37.5[f]	none	74	
POG 8631/ CCG 923[b] (Thomas et al. 2000)	1986–1990	44 44	none none	36 23.4	none none	67±7 52±11	Increased incidence of early, exoprimary neuraxis relapse
HIT '88/'89[f] (Kühl et al. 1998)	1987–1991	55	PCZ/IFOS/VP16/ MTX/CDDP/ ARAC x 2	35.2 (n=34) <30 (n=21)	none	61±7	Results compiled for all patients together
CCG 9892[g] (Packer et al. 1999)	1990–1994	65	none	23.4 + weekly VCR	CCNU/CDDP/ VCR x 8	78±5	23% completed CDDP only with dose reduction and 36% did not complete CDDP because of ototoxicity
HIT '91[h] (Kortmann et al. 2000)	1991–1997	64 94	none IFOS/CDDP/ HD MTX/VP16/ ARAC x 2	35.2 + weekly VCR 35.2	CCNU/CDDP/ VCR x 8 CCNU/CBDCA/ VCR x 8 if incom- plete remission or progressive disease	78%±6% 3-year PFS 65%±5% 3-year PFS nonrandomized patients included	

Study	Years	N	Chemotherapy	RT (Gy)	Chemotherapy	Survival	Results
PNET-3[i] (Taylor et al. 2001)	1992–2000	89 90	none VP16/VCR/CBDCA /CPM x 3	35 35	none none	72% 59%	EFS statistically significant, p=.05
COG A9961[f]	1996–2000			23.4 CSI 23.4 CSI	CCNU/CDDP/ VCR x 8, or CPM/CDDP/VCR x 8		results pending

[a] Posterior fossa boost totaling 50 to 55.2 Gy;
[b] patients classified as low risk;
[c] children 0–3 years included;
[d] children 24–35 months included and received 20 Gy to cranium;
[e] "8-in-1" = methylprednisolone/VCR/CCNU/PCZ/hydroxurea/CDDP/ARAC/CPM;
[f] 23–35 Gy to cranium;
[g] children 3–10 years only;
[h] patients with and without residual disease, M1 patients included, and not all patients randomized to therapy
[i] children 3–16 years included

PCZ=procarbazine; VCR=vincristine; MTX=methotrexate; HD=high dose; IFOS=ifosfamide; VP16=etoposide; CDDP=cisplatin; ARAC=cytarabine; CCHU=lomustine; VCR=vincristine; PFS=progression-free survival; CBDCA=carboplatin; CPM=cyclophosphamide

Table 5.5. Cooperative group studies for high-risk medulloblastoma, age ≥3 years

Study	Years of accrual	Number of eligible patients	Pre-irradiation chemotherapy x cycles	Craniospinal radiotherapy[a] (Gy)	Post-irradiation chemotherapy x cycles	Percent event-free survival	Comments
SFOP M7[b,c] (Gentet et al. 1995)	1985–1988	37	"8-in-1"[d] x 2, HD MTX x 2	30–37.5[e]	"8-in-1" x 4	57 at 5 years	
POG 8695[f] (Mosijczuk et al. 1993)	1986–1990	36	CDDP/VCR x 3; CPM x 2	36	none		PFS 40% at 2 years only 22 of 36 completed therapy, secondary to toxicity; start of radiotherapy delayed in most patients because of myelosuppression
SIOP II[g] (Bailey et al. 1995)	1984–1989	62	PCZ/VCR/MTX x 1	35	CCNU/VCR x 6	56±7 at 5 years	
		71	one	35	CCNU/VCR x 6	53±6 at 5 years	
CCG 921[h] (Zeltzer et al. 1999)	1986–1992	101	none	36 + weekly VCR	CCNU/VCR/PCZ x 8		63%±5% PFS at 5 years
		102	"8-in-1" x 2	36	"8-in-1" x 8		45%±5% PFS at 5 years
HIT '88/'89 (Kühl et al. 1998)	1987–1991	39	PCZ/IFOS/VP16/MTX/CDDP/ARAC x 2	35.2	CCNU/PCZ	33±8 at 5 years	
POG 9031[c] (Tarbell et al. 2000)	1990–1996	114	CDDP/VP16_3	35.2 M0–1; 40 M2–3	CPM/VCR x 8	78±4 at 2 years	Response to chemotherapy correlated with outcome
		112	none	35.2 M0–1; 40 M2–3	CDDP/VP16_3, then CPM/VCR x 8	80±4 at 2 years	

HIT '91 (Kortman et al. 2000)	1991–1997	40[i]	none	35.2 + weekly VCR	CCNU/CDDP/VCR × 8	For all patients 65%±12% PFS for M1, and 30%±15% for M2–3
			IFOS/CDDP/HD MTX/VP16/ARAC × 2	35.2	CCNU/CBDCA/VCR × 8 if incomplete remission or progressive disease	

[a] Posterior fossa boost to 54 to 55.8 Gy;

[b] children >10–35 months included and received 20 Gy to cranium;

[c] brainstem invasion used as a criterion for high risk;

[d] "8-in-1" = methylprednisolone/VCR/CCNU/PCZ/hydroxurea/CDDP/ARAC/CPM;

[e] 22–35 Gy to cranium;

[f] children > 4 years, and brainstem invasion used as an additional criterion for high risk;

[g] children 0–3 years included, and brainstem invasion but not M1 used as a criterion for high risk;

[h] children >1.5 years included and brainstem invasion used as an additional criterion for high risk;

[i] details of which regimen 21 nonrandomized M1 and 19 randomized M2–3 patients not provided

HD MTX=high-dose methotrexate; CDDP=cisplatin; VCR=vincristine; CPM=cyclophosphamide; PFS=progression-free survival; PCZ=procarbazine; CCNU=lomustine; IFOS=ifosfamide; VP16=etoposide; ARAC=cytarabine; CBDCA=carboplatin disease. Secondly, EFS was marginally inferior for the 23.4 Gy group, at 52% at 5 years (*P*=.077). There was an increased rate of early relapse and increased risk of isolated exoprimary recurrence, results contrary to earlier limited institutional experiences (Halberg et al. 1991; Deutsch et al. 1996). In contrast, the subsequent single-arm study CCG 9892, employing 23.4 Gy craniospinal irradiation plus a boost to the posterior fossa totaling 55.2 Gy with concurrent weekly vincristine, followed thereafter by eight courses of lomustine, cisplatin, and vincristine, attained a 5-year EFS of 78%, statistically not different from the POG 8631/CCG 923 benchmark with 36 Gy. While this study accrued just 65 eligible patients, it appears that chemotherapy can be substituted for at least some amount of craniospinal irradiation. Whether greater experience with this approach will demonstrate a change in relapse patterns such as increased isolated exoprimary relapses is uncertain.

In high-risk medulloblastoma studies, and even in some of the average-risk studies, there has been a consistent effort to deliver neoadjuvant chemotherapy, and sometimes post-irradiation chemotherapy (Table 5.5) (Zeltzer et al. 1999; Kortmann et al. 2000; Bailey et al. 1995; Gentet et al. 1995; Mosijczuk et al. 1993; Tarbell et al. 2000). The rationale for neoadjuvant chemotherapy lies in the presumed benefit of unencumbered treatment before radiation, possibly offering better tolerance, less toxicity, and perhaps even increased disease control. To date, few data support such hypothetical advantages. In fact, myelosuppression in some instances has led to delays in initiation of radiotherapy or early disease progression (Kortmann et al. 2000; Mosijczuk et al. 1993). The risk of distant neuraxis relapse also appears to increase with pre-irradiation chemotherapy (Hartsell et al. 1997). It does seem clear that post-irradiation chemotherapy improves survival in patients with high-risk medulloblastoma (Packer et al. 1994). At present, based on all studies, 5-year EFS appears to be at least 50% for high-risk patients. Current trials for these patients are evaluating either chemotherapy concurrent with radiotherapy followed by further adjuvant chemotherapy, or post-irradiation high-dose chemotherapy with blood stem-cell rescue.

5.2.7 Outcome

Data from multiple prospective studies suggests that overall survival for all children with medulloblastoma now approaches 60% at 5 years and at least 40 to 50% at 10 years (Tait et al. 1990; Evans et al. 1990). Relapse beyond 8 years from diagnosis appears unlikely (Belza et al. 1991). While some satisfaction can be derived from these modest improvements in survival, the growing number of children cured of their disease has led to a sobering recognition of the severity of late effects, namely cognitive decline, growth failure, endocrinopathies, hearing loss, CNS vascular disease, and secondary malignancies.

Cranial irradiation has been linked to cognitive decline, with intelligence quotient (IQ) used as a surrogate marker. Cognitive decline appears to be most notable in attention, short-term memory, visual motor processing, spatial relations, and quantitative skills. Whether the additional radiotherapy boost to the posterior fossa with exposure beyond the clinoid processes anteriorly to the hippocampus and forebrain exacerbates this damage is unknown. While data are very limited, children less than age 9 at diagnosis of medulloblastoma who receive 36 Gy craniospinal irradiation, have a full scale IQ approximating 70 six to nine years later; for those receiving 23.4 Gy, IQ averages 85 (Mulhern et al. 1998). Indeed, 100% of children less than age 7 years treated with 24 to 36 Gy craniospinal irradiation go on to require special education services (Radcliffe et al. 1992). For children older than 3 years treated with 23.4 Gy and infants salvaged with a median dosage of 35.2 Gy following relapse after chemotherapy, a striking (and worrying) finding is an approximate 4 point decline in IQ every year following irradiation (Ris et al. 2001; Walter et al. 1999). It is unclear when the IQ decline reaches a plateau.

Growth failure appears to be a nearly universal phenomenon in patients with medulloblastoma, secondary to radiation exposure to the pituitary gland, spinal cord, and vertebral column. Hypothyroidism and gonadal dysfunction are also common. High-frequency hearing loss from both radiation exposure to the cochlea and damage to its hair cells from cisplatin is also quite common. For a fuller discussion of these late effects, the reader is referred elsewhere (Strother et al. 2002). Secondary malignancies from radiotherapy and even chemotherapy are also being increasingly recognized, particularly in children who have Gorlin's syndrome (Stavrou et al. 2001).

5.2.8 Future Directions

Future investigation in medulloblastoma will focus on both the optimal dosage and delivery method for radiotherapy. A single pilot study using 18 Gy craniospinal irradiation followed by lomustine, cisplatin, and vincristine in 10 patients less than age 5 at diagnosis of average-risk medulloblastoma produced 7 long-term survivors four years later with no significant change from baseline IQ (Goldwein et al. 1993). A multi-institution pilot study of this approach is underway, and a COG-sponsored clinical trial is in development to study this dosage in younger children. As for delivery, technological improvements now allow for conformal radiotherapy to limit radiation scatter from the posterior fossa boost, or even to limit the clinical target volume of the boost to the original tumor volume rather than the entire posterior fossa (Freeman et al. 2002). In either instance, conformal techniques promise to limit exposure to the cochlea, hippocampus, forebrain, hypothalamus, and pituitary gland, but possibly carry a risk of increased local recurrence.

5.3 Atypical Teratoid/Rhabdoid Tumor

5.3.1 Epidemiology

Since atypical teratoid/rhabdoid tumor (ATRT) was first described as a distinct entity in the 1980s, measurement of the true incidence is difficult. ATRT constituted 2.1% of primary brain tumors in children 18 years and younger at one institution (Kleihues et al. 2000). Some reports have suggested that up to 1 in 4 embryonal tumors in children less than 3 years old are ATRT (Packer et al. 2002). Indeed, the tumor has a striking predilection for infants, with mean age at diagnosis of 7 months, and 94% of affected children less than 5 years of age (Kleihues et al. 2000; Packer et al. 2002). Boys outnumber girls about 1.5 to 1 (Kleihues et al. 2000; Burger et al. 1998).

5.3.2 Pathology

ATRT is a malignant embryonal tumor containing rhabdoid cells and often additional, disparate components of small embryonal, mesenchymal, and epithelial cells (Fig. 5.9). They contain sheets of rhabdoid cells, which appear as medium-sized, ovoid cells, with an eccentric sometimes reniform nucleus, a prominent nucleolus, and a fine granular homogeneous cytoplasm. These cells almost always express epithelial membrane antigen and vimentin (Burger et al. 1998). Mitoses are abundant. MIB-1 labeling index focally can be up to 80% (Kleihues et al. 2000). Only 10% of tumors are composed strictly of rhabdoid cells, and one-third to one-quarter exhibit an epithelial and/or mesenchymal component (Packer et al. 2002). Epithelial cells may appear adenomatous or squamous, or occur in nests. The epithelial and mesenchymal cells can misleadingly suggest a teratoma, but ATRT is negative for germ cell markers (Packer et al. 2002). Two-thirds of these tumors possess a small-cell component, masquerading as medulloblastoma or other embryonal tumor (Kleihues et al. 2000). All tumors are considered as WHO grade IV.

ATRT appears grossly as a soft, pinkish, bulky tumor demarcated from parenchyma, often with necrosis or sometimes dystrophic calcification, cysts, or hemorrhage. Over half of ATRTs are located in the posterior fossa, with the remainder situated mostly in the supratentorial compartment, sometimes in the pineal region. On MRI, the tumor may appear similar to medulloblastoma, with hypointensity on T1-weighted images and isointensity on T2-weighted images (Fig. 5.10). Enhancement with gadolinium can be inhomogeneous.

Important to the diagnosis of ATRT are cytogenetic and molecular findings. Ninety percent of tumors demonstrate monosomy or a deletion of chromosome 22 by fluorescence in situ hybridization or loss of heterozygosity studies (Burger et al. 1998; Bi-

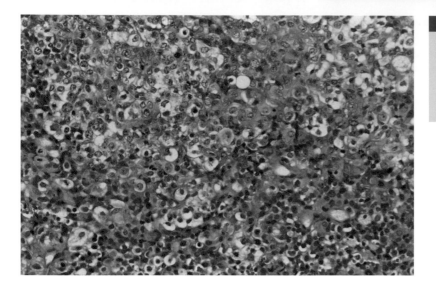

Figure 5.9

Hematoxylin and eosin micrograph of atypical teratoid/rhabdoid tumor, with its disparate small embryonal cell and epithelial and mesenchymal cell components

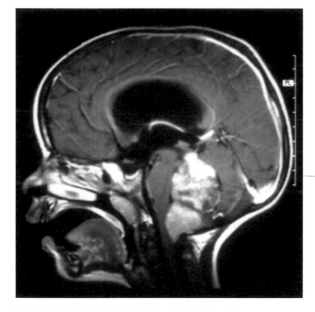

Figure 5.10

Sagittal T1-weighted image of a large midbrain to pontine atypical teratoid/rhabdoid tumor in a 3-month-old boy presenting with a facial palsy

egel et al. 1999). Chromosome 22 abnormalities can be seen in other tumors, and hence this finding is neither sufficient nor necessary for diagnosis. In one study perhaps all ATRTs demonstrate homozygous deletions or mutations of the gene *hSNF5/INI1*, which maps to 22q11.2 (Biegel et al. 1999). While its role in malignant transformation is unknown, *INI1* does appear to be a tumor-suppressor gene involved in rhabdoid tumors of the brain as well as the kidney and other extraneural sites. A fraction of children have germline mutations of *INI1*, which can on rare occasions be transmitted in an autosomal dominant fashion with incomplete penetrance (Biegel et al. 1999; Taylor et al. 2000).

5.3.3 Treatment

Prognosis to date for this tumor has been dismal, and thus optimal therapy unknown. Median survival is less than 10 months, and most children die within a year of diagnosis (Burger et al. 1998; Biegel et al. 1999; Hilden et al. 1998; Olson et al. 1995). Diagnosis is made following a subtotal or gross total surgical resection. Staging studies similar to those in medulloblastoma are reasonable, although ATRT has not been reported to disseminate to bone. Incidence of neuraxis dissemination is uncertain, and reports range from 15% to 40% at diagnosis (Packer et al. 2002; Burger et al. 1998; Hilden et al. 1998). ATRT does not appear to spread outside the neuraxis, and renal rhabdoid tumors do not appear to invade the CNS; thus, abdominal or chest staging is not necessary.

There have been case reports of prolonged survival using high-dose chemotherapy with hematopoietic stem cell rescue or multi-modality treatment with craniospinal irradiation, multiagent chemotherapy, and triple intrathecal chemotherapy, a regimen similar to that seen in the Intergroup Rhabdomyosarcoma Study III guidelines (Hilden et al. 1998; Olson et al. 1995). Other attempts using infant brain tumor chemotherapy regimens with cyclophosphamide, vincristine, cisplatin, and etoposide have led to tumor reduction, but responses do not appear to be sustained (Packere et al. 2002).

5.4 Other Embryonal Tumors

5.4.1 Pineoblastoma

Pineoblastomas are composed of patternless (WHO grade IV) malignant tumors of the pineal region, sheets of densely packed small cells. Homer–Wright rosettes and Flexner–Wintersteiner rosettes, indicating retinoblastic differentiation, may be seen. These tumors account for half of pineal parenchymal tumors, occurring in the first two decades of life slightly more often in males (Kleihues et al. 2000; Schild et al. 1993). Like other embryonal tumors, these have a tendency for neuraxis metastasis. Pineoblastoma can occur with bilateral/familial retinoblastoma, termed "trilateral retinoblastoma," and in such instances has a mean survival of just 11 months (DePotter et al. 1994). Pineoblastoma has also been reported with Turcot's syndrome (Ikeda et al. 1998). Pineoblastoma should be distinguished from pineocytoma or benign pineal cyst.

The mainstay of treatment for pineoblastoma has been irradiation, typically craniospinal, yielding 1-year, 3-year, and 5-year overall survival in older children and adults of 88%, 78%, and 58%, respectively (Schild et al. 1993). Patients with pineoblastoma fare significantly better than those with other supratentorial embryonal tumors (Cohen et al. 1995), and limited prospective data suggest that craniospinal irradiation plus chemotherapy, such as vincristine, lomustine, and prednisone as in CCG 921 may improve overall and progression-free survival in children after 3 years to 73% and 61%, respectively (Jakacki et al. 1995). Chemotherapy alone is insufficient for managing these tumors, especially among infants (Jakacki et al. 1995; Jakacki 1999; Duffner et al. 1995). A residual enhancing mass persisting for as long as 5 years before resolving is not uncommon in pineoblastomas following radiotherapy and chemotherapy, and does not indicate treatment failure (Jakacki et al. 1995).

5.4.2 Other Non-Pineal Embryonal Tumors

Outcome for non-pineal supratentorial embryonal tumors has historically been worse than pineoblastoma or medulloblastoma, with 3-year progression-free survival of 33% following craniospinal irradiation and chemotherapy (Cohen et al. 1995). While these tumors have frequently been treated the same as medulloblastoma, there are no prospective, randomized studies evaluating the role of adjuvant chemotherapy following radiation and no historical data to support this seemingly reasonable approach. Craniospinal irradiation of 35 Gy with an additional boost to at least 54 Gy to the tumor region appear to be necessary (Timmermann et al. 2002). Incomplete resection, tumor dissemination, and younger age appear to be adverse prognostic factors (Albright et al. 1995; Reddy et al. 2000).

Very small numbers of the non-pineal embryonal tumors limit execution of trials aimed specifically at these entities. Additionally, their biologic characterization is incomplete. Analysis by comparative genomic hybridization shows that supratentorial PNET and medulloblastoma have distinctly different patterns of chromosomal gains and losses, suggesting different biologic entities (Russo et al. 1999). Nevertheless, their distinct natural histories and comparably poorer prognosis merit experimental, innovative treatments different from those for medulloblastoma. The reader is referred elsewhere for fuller descriptions of very uncommon tumors such as ependymoblastoma (Dorsay et al. 1995; Robertson et al. 1998; Mørk and Rubinstein 1985), cerebral neuroblastoma (Horton and Rubinstein 1976; Bennett and Rubinstein 1984; Berger et al. 1983), ganglioneuroblastoma, and medulloepithelioma (Molloy et al. 1996).

5.5 Conclusion

Pediatric embryonal malignancies are a clinically and biologically heterogeneous group of tumors. Therapeutic advances in surgery, radiation therapy and chemotherapy have resulted in improved survival for patients with medulloblastoma, but are also associated with increased treatment-related toxicity. Improved understanding of pathologic and biologic features have allowed for identification of atypical teratoid/rhabdoid tumor as a distinct tumor type, separate from medulloblastoma. Although standard-risk medulloblastoma is curable in many patients, most embryonal pediatric CNS tumors have high relapse rates with current treatment strategies. Ongoing investigation is required to better characterize high-risk tumor subtypes and identify better treatment strategies.

References

Albright AL, Wisoff JH, Zeltzer P et al (1995) Prognostic factors in children with supratentorial (nonpineal) primitive neuroectodermal tumors: a neurosurgical perspective from the Children's Cancer Group. Pediatr Neurosurg 22:1–7

Ashley DM, Meier L, Kerby T et al (1996) Response of recurrent medulloblastoma to low-dose oral etoposide. J Clin Oncol 14:1922–1927

Bailey CC, Gnekow A, Wellek S et al (1995) Prospective randomized trial of chemotherapy given before radiotherapy ion childhood medulloblastoma. International Society of Paediatric Oncology (SIOP) and the (German) Society of Paediatric Oncology (GPO): SIOP II. Med Pediatr Oncol 25:166–178

Belza MG, Donaldson SS, Steinberg GK et al (1991) Medulloblastoma: freedom from relapse longer than 8 years – a therapeutic cure? J Neurosurg 75:575–582

Bennett JP, Rubinstein LJ (1984) The biological behavior of primary cerebral neuroblastoma: a reappraisal of the clinical course in a series of 70 cases. Ann Neurol 16:21–27

Berger MS, Edwards MS, Wara WM et al (1983) Primary cerebral neuroblastoma: long-term follow-up, review, and therapeutic guidelines. J Neurosurg 59:418–423

Berger MS, Baumeister B, Geyer JR et al (1991) The risks of metastases from shunting in children with primary central nervous system tumors. J Neurosurg 74:872–877

Biegel JA, Zhou JY, Rorke LB et al (1999) Germ-line and acquired mutations of *INI1* in atypical teratoid and rhabdoid tumors. Cancer Res 59:74–79

Bigner SH, Mark J, Friedman HS et al (1988) Structural chromosomal abnormalities in human medulloblastoma. Cancer Genet Cytogenet 30:91–101

Bouffet E, Bernard JL, Frappaz DL et al (1992) M4 protocol for cerebellar medulloblastoma: supratentorial radiotherapy may not be avoided. Int J Radiat Oncol Biol Phys 24:79–85

Brown HG, Kepner JL, Perlman EJ et al (2000) "Large cell/anaplastic" medulloblastomas: a Pediatric Oncology Group study. J Neuropathol Exp Neurol 10:857–865

Burger PC, Yu IT, Tihan T et al (1998) Atypical teratoid/rhabdoid tumor of the central nervous system: a highly malignant tumor of infancy and childhood frequently mistaken for medulloblastoma: a Pediatric Oncology Group study. Am J Surg Pathol 22:1083–1092

Caputy AJ, McCullough DC, Manz HJ et al (1987) A review of factors influencing the prognosis of medulloblastoma: the importance of cell differentiation. J Neurosurg 66:80–87

Chang CH, Housepian EM, Herbert C (1969) An operative staging system and a megavoltage radiotherapeutic technic for cerebellar medulloblastoma. Radiology 93:1351–1359

Chatty EM, Earle KM (1971) Medulloblastoma: a report of 201 cases with emphasis on the relationship of histologic variants to survival. Cancer 28:977–983

Cohen BH, Zeltzer PM, Boyett JM et al (1995) Prognostic factors and treatment results for supratentorial primitive neuroectodermal tumors in children using radiation and chemotherapy: a Childrens Cancer Group randomized trial. J Clin Oncol 13:1687–1696

DePotter P, Shields CL, Shields JA (1994) Central variations of trilateral retinoblastoma: a report of 13 cases. J Pediatr Ophthalmol Strabismus 31:26–31

Deutsch M, Reigel DH (1980) The value of myelography in the management of medulloblastoma. Cancer 45:2194–2197

Deutsch M, Thomas PRM, Krischer J et al (1996) Results of a prospective randomized trial comparing standard dose neuraxis irradiation (3,600 cGy/20) with reduced neuraxis irradiation (2,340 cGy/13) in patients with low-stage medulloblastoma: a combined Children's Cancer Group-Pediatric Oncology Group study. Pediatr Neurosurg 24:167–177

Dorsay TA, Rovira MJ, Ho VB, Kelley J (1995) Ependymoblastoma: MR presentation. A case report and review of the literature. Pediatr Radiol 25:443–435

Duffner PK, Horowitz ME, Krischer JP et al (1993) Postoperative chemotherapy and delayed radiation in children less than three years of age with malignant brain tumors. N Engl J Med 328:1725–1731

Duffner PK, Cohen ME, Sanford RA (1995) Lack of efficacy of postoperative chemotherapy and delayed radiation in very young children with pineoblastoma. Med Pediatr Oncol 25:38–44

Eberhart CG, Kepner JL, Goldthwaite PT et al (2002) Histopathologic grading of medulloblastomas: a Pediatric Oncology Group study. Cancer 94:552–560

Evans AE, Jenkin RDT, Sposto R et al (1990) The treatment of medulloblastoma: results of a prospective randomized trial of radiation therapy with and without CCNU, vincristine, and prednisone. J Neurosurg 72:572–582

Fine HA (2002) Polyomavirus and medulloblastoma: a smoking gun or guilt by association? J Natl Cancer Inst 94:240–241

Fowler M, Simpson DA (1962) A malignant melanin-forming tumour of the cerebellum. J Pathol Bacteriol 84:307–311

Freeman CR, Taylor RE, Kortmann RD, Carrie C (2002) Radiotherapy for medulloblastoma in children: a perspective on current international clinical research efforts. Med Pediatr Oncol 39:99–108

Gajjar AJ, Heidemann RL, Douglass EC et al (1993) Relation of tumor-cell ploidy to survival in children with medulloblastoma. J Clin Oncol 11:2211–2217

Gajjar AJ, Fouladi M, Walter A et al (1999) Comparison of lumbar and shunt cerebrospinal fluid specimens for cytologic detection of leptomeningeal disease in pediatric patients with brain tumors. J Clin Oncol 17:1825–1828

Gentet JC, Bouffet E, Doz F et al (1995) Preirradiation chemotherapy including "eight drugs in 1 day" regimen and high-dose methotrexate in childhood medulloblastoma: results of the M7 French cooperative study. J Neurosurg 82:608–614

Giangspero F, Rigobello L, Bodily M et al (1992) Large-cell medulloblastomas: a distinct variant with highly aggressive behavior. Am J Surg Pathol 16:687–693

Gilbertson R (2002) Paediatric embryonic tumours: biological and clinical relevance of molecular genetic abnormalities. Eur J Cancer 38:675–685

Gilbertson R, Wickramasinghe C, Hernan R et al (2001) Clinical and molecular stratification of disease risk in medulloblastoma. Br J Cancer 85:705–712

Goldwein JW, Radcliffe J, Packer RJ et al (1993) Results of a pilot study of low-dose craniospinal radiation therapy plus chemotherapy for children younger than 5 years with primitive neuroectodermal tumors. Cancer 71:2647–2652

Gorlin RJ, Goltz RW (1960) Multiple nevoid basal-cell epithelioma, jaw cysts and bifid rib: a syndrome. N Engl J Med 262:908–912

Gorlin RJ, Vickers RA, Kelln E, Williamson JJ (1965) The multiple basal-cell nevi syndrome: an analysis of a syndrome consisting of multiple nevoid basal-cell carcinoma, jaw cysts, skeletal anomalies, medulloblastoma, and hyporesponsiveness to parathormone. Cancer 18:89–104

Grotzer MA, Janss AJ, Fung KN et al (2000) TrkC expression predicts good clinical outcome in primitive neuroectodermal brain tumors. J Clin Oncol 18:1027–1035

Grotzer MA, Geoerger B, Janss AJ et al (2001) Prognostic significance of Ki-67 (MIB-1) proliferation index in childhood primitive neuroectodermal tumors of the central nervous system. Med Pediatr Oncol 36:268–273

Gurney JG, Smith MA, Bunin GR (1999) CNS and miscellaneous intracranial and intraspinal neoplasms. In: Ries LAG, Smith MA, Gurney JG et al (eds) Cancer incidence and survival among children and adolescents: United States SEER Program 1975–1995, National Cancer Institute, SEER Program. NIH Publ no 99–4649. Bethesda, MD

Halberg FE, Wara WM, Fippin LF et al (1991) Low-dose craniospinal irradiation therapy for medulloblastoma. Int J Radiat Oncol Biol Phys 20:651–654

Hamilton SR, Liu B, Parsons RE et al (1995) The molecular basis of Turcot's syndrome. N Engl J Med 332:839–847

Hartsell WF, Gajjar AJ, Heideman RL et al (1997) Patterns of failure in children with medulloblastoma: effects of preirradiation chemotherapy. Int J Radiat Oncol Biol Phys 39:15–24

Haslam RHA, Lamborn KR, Becker LE, Israel MA (1998) Tumor cell apoptosis present at diagnosis may predict treatment outcome for patients with medulloblastoma. J Pediatr Hematol Oncol 20:520–527

Hilden JM, Watterson J, Longee DC et al (1998) Central nervous system atypical teratoid/rhabdoid tumor: response to intensive therapy and review of the literature. J Neurooncol 40:265–275

Honig PJ, Charney EB (1982) Children with brain tumor headaches: distinguishing features. Am J Dis Child 136:121–124

Horten BC, Rubinstein LJ (1976) Primary cerebral neuroblastoma: a clinicopathological study of 35 cases. Brain 99:735–756

Ikeda J, Sawamura Y, van Meir EG (1998) Pineoblastoma presenting in familial adenomatous polyposis (FAP): random association, FAP variant, or Turcot syndrome? Br J Neurosurg 12:576–578

Jakacki RI (1999) Pineal and nonpineal supratentorial primitive neuroectodermal tumors. Childs Nerv Syst 15:586–591

Jakacki RI, Zeltzer PM, Boyett JM et al (1995) Survival and prognostic factors following radiation and/or chemotherapy for primitive neuroectodermal tumors of the pineal region in infants and children: a report of the Childrens Cancer Group. J Clin Oncol 13:1377–1383

Kim JYH, Sutton ME, Lu DJ et al (1999) Activation of neurotrophin-3 receptor TrkC induces apoptosis in medulloblastomas. Cancer Res 59:711–719

Kleihues P, Cavenee WK (2000) Pathology and genetics of tumours of the nervous system. IARC Press, Lyon

Kleinman GM, Hochberg FH, Richardson EP (1981) Systemic metastases from medulloblastoma: report of two cases and review of the literature. Cancer 48:2296–2309

Kortmann RD, Kuhl J, Timmerman B et al (2000) Postoperative neoadjuvant chemotherapy before radiotherapy as compared to immediate radiotherapy followed by maintenance chemotherapy in the treatment of medulloblastoma in childhood: results of the German prospective randomized trial HIT '91. Int J Radiat Oncol Biol Phys 46:269–279

Krischer JP, Ragab AH, Kun L et al (1991) Nitrogen mustard, vincristine, procarbazine, and prednisone as adjuvant chemotherapy in the treatment of medulloblastoma. J Neurosurg 74:905–909

Kühl J, Müller HL, Kortmann RD et al (1998) Preirradiation chemotherapy of children and young adults with malignant brain tumors: results of the German pilot trial HIT '88/'89. Klin Pädiatr 210:227–233

Lee Y, McKinnon PJ (2002) DNA ligase IV suppresses medulloblastoma formation. Cancer Res 62:6395–6399

Levy RA, Blaivas M, Muraszko K, Robertson PL (1997) Desmoplastic medulloblastoma. AJNR 18:1364–1366

Marinesco G, Goldstein M (1933) Sur une forme anatomique, non encore decrite, medullo-myo-blastome. Ann Anat Pathol 10:513–525

McNeil DE, Cote TR, Clegg L, Rorke LB (2002) Incidence and trends in pediatric malignancies medulloblastoma/primitive neuroectodermal tumor: a SEER update. Med Pediatr Oncol 39:190–194

Minn AY, Pollock BH, Garzarella L et al (2001) Surveillance neuroimaging to detect relapse in childhood brain tumors: a Pediatric Oncology Group study. J Clin Oncol 19:4135–4140

Molloy PT, Yachnis AT, Rorke LB et al (1996) Central nervous system medulloepithelioma: a series of eight cases including two arising in the pons. J Neurosurg 84:430–436

Mørk SJ, Rubinstein LJ (1985) Ependymoblastoma: a reappraisal of a rare embryonal tumor. Cancer 55:1536–1542

Morland BJ (1995) Decline in incidence of medulloblastoma in children. Cancer 76:155–156

Mosijczuk AD, Nigro MA, Thomas PRM et al (1993) Preradiation chemotherapy in advanced medulloblastoma: a Pediatric Oncology Group study. Cancer 72:2755–2762

Mulhern RK, Kepner JL, Thomas PR et al (1998) Neuropsychologic functioning of survivors of childhood medulloblastoma randomized to receive conventional or reduced-dose craniospinal irradiation: a Pediatric Oncology Group study. J Clin Oncol 16:1723–1728

Olson TA, Bayar E, Kosnik E et al (1995) Successful treatment of disseminated central nervous system malignant rhabdoid tumor. J Pediatr Hematol Oncol 17:71–75

Packer RJ, Sutton LN, Rorke LB et al (1984) Prognostic importance of cellular differentiation in medulloblastoma of childhood. J Neurosurg 61:296–301

Packer RJ, Sutton LN, Elterman R et al (1994) Outcome for children with medulloblastoma treated with radiation and cisplatin, CCNU, and vincristine chemotherapy. J Neurosurg 81:690–698

Packer RJ, Goldwein J, Nicholson HS et al (1999) Treatment of children with medulloblastoma with reduced-dose craniospinal radiation therapy and adjuvant chemotherapy: a Children's Cancer Group study. J Clin Oncol 17:2127–2136

Packer RJ, Biegel JA, Blaney S et al (2002) Atypical teratoid/rhabdoid tumor of the central nervous system: report on workshop. J Pediatr Hematol Oncol 24:337–342

Pearson ADJ, Ratcliffe JM, Birch JM et al (1982) Two families with the Li-Fraumeni cancer family syndrome. J Med Genet 19:362–365

Pelc K, Vincent S, Ruchoux MM et al (2002) Calbindin-D$_{28 k}$: a marker of recurrence for medulloblastomas. Cancer 95:410–419

Peterson K, Walker RW (1995) Medulloblastoma/primitive neuroectodermal tumor in 45 adults. Neurology 45:440–442

Pietsch T, Waha A, Koch A et al (1997) Medulloblastomas of the desmoplastic variant carry mutations of the human homologue of Drosophila patched. Cancer Res 57:2085–2088

Pomeroy SL, Tamayo P, Gaasenbeek M et al (2002) Prediction of central nervous system embryonal tumour outcome based on gene expression. Nature 415:436–442

Prados MD, Warnick RE, Wara WM, Larson DA, Lamborn K, Wilson C (1995) Medulloblastoma in adults. Int J Radiat Oncol Biol Phys 32:1145–1152

Radcliffe J, Packer RJ, Atkins TE et al (1992) Three- and four-year cognitive outcome in children with noncortical brain tumors treated with whole brain radiotherapy. Ann Neurol 32:551–554

Raffel C, Jenkins RB, Frederick L, Hebrink D, Alderete B, Fults DW, James CD (1997) Sporadic medulloblastomas contain PTCH mutations. Cancer Res 57:842–845

Reddy AT, Janss AJ, Phillips PC et al (2000) Outcome for children with supratentorial primitive neuroectodermal tumors treated with surgery, radiation, and chemotherapy. Cancer 88:2189–2193

Ris MD, Packer R, Goldwein J et al (2001) Intellectual outcome after reduced-dose radiation therapy plus adjuvant chemotherapy for medulloblastoma: a Children's Cancer Group study. J Clin Oncol 19:3740–3746

Roberts RO, Lynch CF, Jones MP, Hart MN (1991) Medulloblastoma: a population-based study of 532 cases. J Neuropathol Exp Neurol 50:134–144

Robertson PL, Zeltzer PM, Boyett JM et al (1998) Survival and prognostic factors following radiation therapy and chemotherapy for ependymomas: a report of the Children's Cancer Group. J Neurosurg 88:695–703

Rogers L, Pattisapu J, Smith RR, Parker P (1988) Medulloblastoma in association with the Coffin-Siris syndrome. Childs Nerv Syst 4:41–44

Rorke LB (1983) The cerebellar medulloblastoma and its relationship to primitive neuroectodermal tumors. J Neuropathol Exp Neurol 42:1–15

Russo C, Pellarin M, Tingby O et al (1999) Comparative genomic hybridization in patients with supratentorial and infratentorial primitive neuroectodermal tumors. Cancer 86:331–339

Scheurlein WG, Schwabe GC, Joos S et al (1998) Molecular analysis of childhood primitive neuroectodermal tumors defines markers associated with poor outcome. J Clin Oncol 16:2478–2485

Schild SE, Scheithauer BW, Schomberg PJ et al (1993) Pineal parenchymal tumors: clinical, pathologic, and therapeutic aspects. Cancer 72:870–880

Shuster J, Hart Z, Stimson CW, Brough AJ, Poulik MD (1966) Ataxia telangiectasia with cerebellar tumor. Pediatrics 37:776–786

Stavrou T, Bromley CM, Nicholson HS et al (2001) Prognostic factors and secondary malignancies in childhood medulloblastoma. J Pediatr Hematol Oncol 23:431–436

Strother DR, Pollock IF, Fisher PG et al (2002) Tumors of the central nervous system: sequelae of treatment. In: Pizzo PA, Poplack DG (eds) Principles and practice of pediatric oncology, 4th edn. Lippincott, Williams and Wilkins, Philadelphia, pp 805–808

Tait DM, Thornton-Jones H, Bollom HJG et al (1990) Adjuvant chemotherapy for medulloblastoma: the first multi-centre control trial of the International Society of Paediatric Oncology (SIOP I). Eur J Cancer 26:464–469

Tarbell NJ, Loeffler JS, Silver B et al (1991) The change in patterns of relapse in medulloblastoma. Cancer 68:1600–1604

Tarbell NJ, Friedman H, Kepner J et al (2000) Outcome for children with high stage medulloblastoma: results of the Pediatric Oncology Group 9031. Int J Radiat Oncol Biol Phys 48 [Suppl 1]:179

Taylor MD, Gokgoz N Andrulis Il et al (2000) Familial posterior fossa brain tumors of infancy secondary to germline mutation of the *hSNF5* gene. Am J Hum Genet 66:1403–1406

Taylor RE, Bailey CC, Lucraft H et al (2001) Results of a randomized study of pre-radiotherapy chemotherapy (carboplatin, vincristine, cyclophosphamide, etoposide) with radiotherapy alone in Chang stage M0/M1 medulloblastoma (SIOP/UKCCSF PNET-3). Med Pediatr Oncol 37:191

Taylor MD, Liu L, Raffel C et al (2002) Mutations in SUFU predispose to medulloblastoma. Nat Genet 31:306–310

Thomas PRM, Deutsch M, Kepner JL et al (2000) Low-stage medulloblastoma: final analysis of trial comparing standard-dose with reduced-dose neuraxis irradiation. J Clin Oncol 18:3004–3011

Thorne RN, Pearson ADJ, Nicoll JAR et al (1994) Decline in incidence of medulloblastoma. Cancer 74:3240–3244

Timmermann B, Kortmann RD, Kühl J et al (2002) Role of radiotherapy in treatment of supratentorial primitive neuroectodermal tumors in childhood: results of the prospective German brain tumor trials HIT 88/89 and 91. J Clin Oncol 20:842–849

Walter AW, Mulhern RK, Gajjar A et al (1999) Survival and neurodevelopmental outcome of young children with medulloblastoma at St Jude Children's Research Hospital. J Clin Oncol 17:3720–3728

Weil MD, Lamborn K, Edwards MSB, Wara W (1998) Influence of a child's sex on medulloblastoma outcome. JAMA 279: 1474–1476

Wetmore C, Eberhart DE, Curran T (2000) The normal patched allele is expressed in medulloblastomas from mice with heterozygous germ-line mutation of patched. Cancer Res 60:2239–2246

Wetmore C, Eberhart DE, Curran T (2001) Loss of p53 but not ARF accelerates medulloblastoma in mice heterozygous for patched. Cancer Res 61:513–516

Wolter M, Reifenberger J, Sommer C et al (1997) Mutations in the human homologue of the Drosophila segment polarity gene patched (*PTCH*) in sporadic basal cell carcinomas of the skin and primitive neuroectodermal tumors of the central nervous system. Cancer Res. 57:2581–2585

Xie J, Johnson RL, Zhang X et al (1997) Mutations of the *PATCHED* gene in several types of sporadic extracutaneous tumors. Cancer Res 57:2369–2372

Zeltzer PM, Boyett JM, Finlay JL et al (1999) Metastasis stage, adjuvant treatment, and residual tumor are prognostic factors for medulloblastoma in children: conclusions from the Children's Cancer Group 921 randomized phase II study. J Clin Oncol 17:832–845

Zerbini C, Gelber RD, Weinberg D et al (1993) Prognostic factors in medulloblastoma, including DNA ploidy. J Clin Oncol 11:616–622

Intracranial Germ Cell Tumors

K. H. Lieuw · D. Haas-Kogan · A. Ablin

Contents

6.1 Introduction

Intracranial germ cell tumors (GCT) are a group of relatively uncommon tumors that display histologic, genetic, biochemical, diagnostic, and therapeutic similarities to the more common GCTs that occur outside the central nervous system. Their extra-embryonic origins in the fetal yolk sac account for their numerous similarities, and subsequent migratory paths early in fetal development underlie their ubiquitous primary sites. Intracranial GCTs most commonly arise from the pineal or suprasellar region and their location has traditionally hampered surgical management. For this reason, radiation alone, frequently encompassing a large treatment volume, has constituted the gold standard for treatment. In the last two decades, effective chemotherapy in combination with improved neurosurgical procedures and radiation techniques have resulted in dramatic improvements in survival. However, the morbidity of radiation therapy in children, particularly craniospinal irradiation (CSI), has prompted many investigators to explore approaches that reduce the volume and dose of radiotherapy while preserving high cure rates (Shirato et al. 1997; Choi et al. 1998; Matsutani et al. 1998; Aoyama et al. 2002).

In this chapter we review the epidemiology of intracranial GCTs, the pathologic features of both benign and malignant GCTs, and their molecular and cytogenetic features. We discuss the clinical features of intracranial GCTs and the role of imaging and laboratory investigations in their diagnoses. In broaching the controversy surrounding diagnostic biopsy, we delineate the salient arguments for and against mandatory biopsy prior to treatment. Finally, we discuss risk stratification to intensify treatment in patients with intracranial GCTs that have a poor prognosis.

6.2 Epidemiology

6.2.1 Anatomical Location

Intracranial GCTs account for less than 4% of pediatric brain tumors in North America. Most intracranial GCTs originate near the third ventricle, extending from the suprasellar cistern to the pineal gland. Pineal region GCTs outnumber those in the suprasellar region by a ratio of 2:1, and in 5 to 10% of cases, the tumor is found in both regions (Jennings et al. 1985b). Whether this is due to bifocal disease or tumor spread remains unknown. Intracranial GCTs occur less commonly in other midline locations such as basal ganglia, thalamus, and ventricles, particularly the fourth ventricle. Intracranial GCTs have also been reported in the cerebellum (Nakase et al. 1994), medulla oblongata (Nakajima et al. 2000), and optic nerves (Iizuka et al. 1996). Germinomas are more frequent in the suprasellar region and in females while nongerminomatous germ cell tumors (NGGCT) are more common in the pineal region and in males.

6.2.2 Age, Sex, and Geographic Variation

In western countries, intracranial GCTs account for 0.4% to 3.4% of all intracranial tumors whereas in Japan and Taiwan, intracranial GCTs are more common and account for 2.1% to 11.1% of brain tumors (Jellinger 1973; Jennings et al. 1985b; Hoffman et al. 1991; Lin et al. 1997). This phenomenon is also seen in testicular GCTs for which the incidence in Japan is far greater than that seen in the United States (Packer et al. 2000). Most intracranial GCTs occur in adolescents and young adults (68%). The peak incidence of intracranial GCTs occurs at 10 to 12 years of age. In particular, most NGGCTs exhibit a predilection for younger children whereas germinomas are most common in teenagers (Jennings et al. 1985b).

Intracranial GCTs exhibit interesting gender propensities. In the United States, between 1986 and 1995, incidence rates were 2.3 per million for males and 0.9 per million for females, representing a male predominance of 2.5:1. When examined by histology, NGGCTs demonstrate a male:female ratio of 3.2:1 while germinomas reveal a male:female ratio of only 1.8:1 (Jennings et al. 1985b). In females, 75% of intracranial GCTs develop in the suprasellar region whereas in males 70% are found in the pineal area. The reason for these sex differences remains unclear. The incidence of intracranial GCTs has increased in the United States from 0.6 per million in 1975 to 1979 to 1.9 per million in 1990 to 1995 (Bernstein et al. 1999).

There are two distinct histological groups within the larger group of intracranial GCTs: germinomas and NGGCTs. Germinomas are more common, accounting for 50 to 70% of the total (Jooma and Kendall 1983; Oi and Matsumoto 1992). NGGCTs represent one third of intracranial GCTs and consist of embryonal carcinoma, endodermal sinus (yolk sac) tumor, choriocarcinoma, teratoma, and GCTs of mixed cellular origin. Jennings et al. (1985b) found that germinomas accounted for 65% of intracranial GCTs followed by teratomas (18%), endodermal sinus tumors (7%), embryonal carcinomas (5%), and choriocarcinomas (5%). Other studies show a higher incidence of mixed tumors ranging from 21% to 32% (Matsutani et al. 1997; Salzman et al. 1997).

6.3 Pathology

6.3.1 Etiology

GCTs can be divided into extragonadal tumors and gonadal tumors, the latter encompassing half of all such tumors. Among extragonadal sites, half are sacrococcygeal and 40% arise intracranially. Rare sites of extragonadal GCTs include midline regions such as the retroperitoneum and nasopharynx. Their sites of origin notwithstanding, the features of GCTs are identical, whether identified by light microscopy, electron microscopy, or enzyme or immunohistochemical assay (Jennings et al. 1985b; Felix and Becker 1990).

The pathogenesis of intracranial GCTs remains elusive. Although gonadotropins have been implicated in the pathogenesis of gonadal GCTs, such evidence for intracranial GCTs is lacking. One hypothesis is that GCTs arise most commonly near centers of gonadotropin regulation because such regions serve as sanctuary sites for undifferentiated germ cells (Jennings et al. 1985b). An additional role for the pineal gland in the neuroendocrine regulation of neoplastic growth has also been suggested (Lapin and Ebels 1981).

The etiology of intracranial GCTs is thought to be mismigration of primordial germ cells during embryonic development followed by malignant transformation. According to the "germ cell theory," primordial germ cells normally develop from the extraembryonic yolk sac endoderm and migrate to the gonadal folds. Germinomas as well as embryonal carcinomas can develop by further differentiation and transformation of the original primordial germ cells. Embryonal carcinomas are composed of pluripotent cells that develop into endodermal sinus tumors, choriocarcinomas, or teratomas depending on the developmental pathway the cells undertake (Teilum 1976). Others have suggested that primordial germ cells can differentiate to yield either embryonal carcinomas or teratomas by differentiation through embryonic pathways, or endodermal sinus tumors or choriocarcinomas by extraembryonic pathways (Takei and Pearl 1981).

The "germ cell theory" is supported by the fact that interaction of the C-kit receptor with its ligand, steel factor (SLF), mediates the migration of primordial germ cells, as lack of C-kit in animal models prevents germ cell migration. The gradient of SLF found from the yolk sac to the gonadal ridge is thought to guide the migration of primordial germ cells, and extragonadal GCTs are thought to arise from such mismigration. The protooncogene *c-kit* encodes a cell-surface receptor that has tyrosine kinase activity in its cytoplasmic demain. The interaction of c-kit with SLF leads to receptor dimerization, kinase activation, and tyrosine phosphorylation of specific cytoplasmic proteins. Mutations in c-kit and SLF have been found that result in a defective signaling pathway leading to

infertility (Loveland and Schlatt 1997; Cushing et al. 2002).

An alternative theory, the "embryonic cell theory," invokes a pluripotent embryonic cell that escapes normal developmental signals and gives rise to GCTs. Finally, a third hypothesis contends that germinoma is the only neoplasm arising from germ cells and other GCTs are due to misfolding and misplacement of embryonic cells into the lateral mesoderm early in embryogenesis leading to the entrapment of these cells into a variety of different brain regions (Sano et al. 1989).

6.3.2 Classification

The current World Health Organization (WHO) classification of GCTs is based on histology and tumor markers such as alpha-feto protein (AFP) and beta-human chorionic gonadotrophin (β-HCG), which have become important in diagnosis as well as prognosis. Table 6.1 lists the various germ cell tumors, separating the malignant from the benign, while Table 6.2 illustrates the classification based on tumor markers. As mentioned above, different GCTs may represent the malignant forms of different stages of normal embryonic development. For example, primordial germ cells result in germinomas, embryonic differentiation gives rise to teratomas and embryonal carcinomas, and extraembryonic derivatives of the yolk sac and trophoblast give rise to endodermal si-

Table 6.1. Classification of GCTs according to benign versus malignant tumors

Benign germ cell tumors	Malignant germ cell tumors
Immature teratoma[a]	Germinoma
Mature teratoma	Embryonal carcinoma
	Endodermal sinus tumor (yolk sac tumor)
	Choriocarcinoma
	Mixed germ cell tumor

[a] May contain rare malignant germ cell elements

Table 6.2. GCTs according to tumor markers

Tumor type	AFP	β-HCG	PLAP
Mature teratoma	–	–	–
Immature teratoma	+/–	+/–	–
Pure germinoma	–	–	+
Endodermal sinus tumor	+	–	–
Choriocarcinoma	–	+	–
Embryonal carcinoma	+	+	–
Mixed germ cell tumor	+/–	+/–	+/–

nus tumors and choriocarcinomas, respectively. Intracranial GCTs can also be classified based on tumor markers found in serum or cerebrospinal fluid (CSF), which can influence diagnoses and prognoses of patients with intracranial GCTs. Typically, germinomas are non-secreting tumors, whereas NGGCTs usually secrete either AFP and/or β-HCG (see Table 6.2).

6.3.3 Histopathology

Intracranial germinomas are histologically identical to dysgerminomas of the ovary and seminomas of the testis (Beeley et al. 1973). Microscopically, they are composed of large monomorphic cells with abundant clear cytoplasm arranged in nests separated by bands of connective tissue. The differential diagnosis includes lymphoma and endodermal sinus tumor. Germinomas can be distinguished from lymphoma by positive placental alkaline phosphatase (PLAP) staining in germinomas, and from endodermal sinus tumor because the latter is positive for AFP while germinomas are not.

Among NGGCTs, teratomas are designated mature or immature based on the absence or presence of differentiated tissues. Mature teratomas contain mature tissues from all three embryonic layers (ectoderm, mesoderm, and endoderm). Immature teratomas are distinguished from mature teratomas by the presence of immature tissues, usually neuroepithelium. Em-

bryonal carcinomas arise from pluripotent embryonic cells and are characterized by large cells with large nuclei and nucleoli with varying amounts of central necrosis. Embryonal carcinomas can produce both AFP and β-HCG. Unlike other GCTs, CD30 (Ki-1 antigen) immunohistochemical staining is positive in embryonal carcinomas. Endodermal sinus tumors arise from differentiated extraembryonic tissue, usually occur as part of mixed GCTs, and produce AFP. Choriocarcinomas arise from placental trophoblastic tissue, also generally occur as part of mixed GCTs, and are characterized by the presence of syncytiotrophoblasts that secrete β-HCG (Felix and Becker 1990; Hawkins 1990; Cushing et al. 2002).

6.3.4 Molecular Biology and Cytogenetics

Multiple complex karyotypes have been reported for intracranial GCTs including loss of chromosomes 4, 9p, 11, 13, and 17p as well as gain of chromosomes 8q, 21, and 1q. In addition, whereas isochromosome 12p seems to be important in the development of testicular tumors, it is less common in extragonadal tumors (de Bruin et al. 1994; Yu et al. 1995; Lemos et al. 1998). A recent study by Rickert et al. (2000), using comparative genomic hybridization to analyze pineal region GCTs, reported various abnormalities including gains on 12p (40%), 8q (27%), and 1q (20%) as well as losses on 13q (47%), 18q (33%), and 9q and 11q (20% each). They also noted different cytogenetic abnormalities based on histology. For example, the most common chromosomal changes in germinomas were –13q and –18q (38% each) whereas in mixed teratomas–germinomas frequent abnormalities included +8q (100%), +12p (75%), –13q (75%), and –9q (50%). Okada et al. (2002) examined 25 intracranial GCTs and found an increased number of X chromosomes in 23/25 cases and noted hypomethylation of the additional X chromosome in 81% of the tumors. Only 20 % of cases had increased copy number of 12p, and 12% had loss of 13q. They concluded that along with the increased incidence of intracranial GCTs in males as well as predisposition in patients with Kleinfelter syndrome, sex chromosome aberrations might have an important role in the development of GCTs.

In addition to cytogenetic changes, some of the genes that may be important in the development of GCTs have been defined. Recently, alterations in the *mdm-2* gene, often amplified in sarcomas, has been implicated in tumorigenesis of some testicular and intracranial GCTs. Mdm-2 is a negative regulator of the p53 tumor-suppressor gene product and is in turn induced by p53. Iwato et al. searched for *p53* mutations and *mdm-2* amplifications in intracranial GCTs and found *mdm-2* amplifications in 19% of intracranial GCTs. Theoretically, increases in mdm-2 protein level would antagonize p53 function (Iwato et al. 2000b).

Iwato et al. (2000a) examined the *INK4a/ARF* locus for alterations in intracranial GCTs and found alterations in 71% of 21 such tumors. The *INK4a/ARF* genes are tumor-suppressor genes and the INK4a protein has been found to inhibit cyclin-dependent kinases and decrease phosphorylation of the retinoblastoma protein, resulting in cell cycle arrest. The ARF protein interacts with mdm-2 and stimulates the latter's degradation. Interestingly, alterations in *INK4a/ARF* were more common in germinomas (90%) than in NGGCTs (55%).

6.4 Clinical Features: Signs and Symptoms

Presenting symptoms of patients with intracranial GCTs depend on tumor location. Pineal region tumors usually present with eye movement disorders or symptoms caused by increased intracranial pressure due to obstructive hydrocephalus. Headache, nausea, and vomiting are the most common symptoms, seen in 56 to 93% of patients. Blurred vision and somnolence are seen in 20 to 54%, while ataxia, seizures, and behavioral disturbances are seen in 10 to 28% (Saitoh et al. 1991; Drummond and Rosenfeld 1999; Steinbok and Cochrane 2001). Involvement of adjacent midbrain structures can result in visual disturbances, such as Perinaud's syndrome, which is seen in 25 to 50% of pineal region GCTs. Perinaud's syndrome is an impairment of upward gaze in combination with dilated pupils that are non-reactive to light but responsive to accommodation. In addition, an attempt at upward gaze may elicit a rhythmic convergence-retraction nystagmus.

On examination, papilledema is present in about half of patients. In patients with pineal region GCTs approximately 80% present with symptoms of increased intracranial pressure (ICP) whereas less than 10% of patients with suprasellar GCTs present with increased ICP. Endocrinopathies such as diabetes insipidus or precocious puberty occur in patients with intracranial GCTs and account for approximately 6 to 12% of presenting symptoms. In fact, patients with suprasellar GCTs most commonly present with endocrinopathies such as diabetes insipidus and manifestations of anterior pituitary dysfunction such as growth failure. These symptoms were seen in 87% of patients versus only 8% of patients with pineal region GCT (Jooma and Kendall 1983; Edwards et al. 1988; Hoffman et al. 1991; Saitoh et al. 1991; Kang et al. 1998; Steinbok and Cochrane 2001).

Intracranial GCTs may infiltrate adjacent structures such as the hypothalamus (11%) and third ventricle (22%) or disseminate throughout the cerebrospinal fluid (10%). For endodermal sinus tumors and choriocarcinomas, dissemination is more common as evidenced by third ventricular involvement in over 40% of cases. Extracranial spread to the lungs and bones has also been reported in approximately 3% of patients (Gay et al. 1985; Jennings et al. 1985a,b).

6.5 Diagnosis

Operative morbidity and mortality prior to the 1980s was high and impeded histological diagnoses of many intracranial GCTs. Therefore, radiodiagnostic trials of 20 Gy historically functioned as surrogates for a histological diagnosis of germinoma, since these tumors were characteristically radioresponsive. Poor response to 20 Gy indicated an alternate diagnosis such as NGGCT or glioma. A robust response to 20 Gy suggested a histological diagnosis of germinoma, and treatment was continued to 50 Gy for definitive treatment. In light of the advances in neurosurgical techniques as well the ability to differentially treat with chemotherapy, surgical biopsy in the modern era is generally much safer and usually recommended prior to treatment. However, controversy remains whether biopsy is indicated for these tumors. This primary decision determines the management plan.

6.5.1 Laboratory Investigations

AFP is normally expressed during embryonic development. It is the earliest serum binding protein in the fetus and reaches peak concentration at 12 to 14 weeks of gestation then gradually falls to reach adult levels of 10 ng/dl at 1 to 2 years of age. As AFP levels decline during fetal development, albumin becomes the predominant binding protein. The presence of AFP (>25 ng/ml) indicates that there are malignant components in the tumor consisting of yolk sac elements or embryonal carcinoma. The half life of AFP is 5 to 7 days and is a useful marker to follow, with one caveat: due to the variable rates of AFP levels in infants, AFP levels are less informative in this very young age group. Of note is the phenomenon of increasing AFP levels due to chemotherapy-induced tumor lysis and not necessarily due to disease progression. β-HCG is produced by syncytiotrophoblasts during pregnancy to maintain the corpus luteum, and minute amounts are found in normal adults. Pathologic elevations of β-HCG (>50 IU/L) are found when there is a clonal disorder of syncytiotrophoblasts such as in choriocarcinoma or syncytiotrophoblastic giant cells found in embryonal carcinomas. Therefore, when an elevation of one of these tumor markers is present, it is highly suggestive of the histological diagnosis.

Embryonal carcinomas secrete both AFP and β-HCG while endodermal sinus tumors and choriocarcinomas secrete only AFP and β-HCG, respectively (see Table 6.2). However, in as many as 30 % of GCTs, more than one histologic subtype is found (Matsutani et al. 1997). The most useful laboratory values for the diagnosis of GCTs are elevations of AFP and/or β-HCG in serum or CSF. It is important to sample both serum and CSF, as serum levels can be normal in the presence of elevated CSF levels. If present, the protein levels can serve as useful tumor markers since they decrease as tumor burden decreases. GCTs that have elevations of these tumor markers show worse prognosis when matched with patients with identical histologic diagnoses but normal marker levels (Itoyama et al. 1995; Nishizaki et al. 2001). AFP can be used as a tumor marker in endodermal sinus tumors and β-HCG is useful in choriocarcinoma. Embryonal carcinomas can secrete both AFP and β-HCG.

Another helpful tumor marker is placental alkaline phosphatase (PLAP), which is a fetal isoenzyme of alkaline phosphatase and is almost always elevated in germinomas (Cushing et al. 2002). Therefore, one controversial option in patients with elevated PLAP but normal β-HCG and AFP would be to assume the diagnosis is germinoma and treat accordingly (Steinbok 2001). However, PLAP is not readily available as a test in many institutions and such empiric diagnoses are extraordinarily rare. Another marker for germinoma that has recently been investigated is the soluble isoform of C-kit (S-kit). Elevations of S-kit were found in the CSF of patients with germinoma and also correlated with the patient's clinical course. Moreover, the level of S-kit was remarkably higher in patients with tumor dissemination and suggests that S-kit may be another useful tumor marker (Miyanohara et al. 2002).

6.5.2 Diagnostic Imaging

As in the diagnosis of other brain tumors, computed tomography (CT) and magnetic resonance imaging (MRI) are the most common modalities used to diagnose intracranial GCTs. Of historic interest only, pineal region tumors can be detected on plain skull films by the presence of calcifications. MRI is the study of choice although CT has an advantage over MRI in identifying calcifications. The identification of calcification in the pineal gland in a child younger than 6 years old is an indication for an MRI even when no mass is apparent on CT (Zimmerman and Bilaniuk 1982; Steinbok 2001).

Findings on CT or MRI are almost never sufficient for the diagnosis of GCTs. Germinomas are usually diffusely enhancing on CT and MRI whereas NG-GCTs are more likely to be heterogeneous in part due to hemorrhage. Larger germinomas can also have a heterogeneous appearance (Fig. 6.1). A tumor in the suprasellar region in association with a pineal tumor

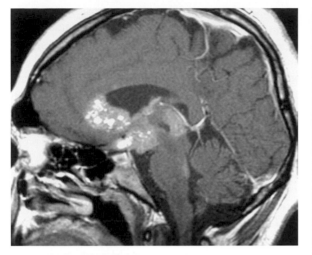

Figure 6.1

A sagittal T1-weighted image following contrast administration shows an extensive heterogeneous suprasellar mass with multiple cysts within the tumor. The tumor fills the anterior portion of the third ventricle and extends posteriorly into the pineal region

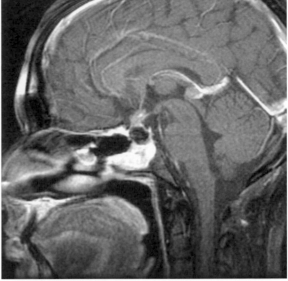

Figure 6.3

A sagittal T1-weighted MR image following contrast shows an unusual case of a mixed germ cell tumor containing both germinoma and teratoma located in both the suprasellar, sellar, and pineal regions. The sellar component was biopsied through a transsphenoidal approach. The area of low signal intensity within the sella represents a fat patch to prevent a postoperative CSF leak

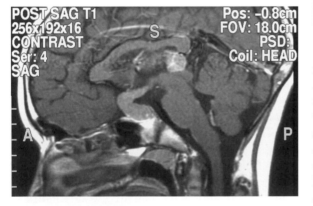

Figure 6.2

A sagittal T1-weighted MR image following contrast administration shows an anterior third ventricle mass and a pineal region mass that both enhance relative to the normal brain. This tumor was diagnosed after biopsy as a germinoma. Pineoblastoma, a malignant undifferentiated pineal tumor, can also present with dissemination along the CSF pathways

is usually a GCT, most likely a germinoma (Fig. 6.2). A bifocal location is not guaranteed to be a germinoma as GCTs with mixed elements can also appear in two locations (Fig. 6.3). A recent or old hemorrhage seen in the tumor suggests an NGGCT, particularly common with choriocarcinoma (Fig. 6.4). Intracranial teratomas tend to be well circumscribed and have large cysts and calcifications within the tumor, which can be helpful in distinguishing them from germinomas. Immature teratomas tend to have fewer cysts and calcifications and may secrete tumor markers if microscopic malignant germ cell elements are present (Fujimaki et al. 1994).

In addition to GCT, the differential diagnosis of a pineal lesion includes pineoblastoma, trilateral retinoblastoma in a patient with bilateral retinoblastoma, pineocytoma, glioma, meningioma, lymphoma, or a

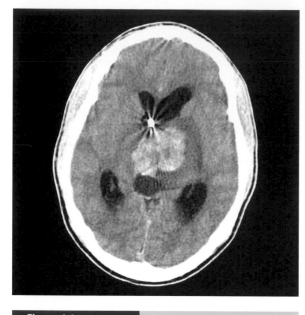

Figure 6.4

An axial CT image from a teenage boy who presented with headaches and a change in mental status. A large, partially hemorrhagic tumor is seen extending into the lateral ventricles. An endoscopic biopsy was consistent with choriocarcinoma. β-HCG as measured in the CSF was 88,767 IU/L (normal: <1.5). Hydrocephalus is present and an external ventricular catheter has been inserted into the anterior portion of the ventricle

ommended histological diagnoses as the initial management of pineal region tumors. This discrepancy may be due to the fact that pineal region tumors are much more common in Japan and the incidence of germinomas in particular is higher (Oi and Matsumoto 1992). A follow-up study by Oi et al. showed that by 1998, radical resection of the tumor was recommended as the initial procedure by only 22% of Japanese neurosurgeons with 39% recommending biopsy and 39% recommending radiation therapy. The authors suggested that tissue diagnosis by ventriculoscopic or stereotactic approach as the most appropriate initial step for the treatment planning of pineal region tumors (Oi et al. 1998).

Although a definitive conclusion cannot be reached, a prudent strategy would be to utilize a safe and minimally invasive technique to obtain tissue for histologic analysis. Such techniques would include endoscopic biopsy at the time of third ventriculostomy or aqueductoplasty, or stereotactic biopsy. A review of 370 cases of stereotactic biopsies in France reported only 1.3% mortality and 1% major morbidity rates (Regis et al. 1996). Despite these relatively low rates, most surgeons are more comfortable with open biopsy in this region due to the close proximity of deep cerebral veins. One of the advantages of open biopsy is that sampling error can be minimized by taking several biopsies. This is particularly important since mixed GCTs are commonly encountered. Advances in surgical techniques allow open procedures to access the pineal region without major morbidity.

6.6 Treatment

6.6.1 Role of Surgery

Prior to 1970, surgery resulted in 25 to 70% morbidity and mortality rates and led to radiotherapy becoming the treatment of choice with 60 to 80% 5-year survival rates. In Japan, the standard of care was administration of a radiodiagnostic trial of 20 Gy followed by definitive doses of radiation if 20 Gy induced a tumor response (Handa and Yamashita 1981). Conventional radiotherapy for CNS germinomas involved 30 Gy of craniospinal irradiation (CSI)

benign lesion such as a cyst. Benign cysts can be generally distinguished from malignant cystic neoplasms by the lack of enhancement, or by a very thin rim of enhancement surrounding a hypointense center (Steinbok 2001).

6.5.3 Obtaining Tissue Diagnosis

There is geographic variation in management strategies. In 1992, Oi and Matsumoto noted that the majority (84%) of Japanese neurosurgeons were comfortable using a radiodiagnostic trial of 20 Gy in lieu of histological confirmation of a germinoma. In contrast, the majority (78%) in Western countries rec-

followed by a boost to the primary disease site to a total dose of 50 Gy. The main role of surgery at that time was for treatment of hydrocephalus by placement of ventriculo–peritoneal shunts, which resulted in peritoneal metastases at times (Brandes et al. 2000).

Chemotherapy was incorporated into the treatment of intracranial GCTs after agents known to have activity against testicular GCTs were shown to cross the blood-brain barrier (Ginsberg et al. 1981; Brandes et al. 2000). The next logical step in the treatment of intracranial GCTs incorporated chemotherapy administered prior to irradiation (neoadjuvant chemotherapy) in an attempt to reduce the doses and volumes of radiation and the resulting toxicity (Allen et al. 1987). Chemotherapy without radiation, however, does not provide as durable a response to treatment. One study reported that of 13 AFP- and β-HCG-secreting GCTs treated by chemotherapy and surgery alone, 12 relapsed (Baranzelli et al. 1998). Approximately 50% of these patients could be salvaged by radiation therapy. The authors concluded that focal radiotherapy should be part of the treatment of these tumors.

As chemoradiation emerged as the standard of care for intracranial NGGCTs, the role of surgery remained controversial. In a study by Weiner et al., radical resection in addition to chemotherapy improved prognosis for patients with intracranial NGGCT. They recommended delayed surgical resection for patients who have normalized tumor markers with persistent radiographic abnormalities after three cycles of initial chemotherapy in order to avoid unnecessary radiation or further chemotherapy (see also Chap. 13; Balmaceda et al. 1996; Weiner et al. 2002). Most centers continue to use chemoradiation as the mainstay of treatment with surgery reserved for residual disease. A clear indication for surgery is in mature teratoma where surgical resection is generally accepted as sufficient for cure. In immature teratomas, chemoradiotherapy should be utilized if tumor markers are present since it may be presumed that malignant germ cell elements have been missed. For completely resected non-secreting immature teratomas, there is still a risk of relapse without adjuvant therapy (Sawamura et al. 1998b).

6.6.2 Chemotherapy

With the recognition of chemosensitivity of intracranial GCTs, a number of agents were evaluated. As single agents, actinomycin-D, vinblastine, bleomycin, doxorubicin, cisplatin, carboplatin, etoposide, ifosfamide, and cyclophosphamide are active against GCTs, and combinations of these agents are the basis for treatment regimens. The most common combinations currently in use incorporate cisplatin with etoposide and bleomycin (PEB), with alternatives such as PVB containing vinblastine instead of etoposide, and JEB containing carboplatin instead of cisplatin (Hawkins et al. 1986; Pinkerton et al. 1990; Einhorn and Donohue 1997; Cushing et al. 2002). In addition, ifosfamide has been found to be the third most active agent against GCTs following cisplatin and etoposide and was investigated as salvage therapy in patients with refractory disease (Nichols 1996).

Recent studies have supported distinct therapeutic approaches for germinomas and NGGCTs as NGGCT clearly have worse prognoses than germinomas. For NGGCTs, radiation alone produces 5-year survival rates of only 30 to 40%. Excellent response rates to chemotherapy have shifted the standard treatment of NGGCT to combined modality therapy consisting of chemotherapy and radiation. For mixed GCTs, treatment is directed at the most malignant element. Because histology will influence the choice of treatment, and coincident with improved surgical techniques, the need for obtaining tumor histology is now recognized (Aydin et al. 1992; Sawamura et al. 1997).

Calaminus et al. (1997) reported promising results with four courses of PEI [cisplatin (20 mg/m^2 day 1 to 5), VP16 (100 mg/ m^2 day 1 to 3), and ifosfamide (1.5 g/ m^2 day 1 to 5)], resection of the residual tumor if feasible, followed by radiation consisting of 30 Gy CSI and an additional 24 Gy boost to the primary site. Event free survival (EFS) was 81% with 11 months follow-up, representing a significant improvement from previous studies. Robertson et al. (1997) reported improved outcome for intracranial NGGCTs utilizing a treatment plan of initial radical surgical resection followed by three or four cycles of adjuvant chemotherapy with cisplatin (100 mg/ m^2/cycle) and VP-16 (500 mg/m2/cycle), followed by radiotherapy and finally four additional cycles of post-radiation chemotherapy. Four-year actuarial EFS and overall survival were 67% and 74%, respectively. It remains to be seen whether further intensification using myeloablative chemotherapy with autologous stem-cell rescue has a role in patients with poor-prognosis GCTs or relapsed GCTs.

6.6.3 Radiation Therapy

The extent of the radiation field in the treatment of localized NGGCT remains unclear. There is little literature addressing the appropriate radiation field for localized NGGCT, and only small patient numbers. In a study by the French Society of Pediatric Oncology chemotherapy and focal radiation resulted in 5 relapses among 24 patients with localized NGGCTs (Bouffet et al. 1999). A similar regimen in a separate study resulted in 3 of 18 patients experiencing disease recurrence, 2 with isolated spinal relapses (Robertson et al. 1997).

Recommendations for the multimodality approach to NGGCT have emerged from recent studies. For patients with NGGCTs and complete responses to chemotherapy, Buckner recommends 54 Gy limited-field irradiation and 30 Gy CSI if the spinal axis is involved; in patients with partial response, 59.4 Gy limited field was recommended with 36 Gy CSI if spinal involvement is evident (Buckner et al. 1999).

Of the various histologic subtypes of intracranial GCTs, germinoma represents the most common and prognostically most favorable subgroup. The roles of surgery, chemotherapy, and radiation are constantly evolving. Other than as a diagnostic tool, surgery has no proven role in the treatment of intracranial germinomas. Several studies have shown no benefit to radical surgical resection in overall survival for germinoma patients (Sawamura et al. 1997). Unlike surgery, radiation remains a critical component of the treatment of intracranial germinomas. In fact, the gold standard against which all new approaches must be measured remains radiotherapy alone. Controversy persists regarding the appropriate fields and volumes for irradiation, particularly for localized, non-disseminated germinomas. A key point

of controversy involving radiation for localized germinomas has been the need for CSI. Current evidence substantiates omitting CSI from the treatment of localized germinoma. Spinal failure rates of less than 10% in the absence of CSI, reported in most contemporary series, do not justify routine incorporation of CSI into treatment strategies for localized germinoma. Since CSI is no longer indicated for localized pure germinomas, the value of whole brain irradiation and whole ventricular radiation have been questioned as well.

Although most investigators now omit whole brain radiation, several studies have reported higher recurrence rates associated with radiation targeting the tumor volume only (Uematsu et al. 1992; Shibamoto et al. 1994; Wolden et al. 1995; Brandes et al. 2000). Specifically, tumor recurrences following radiation fields confined to only the primary tumor result in disease failure within adjacent brain parenchyma and ventricles. Therefore, investigators have recommended initial inclusion of the entire ventricular field followed by a boost to the primary tumor to a total dose of 45 Gy for tumors less than 4 cm in size, and 20 Gy for spinal prophylaxis in case of positive cytology (Uematsu et al. 1992; Shibamoto et al. 1994). Shibamoto et al. suggested modulating the radiotherapy dose according to tumor diameter, with 40 Gy for tumors up to 2.5 cm, 45 Gy for tumors between 2.5 to 4 cm, and 50 Gy for tumors over 4 cm (Shibamoto et al. 1994). Dissemination to hypothalamus, third ventricle, or spinal cord identifies a high-risk group that warrants consideration of CSI with systemic chemotherapy (Jennings et al. 1985b).

We recommend whole ventricular irradiation, followed for localized germinoma by a boost to the primary tumor when using radiation alone. Some question the rationale of whole ventricular irradiation given the continuity of CSF space throughout the entire central nervous system. We argue that the natural history of germinomas is characterized by multifocality and intracranial relapses at foci separate from the primary tumor with lesser propensity for diffuse CNS involvement. These features distinguish germinomas from other CNS malignancies, such as medulloblastoma, that require CSI for cure. Whether more generous local radiation fields sterilize occult multifocal disease or target direct ventricular invasion, a role appears to exist for whole ventricular irradiation in the treatment of localized germinoma. As for dose, the literature supports ≥45 Gy to the primary tumor for germinomas treated with radiation alone.

6.6.4 Combined-Modality Treatment

Historically, intracranial germinomas have been treated with radiation alone, producing excellent cure rates. The significant long-term toxicity of radiation, particularly in children, has prompted investigations into alternative treatments that minimize the dose and volume of irradiation. However, these alternative approaches must be required to preserve the high cure rates established with radiation alone. Combined-modality approaches in which chemotherapy precedes radiation have gained credence and are now considered a standard alternative to radiation alone.

Several series have reported excellent clinical outcome with pre-irradiation chemotherapy followed by focal irradiation. Buckner et al. and Sawamura et al. reported 100% survival with median follow-ups of 51 and 24 months respectively (Sawamura et al. 1998c; Buckner et al. 1999). Buckner et al. treated 9 patients with germinomas and 8 with mixed GCTs. Treatment consisted of etoposide (100 mg/ m^2/d) plus cisplatin (20 mg/ m^2/d) daily for 5 days every 3 weeks for four cycles, followed by radiation therapy. They recommend that germinoma patients with complete responses after standard chemotherapy receive 30 Gy to a limited field with the addition of 20 Gy CSI for disseminated disease. For patients with partial responses, dose of 54 Gy were recommended with 30 Gy CSI for disseminated disease.

A recent study by Aoyama et al. (2002) reported excellent results for chemoradiation. Patients with pure germinomas were treated with EP (etoposide 100 mg/m^2 and cisplatin 20 mg/m^2) given for 5 days every 4 weeks for 4 four cycles; patients with other pathologic types were treated with ICE (ifosfamide 900 mg/m^2, cisplatin 20 mg/m^2, and etoposide 60 mg/m^2) for 5 consecutive days every 4 weeks for up to six cycles depending on chemoresponsiveness, extent of surgical resection, and tumor marker levels. At 5 years, they observed overall survival rate of 100% with relapse-free survival rate of 90% for germinoma patients and 44% for β–HCG secreting germinomas, which represent a mixed germ cell tumor with β–HCG secreting syncytiotrophoblastic giant cells. This is additional evidence that treatment should be directed at the most malignant element. The 5-year overall survival rates were 93% for non-β–HCG secreting germinomas and 75% for β-HCG-secreting germinomas. The Aoyama group recommend, following EP chemotherapy, that dose and volume can be reduced to 24 Gy in 12 fractions for non-β–HCG-secreting germinomas, but higher radiation doses maintained for β–HCG secreting germinomas.

Sawamura et al. (1998a) have recommended further risk stratification of patients into three categories. They have categorized pure germinoma and mature teratoma as the good-prognosis group with the poor-prognosis group including embryonal carcinoma, yolk sac tumor, choriocarcinoma, and mixed germ cell tumor containing any embryonal carcinoma, yolk sac tumor, or choriocarcinoma elements. Finally, their intermediate-prognosis group includes germinomas with elevated β–HCG, immature teratoma, extensive/multifocal germinoma, and mixed germ cell tumor containing only germinoma with teratoma elements. Further therapeutic studies incorporating this type of risk stratification is warranted to determine if prognosis can be improved in the poor-risk group while minimizing the therapy-induced physical or cognitive sequelae.

The chemoresponsiveness of intracranial GCTs prompted regimens using chemotherapy alone. However, efforts to omit radiation and treat intracranial GCTs with chemotherapy alone have not been promising. Yoshida et al. saw a response rate of 80 to 85% in patients treated with a combination regimen with cisplatin and etoposide but survival times at 2 years were 88% in germinomas and 48% in NGGCTs. Baranzelli et al. used six cycles of chemotherapy followed by surgery in case viable residual tumor was found on imaging, and radiation was further delivered in case viable residual tumor was found on pathology. They reported 66% cure rate; however, patients who did not receive radiation relapsed. Thus, chemotherapy alone does not provide comparable cure rates (Yoshida et al. 1993; Balmaceda et al. 1996; Baranzelli et al. 1998).

6.6.5 Treatment of Recurrent Disease

As with most malignancies, relapse poses a formidable problem. For patients who relapse with intracranial GCTs, salvage therapy using the same chemotherapy regimen followed by radiotherapy has been effective (Sawamura et al. 1999). Kobayashi et al. (1989) used combinations of cisplatin and etoposide in four cases of recurrent intracranial germ-cell tumor (three malignant teratomas and one germinoma) with a response rate of 100%. Aoyama et al. successfully treated recurrent germinomas with further chemotherapy and re-irradiation (Aoyama et al. 2002). However, improving prognosis for NGGCTs remains a concern. Encouraging results from Tada et. al. (1999) used high-dose chemotherapy (200 mg/ m^2 cisplatin, 1250 mg/ m^2 etoposide, and 150 mg/ m^2 ACNU) with autologous stem-cell rescue in six patients with high-risk intracranial nongerminomatous germ cell tumor and reported 100% survival with 1 to 7-year follow-up (Tada et al. 1999). Although trials using high-dose chemotherapy with stem-cell rescue seem to be showing promise in relapsed extracranial GCTs, it remains to be seen whether myeloablative consolidation therapy has a role in the treatment of intracranial GCTs.

6.7 Outcome

The outcome for patients with pure intracranial germinoma is significantly better than for NGGCT. Cure rates above 90% with radiation alone establish radiation as the benchmark against which combined-modality therapy must be compared. Comparable outcomes are achieved in patients with intracranial teratoma. Prognosis for NGGCTs other than teratoma is poorer than for germinomas with historically 20 to 49% 5-year survival rates (Jennings et al. 1985b;

Schild et al. 1996; Matsutani et al. 1997; Drummond and Rosenfeld 1999; Jaing et al. 2002). However, it is clear that combined-modality therapy has dramatically improved these historically poor clinical outcomes of patients with NGGCTs. The roles of surgical resection and high-dose chemotherapy with stem-cell rescue for patients with NGGCTs are currently under investigation.

Given higher cure rates for patients with intracranial GCTs, long-term toxicities are clearly evident. Sawamura et al. (1998a) reported a variety of late adverse effects of therapy including stroke, secondary malignancy, and cognitive, endocrinologic, auditory, and visual dysfunctions. Of 85 patients, 58 required hormone replacement therapy and 26 patients showed poor performance status. Young patients are at increased risk of physical as well as neuropsychological deficits. As expected, patients who received less than 55 Gy showed higher Karnofsky scores (Ono et al. 1994).

Sands et al. (2001) reported the results of quality of life and neuropsychological functioning in patients enrolled in the First International CNS Germ Cell Tumor Study. Patients who received CNS radiation therapy had worse physical health but similar psychosocial health. Patients with germinomas significantly outperformed those with NGGCTs on all neuropsychological measures, and younger patients were at increased risk for psychosocial and physical problems as well as neuropsychologic deficits. In the study by Aoyama et. al. (2002) using chemotherapy followed by low-dose involved-field radiotherapy, the authors noted no remarkable deterioration in quality of life or neurocognitive function.

Combination chemoradiotherapy regimens with risk stratification and dose adjustments will likely decrease the long-term side effects of therapy while improving the prognosis for those with the poor-risk intracranial GCTs. New approaches hold promise as well. Osada et al. (2001) provide a case report of utilizing dendritic-cell based immunotherapy in a patient with relapsed, resistant intracranial germ cell tumor who had significant tumor shrinkage as well as decrease in tumor markers after four infusions of peripheral blood dendritic cells followed by monocyte-derived dendritic cells.

6.8 Conclusion

In this chapter, we have reviewed the epidemiology, pathology, clinical features, diagnosis, and treatment of intracranial germ cell tumors. The utilization of tumor markers, improved imaging technologies, and safer biopsy techniques has made the diagnosis of intracranial germ cell tumors relatively straightforward. Mixed GCTs remain a diagnostic challenge. The outcomes of patients with GCTs have paralleled the success that has been achieved in other types of pediatric cancers with the advances in combinatorial regimens and intensification of treatments. As with other pediatric malignancies, the challenge is to distinguish the patients who require more intensive therapy from those needing standard treatment. Risk-stratified treatment protocols individualized to a patient's tumor profile are clearly the next step. Technological advances in the field of neurosurgery and radiation oncology continue to further treatment success and decrease long-term sequelae of our therapies. Further understanding of the biology of intracranial GCTs should result in novel, targeted, and less toxic therapeutics.

References

Allen JC, Kim JH, Packer RJ (1987) Neoadjuvant chemotherapy for newly diagnosed germ-cell tumors of the central nervous system. J Neurosurg 67:65–70

Aoyama H, Shirato H, Ikeda J et al (2002) Induction chemotherapy followed by low-dose involved-field radiotherapy for intracranial germ cell tumors. J Clin Oncol 20:857–865

Aydin F, Ghatak NR, Radie-Keane K et al (1992) The short-term effect of low-dose radiation on intracranial germinoma. A pathologic study. Cancer 69:2322–2326

Balmaceda C, Heller G, Rosenblum M et al (1996) Chemotherapy without irradiation – a novel approach for newly diagnosed CNS germ cell tumors: results of an international cooperative trial. The First International Central Nervous System Germ Cell Tumor Study. J Clin Oncol 14:2908–2915

Baranzelli MC, Patte C, Bouffet E et al (1998) An attempt to treat pediatric intracranial alphaFP and betaHCG secreting germ cell tumors with chemotherapy alone. SFOP experience with 18 cases. Societe Francaise d'Oncologie Pediatrique. J Neurooncol 37:229–239

Beeley JM, Daly JJ, Timperley WR et al (1973) Ectopic pinealoma: an unusual clinical presentation and a histochemical comparison with a seminoma of the testis. J Neurol Neurosurg Psychiatry 36:864–873

Bernstein L, Smith MA, Liu L et al (1999) Germ cell, trophoblastic, and other gonadal neoplasms in cancer incidence and survival among children and adolescents: US SEER program 1975–1995. National Cancer Institute, Bethesda, Maryland, pp 125–137

Bouffet E, Baranzelli MC. Patte C et al (1999) Combined treatment modality for intracranial germinomas: results of a multicentre SFOP experience. Societe Francaise d'Oncologie Pediatrique. Br J Cancer 79:1199–1204

Brandes AA, Pasetto LM, Monfardini S (2000) The treatment of cranial germ cell tumours. Cancer Treat Rev 26:233–242

Buckner JC, Peethambaram PP, Smithson WA et al (1999) Phase II trial of primary chemotherapy followed by reduced-dose radiation for CNS germ cell tumors. J Clin Oncol 17:933–940

Calaminus G, Andreussi L, Garre ML et al (1997) Secreting germ cell tumors of the central nervous system (CNS). First results of the cooperative German/Italian pilot study (CNS sGCT). Klin Padiatr 209:222–227

Choi JU, Kim DS, Chung SS et al (1998) Treatment of germ cell tumors in the pineal region. Childs Nerv Syst 14:41–48

Cushing B, Perlman EJ, Marina NM et al (2002) Germ cell tumors. In: Pizzo PA, Poplack DG (eds) Principles and practice of pediatric oncology, vol 1. Lippincott Williams and Wilkins, Philadelphia, PA, pp 1091–1113

de Bruin TW, Slater RM, Defferrari R et al (1994) Isochromosome 12p-positive pineal germ cell tumor. Cancer Res 54:1542–1544

Drummond KJ, Rosenfeld JV (1999) Pineal region tumours in childhood. A 30-year experience. Childs Nerv Syst 15:119–126; discussion 127

Edwards MS, Hudgins RJ, Wilson CB et al (1988) Pineal region tumors in children. J Neurosurg 68:689–697

Einhorn LH, Donohue J (1997) Cis-diamminedichloroplatinum, vinblastine, and bleomycin combination chemotherapy in disseminated testicular cancer. J Urol 167:928–932; discussion 933

Felix I, Becker LE (1990) Intracranial germ cell tumors in children: an immunohistochemical and electron microscopic study. Pediatr Neurosurg 16:156–162

Fujimaki T, Matsutani M, Funada N et al (1994) CT and MRI features of intracranial germ cell tumors. J Neurooncol 19:217–226

Gay JC, Janco RL, Lukens JN (1985) Systemic metastases in primary intracranial germinoma. Case report and literature review. Cancer 55:2688–2690

Ginsberg S, Kirshner J, Reich S et al (1981) Systemic chemotherapy for a primary germ cell tumor of the brain: a pharmacokinetic study. Cancer Treat Rep 65:477–483

Handa H, Yamashita J (1981) Current treatment of pineal tumors (author's translation). Neurol Med Chir (Tokyo) 21:147–154

Hawkins EP (1990) Pathology of germ cell tumors in children. Crit Rev Oncol Hematol 10:165–179

Hawkins EP, Finegold MJ, Hawkins HK et al (1986) Nongerminomatous malignant germ cell tumors in children. A review of 89 cases from the Pediatric Oncology Group, 1971–1984. Cancer 58:2579–2584

Hoffman HJ, Otsubo H, Hendrick EB et al (1991) Intracranial germ-cell tumors in children. J Neurosurg 74:545–551

Iizuka H, Nojima T, Kadoya S (1996) Germinoma of the optic nerve: case report. Noshuyo Byori 13:95–98

Itoyama Y, Kochi M, Kuratsu J et al (1995) Treatment of intracranial nongerminomatous malignant germ cell tumors producing alpha-fetoprotein. Neurosurgery 36:459–464; discussion 464–466

Iwato M, Tachibana O, Tohma Y et al (2000a) Alterations of the INK4a/ARF locus in human intracranial germ cell tumors. Cancer Res 60:2113–2115

Iwato M, Tachibana O, Tohma Y et al (2000b) Molecular analysis for p53 and mdm2 in intracranial germ cell tumors. Acta Neuropathol (Berl) 99:21–25

Jaing TH, Wang HS, Hung IJ et al (2002) Intracranial germ cell tumors: a retrospective study of 44 children. Pediatr Neurol 26:369–373

Jellinger K (1973) Primary intracranial germ cell tumours. Acta Neuropathol 25:291–306

Jennings CD, Powell DE, Walsh JW et al (1985a) Suprasellar germ cell tumor with extracranial metastases. Neurosurgery 16:9–12

Jennings MT, Gelman R, Hochberg F (1985b) Intracranial germ-cell tumors: natural history and pathogenesis. J Neurosurg 63:155–167

Jooma R, Kendall BE (1983) Diagnosis and management of pineal tumors. J Neurosurg 58:654–665

Kang JK, Jeun SS, Hong YK et al (1998) Experience with pineal region tumors. Childs Nerv Syst 14:63–68

Kobayashi T, Yoshida J, Ishiyama J et al (1989) Combination chemotherapy with cisplatin and etoposide for malignant intracranial germ-cell tumors. An experimental and clinical study. J Neurosurg 70:676–681

Lapin V, Ebels I (1981) The role of the pineal gland in neuroendocrine control mechanisms of neoplastic growth. J Neural Transm 50:275–282

Lemos JA, Barbieri-Neto J, Casartelli C (1998) Primary intracranial germ cell tumors without an isochromosome 12p. Cancer Genet Cytogenet 100:124–128

Lin IJ, Shu SG, Chu HY et al (1997) Primary intracranial germ-cell tumor in children. Zhonghua Yi Xue Za Zhi (Taipei) 60:259–264

Loveland KL, Schlatt S (1997) Stem cell factor and c-kit in the mammalian testis: lessons originating from Mother Nature's gene knockouts. J Endocrinol 153:337–344

Matsutani M, Sano K, Takakura K et al (1997) Primary intracranial germ cell tumors: a clinical analysis of 153 histologically verified cases. J Neurosurg 86:446–455

Matsutani M, Sano K, Takakura K et al (1998) Combined treatment with chemotherapy and radiation therapy for intracranial germ cell tumors. Childs Nerv Syst 14:59–62

Miyanohara O, Takeshima H, Kaji M et al (2002) Diagnostic significance of soluble c-kit in the cerebrospinal fluid of patients with germ cell tumors. J Neurosurg 97:177–183

Nakajima H, Iwai Y, Yamanaka K et al (2000) Primary intracranial germinoma in the medulla oblongata. Surg Neurol 53:448–451

Nakase H, Ohnishi H, Touho H et al (1994) Cerebellar primary germ-cell tumor in a young boy. Brain Dev 16:396–398

Nichols CR (1996) Ifosfamide in the treatment of germ cell tumors. Semin Oncol 23 [Suppl 6]:65–73

Nishizaki T, Kajiwara K, Adachi N et al (2001) Detection of craniospinal dissemination of intracranial germ cell tumours based on serum and cerebrospinal fluid levels of tumour markers. J Clin Neurosci 8:27–30

Oi S, Matsumoto S (1992) Controversy pertaining to therapeutic modalities for tumors of the pineal region: a worldwide survey of different patient populations. Childs Nerv Syst 8:332–336

Oi S, Matsuzawa K, Choi JU et al (1998) Identical characteristics of the patient populations with pineal region tumors in Japan and in Korea and therapeutic modalities. Childs Nerv Syst 14:36–40

Okada Y, Nishikawa R, Matsutani M et al (2002) Hypomethylated X chromosome gain and rare isochromosome 12p in diverse intracranial germ cell tumors. J Neuropathol Exp Neurol 61:531–538

Ono N, Kakegawa T, Zama A et al (1994) Factors affecting functional prognosis in survivors of primary central nervous system germinal tumors. Surg Neurol 41:9–15

Osada T, Fujimaki T, Takamizawa M et al (2001) Dendritic cells activate antitumor immunity for malignant intracranial germ cell tumor: a case report. Jpn J Clin Oncol 31:403–406

Packer RJ, Cohen BH, Cooney K (2000) Intracranial germ cell tumors" Oncologist 5:312–320

Pinkerton CR, Broadbent V, Horwich A et al (1990) 'JEB'–a carboplatin based regimen for malignant germ cell tumours in children. Br J Cancer 62:257–262

Regis J, Bouillot P, Rouby-Volot F et al (1996) Pineal region tumors and the role of stereotactic biopsy: review of the mortality, morbidity, and diagnostic rates in 370 cases. Neurosurgery 39:907–912; discussion 912–914

Rickert CH, Simon R, Bergmann M et al (2000) Comparative genomic hybridization in pineal germ cell tumors. J Neuropathol Exp Neurol 59:815–821

Robertson PL, DaRosso RC, Allen JC (1997) Improved prognosis of intracranial non-germinoma germ cell tumors with multimodality therapy. J Neurooncol 32:71–80

Saitoh M, Tamaki N, Kokunai T et al (1991) Clinico-biological behavior of germ-cell tumors. Childs Nerv Syst 7:246–250

Salzman KL, Rojiani AM, Buatti J et al (1997) Primary intracranial germ cell tumors: clinicopathologic review of 32 cases. Pediatr Pathol Lab Med 17:713–727

Sands SA, Kellie SJ, Davidow AL et al (2001) Long-term quality of life and neuropsychologic functioning for patients with CNS germ-cell tumors: from the First International CNS Germ-Cell Tumor Study. Neuro-oncology 3:174–183

Sano K, Matsutani M, Seto T (1989) So-called intracranial germ cell tumours: personal experiences and a theory of their pathogenesis. Neurol Res 11:118–126

Sawamura Y, de Tribolet N, Ishii N et al (1997) Management of primary intracranial germinomas: diagnostic surgery or radical resection? J Neurosurg 87:262–266

Sawamura Y, Ikeda J, Shirato H et al (1998a) Germ cell tumours of the central nervous system: treatment consideration based on 111 cases and their long-term clinical outcomes. Eur J Cancer 34:104–110

Sawamura Y, Kato T, Ikeda J et al (1998b) Teratomas of the central nervous system: treatment considerations based on 34 cases. J Neurosurg 89:728–737

Sawamura Y, Shirato H, Ikeda J et al (1998c) Induction chemotherapy followed by reduced-volume radiation therapy for newly diagnosed central nervous system germinoma. J Neurosurg 88:66–72

Sawamura Y, Ikeda JL, Tada M et al (1999) Salvage therapy for recurrent germinomas in the central nervous system. Br J Neurosurg 13:376–381

Schild SE, Haddock MG, Scheithauer BW et al (1996) Nongerminomatous germ cell tumors of the brain. Int J Radiat Oncol Biol Phys 36:557–563

Shibamoto Y, Oda Y, Yamashita J et al (1994) The role of cerebrospinal fluid cytology in radiotherapy planning for intracranial germinoma. Int J Radiat Oncol Biol Phys 29:1089–1094

Shibamoto Y, Takahashi M, Abe M (1994) Reduction of the radiation dose for intracranial germinoma: a prospective study. Br J Cancer 70:984–989

Shirato H, Nishio M, Sawamura Y et al (1997) Analysis of long-term treatment of intracranial germinoma. Int J Radiat Oncol Biol Phys 37:511–515

Steinbok P (2001) Management of malignant pineal germ cell tumors with residual mature teratoma. Neurosurgery 49:1271

Steinbok P, Cochrane DD (2001) Pineal region and intracranial germ cell tumors. In: McLone DG (ed) Pediatric neurosurgery: surgery of the developing nervous system. Saunders, Philadelphia, pp 711–724

Tada T, Takizawa T, Nakazato F et al (1999) Treatment of intracranial nongerminomatous germ-cell tumor by high-dose chemotherapy and autologous stem-cell rescue. J Neurooncol 44:71–76

Takei Y, Pearl GS (1981) Ultrastructural study of intracranial yolk sac tumor: with special reference to the oncologic phylogeny of germ cell tumors. Cancer 48:2038–2046

Teilum G (1976) Special tumors of ovary and testis and related extragonadal lesions: comparative pathology and histological identification. Munksgaard, Copenhagen; Lippincott, Philadelphia

Uematsu Y, Tsuura Y, Miyamoto K et al (1992) The recurrence of primary intracranial germinomas. Special reference to germinoma with STGC (syncytiotrophoblastic giant cell). J Neurooncol 13:247–256

Weiner HL, Lichtenbaum RA, Wisoff JH et al (2002) Delayed surgical resection of central nervous system germ cell tumors. Neurosurgery 50:727–733; discussion 733–734

Wolden SL, Wara WM, Larson DA et al (1995) Radiation therapy for primary intracranial germ-cell tumors. Int J Radiat Oncol Biol Phys 32:943–949

Yoshida J, Sugita K, Kobayashi T et al (1993) Prognosis of intracranial germ cell tumours: effectiveness of chemotherapy with cisplatin and etoposide (CDDP and VP-16). Acta Neurochir (Wien) 120:111–117

Yu IT, Griffin CA, Phillips PC et al (1995) Numerical sex chromosomal abnormalities in pineal teratomas by cytogenetic analysis and fluorescence in situ hybridization. Lab Invest 72:419–423

Zimmerman RA, Bilaniuk LT (1982) Age-related incidence of pineal calcification detected by computed tomography. Radiology 142:659–662

Craniopharyngioma

R. Du · R. H. Lustig · B. Fisch
M. W. McDermott

Contents

7.1 Introduction

Craniopharyngiomas are histologically benign neuroepithelial tumors that arise from squamous cell rests found along the path of the primitive craniopharyngeal duct and adenohypophysis. They frequently involve vital structures in the sellar region including the optic apparatus and the pituitary, and often lead to visual, endocrine, and mental disturbances. Thus, despite their benign histology, the involvement of various neural structures in the suprasellar region makes the treatment and management of craniopharyngiomas difficult. There is an ongoing controversy regarding optimal treatment of craniopharyngiomas. The debate revolves around the risks and benefits of attempted gross total resection as compared to subtotal resection or biopsy followed by adjunctive therapy such as external beam radiotherapy, radiosurgery, intracavitary radiation, and/or chemotherapy.

7.2 Epidemiology

The incidence of craniopharyngioma is 1.3 per 1,000,000 person years and does not vary with gender or race. There is a bimodal distribution with peak rates during childhood (5 to 14 years) and in older adults [65 to 74 years in the Central Brain Tumor Registry of the United States (CBTRUS) and 50 to 74 years in the Los Angeles County Cancer Surveillance Program; Bunin et al. 1998]. Craniopharyngiomas account for 5 to 10 % of pediatric brain tumors and 1 to 4 % of adult brain tumors (Kernohan 1971; Samii and Tatagiba 1997; Bunin et al. 1998; Moore and Couldwell 2000). It is the most common neuroepithelial intracranial tumor in children and accounts for 56% of pediatric sellar and suprasellar tumors (Miller 1994). One should note, however, that the majority of craniopharyngiomas occur in adults because the overall incidence of brain tumors in adults is much greater than in children.

7.3 Pathology

7.3.1 Etiology

In the middle of the fourth week of gestation, Rathke's pouch projects upwards from the roof of the stomodeum (oral cavity) and grows towards the infundibulum, a downward growth from the diencephalon (Fig. 7.1). During the sixth week of gestation, the connection between Rathke's pouch and the oral cav-

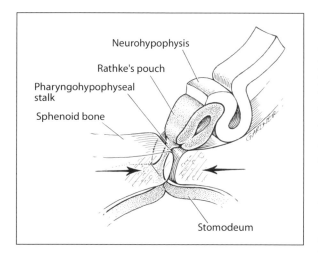

Figure 7.1

Rathke's pouch projects from the roof of the stomodeum and grows towards the infundibulum during the fourth week of gestation. During the sixth week of gestation, the connection between Rathke's pouch and the pharyngohypophyseal stalk disappears. Rathke's pouch then develops into the adenohypophysis. Craniopharyngiomas are generally believed to develop from squamous cell rests along the path of the primitive craniopharyngeal duct and adenohypophysis (Reprinted by permission)

ity (the pharyngohypophyseal stalk) disappears. Rathke's pouch then develops into the pars distalis, pars intermedia, and pars tuberalis, which make up the adenohypophysis (Moore and Persaud 1993; Miller 1994; Samii and Tatagiba 1997). Craniopharyngiomas are generally believed to develop from squamous cell rests found along the path of the primitive craniopharyngeal duct and adenohypophysis (Donovan and Nesbit 1996; Moore and Couldwell 2000). A metaplastic origin from adenohypophyseal cells has been proposed for the papillary subtype of craniopharyngioma, but the exact origin of these tumors remains controversial (Miller 1994).

7.3.2 Classification

Craniopharyngiomas are divided anatomically into four groups depending on the relationship of the tumor to the optic chiasm: prechiasmatic, retrochiasmatic, subchiasmatic, and laterally expansile (Hoffman et al. 1999). Most craniopharyngiomas are both intra- and extrasellar (75%), but some are purely suprasellar (20%) or purely intrasellar (5%). Thirty percent extend anteriorly, 25% extend laterally into the middle fossa, and 20% are retroclival. Intraventricular craniopharyngiomas, which arise within the third ventricle and extend downward through the sphenoid bone into the nasopharynx, are very uncommon (Harwood-Nash 1994).

7.3.3 Histopathology

Craniopharyngiomas can also be classified by pathologic type: adamantinomatous, papillary, and mixed. The adamantinomatous type is the most common; it is cystic and filled with dark brown fluid (Sidawy and Jannotta 1997). The epithelium resembles tumors of tooth-forming tissues or ameloblastomas, and less commonly of long-bone tumors known as adamantinomas, thereby giving these the name "adamantinomatous craniopharyngiomas." Microscopically, the epithelium consists of a basal layer of small basophilic cells, followed by an intermediate layer of variable thickness composed of a loose collection of stel-

Figure 7.2

Adamantinomatous craniopharyngioma showing palisading basal squamous epithelium surrounding loosely arranged epithelial cells (stellate reticulum) and nodules of eosinophilic keratinized cells

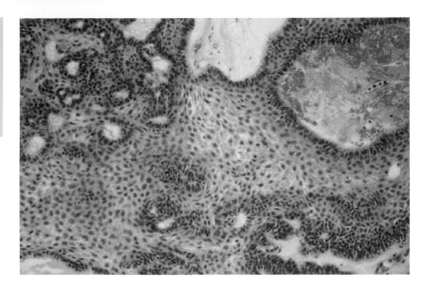

late cells whose processes traverse the intercellular spaces (Fig. 7.2). The top layer consists of keratinized squamous cells that desquamate as stacks of flat keratin plates into the cyst cavity. The cyst fluid is therefore rich in membrane lipids such as cholesterol, as well as in keratin from the cytoskeleton, and can cause chronic inflammation within the cyst walls. The desquamated cells often calcify but rarely progress to metaplastic bone formation (Miller 1994).

Squamous papillary craniopharyngiomas, the second variety, are composed of stratified squamous epithelium that has papillary projections of epithelial cords into the surrounding tissues. These tumors rarely calcify or desquamate, the cell layers being solid and compact with no stellate regions. These tumors occur mostly in adults. Mixed craniopharyngiomas, the third type, have features of both the adamantinomatous and papillary types.

While the adamantinomatous type is common in all age groups, the squamous papillary type is rare in children. In pediatric patients, 92 to 96% have been found to be adamantinomatous, 0% squamous papillary, 0 to 4% mixed, and 4% not classified (Miller 1994; Weiner et al. 1994). In adults, 63 to 66% were adamantinomatous, 27 to 28% squamous papillary, 6 to 7% mixed, and 3% not classified. However, one pure squamous papillary tumor has been found in a child, showing that while these are rare in children, they are not exclusive to adults.

7.3.4 Tumor Biology

Raghavan et al. (2000) have measured the proliferative activity of craniopharyngiomas based on their MIB-1 immunostaining for the Ki-67 nuclear antigen, but found no correlation with morphological features or clinical outcomes. Thapar et al. (1994) demonstrated the expression of estrogen-receptor gene in the proliferative epithelial component of 19 adamantinomatous and 4 papillary craniopharyngiomas, which suggested hormonal involvement in the genesis or progression of craniopharyngiomas. However, there was no correlation between the presence of estrogen-receptor mRNA hybridization signal and the clinical outcome. Barbosa et al. (2001) several different types of brain tumors and found a high level of acetylcholinesterase activity and a low level of butyrylcholinesterase activity in all three craniopharyngiomas studied. Low levels of butyrylcholinesterase were correlated with slow growth in the tumors studied but the correlation between the level of this enzyme and clinical outcome was not studied. Vidal et al. (2002) found strong cytoplasmic immunoreactivity for vascular endothelial growth factor (VEGF) in epithelial cells of both adamantinomatous and papillary craniopharyngiomas and that microvessel density, a measure of angiogenesis, correlated with an increased risk of recurrence. However, not every recurrent tumor had a high microvessel density, indicating that other factors are involved in the prognosis of these tumors.

Little is known about the genetic basis for the development of craniopharyngiomas. Sarubi et al. (2001) studied 22 adamantinomatous craniopharyngiomas for mutations in three genes associated with odontogenic tumors, $Gs\alpha$, $Gi2\alpha$, and *patched* (*PTCH*). No mutations were detected in any of the three. Matsuo et al. (2001) demonstrated the expression of prostaglandin H synthetase-2 (PHS-2) in a variety of brain tumors, including 2 out of 4 craniopharyngiomas, suggesting that PHS-2 may play a role in tumorigenesis, but the significance of this isolated finding remains unclear. Nozaki et al. (1998) studied the occurrence of *p53* mutations in a variety of tumors, but found no evidence of *p53* mutations in any of four craniopharyngiomas. Overall, these data demonstrate that the genetic and molecular basis for craniopharyngiomas remains poorly understood, in contrast to the advances that have been made in understanding the oncogenesis of many malignant tumors. Further experimental studies are clearly required if specific biological therapies are to be developed.

7.4 Clinical Features

7.4.1 Signs and Symptoms

The sellar/suprasellar location of craniopharyngiomas can cause compression or destruction of the optic chiasm, nerves, and/or tracts, hypothalamus, pituitary stalk, and/or adjacent vascular structures, leading to the typical clinical picture of progressive visual loss, headaches, and/or endocrine abnormalities (Miller 1994). The exact position of the tumor can influence the clinical picture. Retrochiasmatic tumors extend posteriorly and push the chiasm anteriorly against the tuberculum sella. These tumors tend to

fill the third ventricle and cause hydrocephalus, which typically presents as headache, nausea, and vomiting (Sanford and Muhlbauer 1991; Hoffman et al. 1999). Lateral extension of the tumor can cause displacement of internal carotid arteries and posterior communicating arteries. Posterior extension of the tumor can displace the tip of the basilar artery, posterior cerebral arteries, oculomotor nerves, and rostral brainstem (Miller 1994). Regardless of the exact origin, large tumors can compress the pituitary stalk or adenohypophysis leading to a variety of endocrine abnormalities such as diabetes insipidus, hyperprolactinemia, and/or panhypopituitarism. Subtle endocrinopathies often escape clinical detection for long periods of time and are only apparent in hindsight.

Visual and endocrine abnormalities are the most common symptoms at presentation. In a retrospective study of 72 patients treated with radiation therapy at the University of California at San Francisco (UCSF) from 1972 to 1999, 56% had visual defects and 50% had endocrine abnormalities prior to treatment (unpublished results). Other presenting symptoms included behavioral abnormalities (28%), increased intracranial pressure or hydrocephalus (19%), and headaches alone (4%). For 36 patients with recurrent disease, 61% were asymptomatic at the time of detection, 28% had deterioration of visual function, and 22% had worsening headaches.

Although the classic sellar mass will typically present with a superior temporal field cut, the eccentric growth of craniopharyngioma can lead to patterns of visual loss that vary in type and severity. These include decreased acuity, diplopia, blurred vision, and subjective visual field deficits, and cases have even been reported of unilateral or bilateral blindness (Hoffman et al. 1999). Eighty percent of adults have visual disturbance while only 20 to 63% of children do (Fisher et al. 1998; Moore and Couldwell 2000). This discrepancy may be due to the lack of awareness amongst children of a progressive narrowing of the peripheral fields. Toddlers, in particular, can become virtually blind before the extent of visual loss becomes apparent.

Elevated intracranial pressure (ICP) results from hydrocephalus or from mass effect. As expected, headache is the most common complaint in all age groups with high ICP. Children are more likely to present with headache and vomiting than with visual disturbances, and twenty percent of children have papilledema at presentation (Moore and Couldwell 2000).

7.4.2 Endocrine Abnormalities

Hormonal abnormalities occur in 43 to 90% of patients at presentation (Moore and Couldwell 2000). Pure intrasellar craniopharyngiomas are rare so the loss of hormone secretion usually results from direct compression or destruction of the hypothalamus and/or pituitary stalk. Virtually all of the adenohypophyseal hormones can be affected including growth hormone (75%), luteinizing hormone or follicle stimulating hormone (40 to 44%), adrenocorticotropic hormone (25 to 56%), and thyroid stimulating hormone (25 to 64%). Hyperprolactinemia occurs in 1 to 20% of cases from impingement on the pituitary stalk (the "stalk effect") and from reduced amounts of prolactin inhibitory factor (mainly dopamine) reaching the prolactin-secreting cells of the anterior pituitary. Diabetes insipidus is reported to occur in 9 to 17% of patients prior to surgery, but mainly develops postoperatively after removal of large tumors involving the third ventricle (Sanford and Muhlbauer 1991; Moore and Couldwell 2000; B. Fisch 2002, personal communication). Deficiencies in LH and FSH lead to delayed or arrested puberty in adolescents, and loss of libido or secondary amenorrhea in adults.

Short stature, hypothyroidism, and diabetes insipidus (DI) are the three most common endocrine abnormalities at presentation in children (Sanford and Muhlbauer 1991). These in turn can lead to a constellation of other clinical features. Low growth-hormone levels will result in growth retardation and delayed bone age. Hypothyroidism leads to poor growth, weight gain, cold intolerance, and fatigability. Forty percent of children demonstrate decreased height velocity or short stature at presentation, either from growth hormone deficiency, central hypothyroidism, delayed puberty, or a combination of these three. Lastly, many of these children are obese at pre-

sentation, due to damage of the ventromedial hypothalamus (VMH), with resultant dysregulation of energy balance, termed "hypothalamic obesity" (Hoffman et al. 1999; Lustig 2002; Lustig et al. 2003).

Mental status changes are unusual in children but occur in 25% of adults. Tumor growth involving the frontal lobe can lead to dementia, apathy, and abulia. Temporal lobe involvement can lead to seizures and amnesia (Moore and Couldwell 2000).

7.5 Natural History

Craniopharyngiomas are histologically and cytologically benign but locally aggressive and tend to recur. The rate of recurrence with any form of treatment is 8 to 26% at 5 years and 9 to 100% at 10 years. If recurrence cannot be controlled, local invasion and growth can result in death. Malignant change, however, is extremely rare, only a handful of cases having been reported in the literature. One was of an adamantinomatous craniopharyngioma in a patient who underwent surgical resections and three courses of radiotherapy with subsequent transition of the craniopharyngioma to a moderately differentiated squamous cell carcinoma (Kristopaitis et al. 2000). Other cases reported in the literature were presumably from transplantation of tumor fragments during surgery or from meningeal seeding (Barloon et al. 1988; Ragoowansi and Piepgras 1991; Malik et al. 1992; Israel and Pomeranz 1995; Gupta et al. 1999; Lee et al. 1999; Ito et al. 2001).

7.6 Diagnosis and Imaging

7.6.1 Computed Tomography and Magnetic Resonance Imaging

Modern imaging studies used for diagnosing craniopharyngiomas include CT and MRI. Plain radiographs are rarely used for diagnosis, but if performed will demonstrate sellar changes and associated calcifications (Harwood-Nash 1994). Sixty-six percent of adults and 90% of children will have abnormalities such as sellar enlargement, erosion of the clinoid pro-

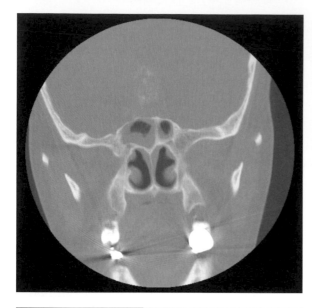

Figure 7.3
CT scan (coronal view) showing punctate calcifications within a tumor

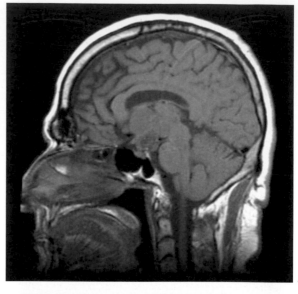

a

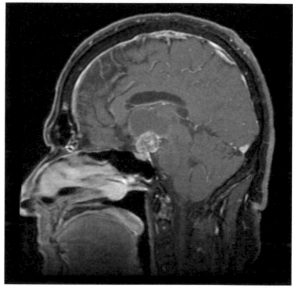

b

Figure 7.4 a,b

Multiple MRI sequences of a typical cystic craniopharyngioma: a Sagittal T1-weighted image without contrast. A multilobulated mass is seen in the suprasellar region. b Sagittal T1-weighted image following gadolinium. The suprasellar solid component enhances while the cystic area above it does not. ▶

cesses or dorsum sella, or calcifications on plain radiographs. Tumor-associated calcification is seen in 40% of adults and 80% of children (Moore and Couldwell 2000). Sellar enlargement is seen in 65% of patients while sellar erosion is seen in 44% (Donovan and Nesbit 1996).

Calcifications, particularly in the suprasellar region, are best demonstrated by CT. The presence of abundant suprasellar calcification is important information for the surgeon as these tumors are extremely difficult to remove. The calcification can be obvious with large confluent areas or small punctuate or curvilinear areas (Fig. 7.3). Sellar enlargement and erosion are also well seen on CT. The tumor often appears as a lobulated, heterogeneous, and cystic suprasellar mass. The cyst fluid is isodense or hypodense, and the solid portion and cyst capsule enhance with contrast (Harwood-Nash 1994; Moore and Couldwell 2000).

Calcification is more difficult to detect on MRI, but MRI provides far more detail regarding the relationship of the tumor to adjacent anatomical and vascu-

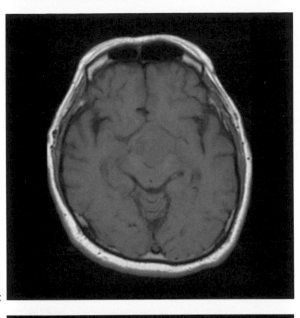

c

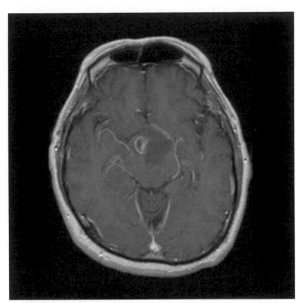

d

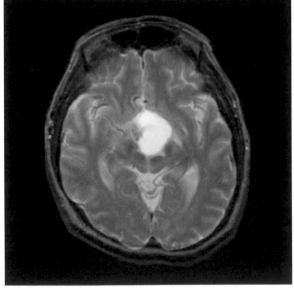

e

Figure 7.4 c–e

c Axial T1-weighted image without contrast. d Axial T1-weighted image with gadolinium. e Axial T2-weighted image

lar structures. High-resolution sequences of the sellar region, with and without contrast enhancement, should be obtained in all cases. The signal characteristics of craniopharyngiomas on MRI scans are typically heterogeneous and depend upon the amount of cystic and solid components, as well as the amount of cholesterol, keratin, hemorrhage, and calcification (Figs. 7.4, 7.5). On T1-weighted images, the cystic component is hypointense while the cyst rim enhances following contrast administration. The solid component is isointense but enhances with contrast (Moore and Couldwell 2000). The tumor is almost always hyperintense on T2-weighted images (Donovan and Nesbit 1996).

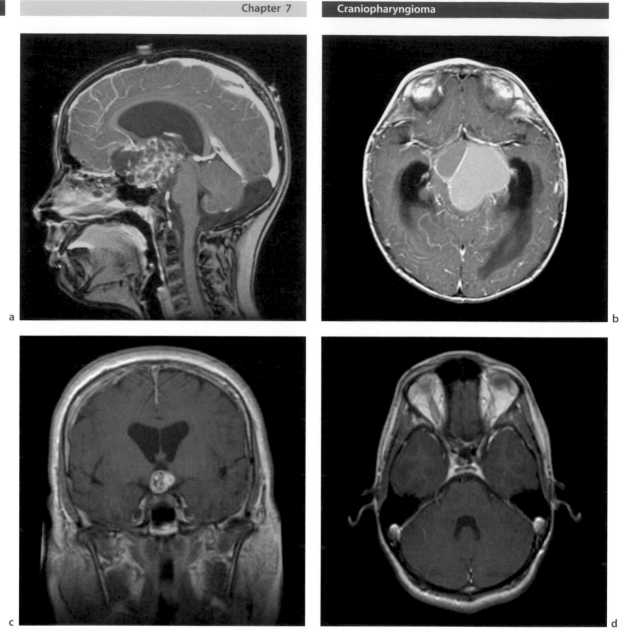

a   b
c   d

Figure 7.5 a–d

Other examples of craniopharyngiomas: a Sagittal T1-weighted image with contrast showing a large mixed solid and cystic craniopharyngioma. b Axial T1-weighted image with contrast showing a large cystic craniopharyngioma with two major compartments. c Coronal T1-weighted image with contrast showing a small solid suprasellar craniopharyngioma. d Axial T1-weighted MRI with contrast showing a small recurrent craniopharyngioma within the sella

The differential radiographic diagnosis of cystic suprasellar masses include Rathke's cleft cyst (no solid component, not lobulated, nonenhancing, more homogeneous), pituitary adenomas (enlarges sella, more homogeneous, less cystic), meningiomas (rarely cystic, isointense on T1- and T2-weighted images), optic pathway gliomas (usually not calcified), and aneurysms (laminated thrombus; Donovan and Nesbit 1996; Fischbein et al. 2000).

7.6.2 Clinical Evaluation

The evaluation and management of patients with craniopharyngiomas requires a multidisciplinary team approach with the active participation of subspecialties such as neurosurgery, radiation and medical oncology, neuroophthalmology, endocrinology, and psychology. All patients with craniopharyngiomas should have assessment of visual acuity and a complete visual field examination prior to treatment and then at intervals after treatment as follow-up.

Any hormonal deficiency should be evaluated and treated prior to definitive treatment (Wilson et al. 1998). A complete endocrinologic assessment is often necessary prior to surgery and is invaluable if and when any endocrine dysfunction develops (Table 7.1). All patients should get stress-dose steroids prior to surgery on the assumption that normal ACTH regulation is blunted (Samii and Tatagiba 1997). Hypothyroidism can take several days to correct and treatment should begin preoperatively. However, adrenocorticoid insufficiency can be precipitated if thyroid replacement is begun before steroid is given (Moore and Couldwell 2000). Finally, any electrolyte abnormalities should be identified and corrected prior to surgery.

Table 7.1. Endocrinologic evaluation

Pituitary function	Tests
Adrenal axis	Morning cortisol level 24-hour urine free cortisol level Cosyntropin stimulation test in questionable cases
Thyroid axis	Free T4 level Thyroid stimulating hormone level Thyrotropin releasing hormone stimulation test in questionable cases
Gonadal axis	Follicle stimulating hormone level Luteinizing hormone level Sex steroids: estradiol in women, testosterone in men
Growth hormone	Somatomedin-C (IGF-1) level (growth hormone level is pulsatile so a single random level is not reliable) IGF binding protein-3
Prolactin	Prolactin level
Antidiuretic hormone (ADH)	Serum sodium Serum osmoles Urine sodium Urine osmoles Fluid intake and urine output

7.7 Treatment

The overall treatment philosophy for craniopharyngioma is controversial and remains the subject of ongoing debate. The individual modalities of treatment include surgical resection, cyst aspiration, radiation therapy, stereotactic radiosurgery, intracavitary irradiation, and new approaches such as chemotherapy and use of interferon alpha. Mainly due to strongly held opinions and a lack of randomized clinical trial data, one camp views radical resection as offering the best chance for long-term survival while the opposite camp feels that radical resection leads to unacceptable long-term morbidity. The various treatment modalities and their associated complications will be described in the following sections.

7.7.1 Surgery

7.7.1.1 Surgical Indications

There are three surgical goals in the treatment of craniopharyngioma: diagnosis, decompression, and prevention of recurrence (van Effenterre and Boch 2002). Hydrocephalus and endocrine abnormalities are associated with high perioperative morbidity and must be treated first. Hydrocephalus can be treated acutely with either an external ventricular drain or a ventriculoperitoneal shunt prior to definitive surgery. Patients with craniopharyngiomas who present with acute visual deterioration or symptoms of elevated intracranial pressure from tumor-associated mass effect also require urgent surgical decompression. Since endocrine abnormalities such as hypothyroidism may take several days to correct, a patient who is stable should have surgery performed electively after all endocrine abnormalities are controlled. Those patients with large tumors and cerebral edema will benefit from dexamethasone.

7.7.1.2 Surgical Approaches

The surgical approach is determined by the anatomic location and the consistency of the tumor (cystic vs. solid). The most common approaches are bifrontal/extended frontal, unilateral subfrontal, pterional, transsphenoidal, transcallosal/transventricular, and subtemporal. Each of these approaches has its advantages and disadvantages although some are better suited for tumors in specific locations.

The bifrontal and subfrontal approach are used for primarily suprasellar tumors such as prechiasmatic and large retrochiasmatic lesions that extend anteriorly and fill the third ventricle (Samii and Tatagiba 1997; Moore and Couldwell 2000). The bifrontal/extended frontal approach is the preferred approach at our institution. A bifrontal craniotomy is followed by an extradural bilateral supraorbital osteotomy from the frontozygomatic processes laterally, through the roof of both orbits and the frontonasal suture in the midline. It is considered excessive by some, but the extent of frontal lobe retraction following removal of the supraorbital ridge is minimized and the visualization of the tumor is improved.

The unilateral subfrontal approach also allows good visualization of the optic nerves, the internal carotid arteries, and access to the third ventricle via the lamina terminalis (Moore and Couldwell 2000). Although it gives good exposure of both optic nerves, it does not provide access to the contralateral nerve and tract and lateral exposure of the suprasellar region behind the supraclinoid carotid is limited (Einhaus and Sanford 1999). For retrochiasmatic tumors the majority of the tumor must be removed via the lamina terminalis.

The pterional approach allows a more lateral view than the subfrontal approach and is used for large retrochiasmatic tumors with both anterior and posterior extensions (Samii and Tatagiba 1997; Moore and Couldwell 2000). This approach can be combined with the unilateral subfrontal approach (Einhaus and Sanford 1999).

The transsphenoidal approach is used for cystic infradiaphragmatic lesions, for symmetrical and well-defined suprasellar and retrosellar lesions with an enlarged sella, and for tumors without calcification that are not adherent to parasellar structures (Norris et al. 1998; de Divitiis et al. 2000; Moore and Couldwell 2000). The transsphenoidal approach results in lower surgical morbidity and postoperative visual loss as compared to the various intracranial routes (Rilliet et al. 1999). In two recent studies involving 45 patients, no patient had a deterioration in vision after transsphenoidal surgery (Fahlbusch et al. 1999; Rilliet et al. 1999). The disadvantages include the limited lateral exposure and the possibility of a cerebrospinal leak. If suprasellar calcifications are found, complete tumor removal is unlikely via the transsphenoidal approach and a subfrontal approach is necessary (Samii and Tatagiba 1997).

For purely intraventricular tumors, an interhemispheric transcallosal approach is used (Samii and Tatagiba 1997; Moore and Couldwell 2000). For this approach, a major portion of the tumor lies within the third ventricle, which is expanded, and the foramen of Munro is usually found to be enlarged. A staged surgical approach can also be used to combine the intraventricular approach with the subfrontal or pterional approach at a later date to resect portions of the tumor within the sella.

For tumors that are mainly cystic, stereotactic cyst aspiration followed by tumor resection or radiotherapy with instillation of radioisotopes into the cyst cavity may be successful (Samii and Tatagiba 1997; Hayward 1999; Nakamizo et al. 2001). Cyst aspiration can also relieve hydrocephalus (Hayward 1999). Regardless of surgical approach, any open procedure should be followed by a postoperative MRI scan to document the degree of resection. This study should be done within 48 hours of surgery before postoperative enhancement appears and confuses interpretation (Harwood-Nash 1994).

7.7.2 Radiotherapy

7.7.2.1 Conventional Radiotherapy

Radiation therapy is often used as an adjuvant to partial resection of the tumor or in cases of tumor recurrence. Different modalities of radiation therapy include external-beam fractionated radiotherapy, ster-

eotactic fractionated radiotherapy, stereotactic radiosurgery, and intracavitary irradiation.

Conventional fractionated external-beam radiation results in the delivery of a high dose of radiation to the target by dividing the treatment into multiple daily doses. Total doses typically range from 50 to 65 Gy divided into fractionated doses of 180 to 200 cGy/d (Einhaus and Sanford 1999). Doses less than 54 Gy have been associated with a 50% recurrence rate in children and a 33% recurrence rate in adults while doses greater than 54 Gy have a 15% recurrence rate in children and a 17% recurrence rate in adults (Regine et al. 1993). Obvious tissue necrosis occurs at threshold doses of 45 Gy in 10 fractions and 60 Gy in 35 fractions (Sheline et al. 1980).

7.7.2.2 Fractionated Stereotactic Radiotherapy

Fractionated stereotactic radiotherapy is similar to conventional external fractionated radiation but also utilizes stereotactic guidance. It has the advantage of treating tumors greater than 3 cm in size and those that are close to important structures (Tarbell et al. 1994; Moore and Couldwell 2000). It spares the frontal and temporal lobes, presumably reducing the risk of mental retardation and behavioral problems in children as well as the risk of radiation-induced neoplasms (Einhaus and Sanford 1999). Experience with this modality is limited.

7.7.2.3 Radiosurgery

Radiosurgery employs a single treatment session and uses multiple intersecting beams to concentrate the radiation and reduce the dose of radiation to the adjacent vital structures. The radiation source is either a linear accelerator (LINAC) or multiple cobalt-60 sources (Gamma Knife, Elekta AB, Stockholm). In stereotactic radiosurgery, the radiation dose can be tailored to the tumor with minimal radiation exposure to the hypothalamic–pituitary axis and the optic apparatus (Mokry 1999), and is the favored modality at our institution. Two features that limit radiosurgery are large tumor volume and inability to distinguish a boundary between the tumor and a critical structure such as the optic nerve. Other treatment steps can sometimes lead to a more amenable situation for radiosurgery. For example, when the bulk of the tumor is cystic, it can be aspirated so as to allow delineation of those structures and subsequent treatment with stereotactic radiosurgery (Chung et al. 2000). Stereotactic radiosurgery has mainly been used as an adjunct therapy to surgery, cyst aspiration, and conventional radiotherapy. It is often used in cases of recurrent craniopharyngiomas.

Historically, the total radiation dose used is determined by balancing the dose required to control the tumor against that which will avoid damage to the optic apparatus. The doses used for the tumor margins have varied from 9.5 to 16.5 Gy, as reported in a number of recent series (Regine et al. 1993; Kobayashi et al. 1994; Mokry 1999; Chung et al. 2000; Chiou et al. 2001). The optic apparatus in these reports received 13 Gy or less, but in more recent studies this has been further reduced to 8 Gy or less (Kobayashi et al. 1994; Mokry 1999; Chung et al. 2000; Chiou et al. 2001). With radiosurgery, tumor control rates range from 70 to 92%, although mean follow-up periods of 6 months to 28 months are too short to state the long-term effect with confidence (Table 7.2) (Kobayashi et al. 1994; Mokry 1999; Chung et al. 2000; Yu et al. 2000; Chiou et al. 2001). Chung et al. (2000) reported on three patients who developed enlargement of the cystic portion of the tumor 5 to 17 months after Gamma Knife (Elekta AB, Stockholm) radiosurgery and required cyst aspiration. The mechanism of the cyst enlargement remains unclear. Smaller tumors were found to be more likely to respond (Mokry 1999).

With respect to outcome, a majority of patients retained good function after treatment with stereotactic radiosurgery. Diabetes insipidus, panhypopituitarism, and visual loss were reported to occur, respectively, in 0 to 4%, 0 to 2%, and 0 to 4% of patients who underwent radiosurgery (Mokry 1999; Chung et al. 2000; Yu et al. 2000). Chung et al. (2000) reported good to excellent outcomes (independent living) in all patients with mainly solid or cystic tumors and in 50% of those with mixed solid and cystic tumors. Visual deterioration occurred in 10 to 66% of patients (Kobayashi et al. 1994; Einhaus and Sanford 1999). Given its effects on vision, stereotactic radiosurgery should be applied only to small tumors less than 2 cm in size and more than 4 to 5 mm away from the optic apparatus (Lunsford et al. 1994).

7.7.3 Intracavitary Therapy

Intracavitary therapy of cystic craniopharyngiomas, first reported by Leksell and Liden in 1952, has been used both as a primary mode of therapy as well as an adjunctive therapy for recurrent cases. Intracavitary therapy refers to the instillation of a radioisotope such as yttrium-90, phosphorus-32, or rhenium-186 through an indwelling catheter into the tumor cyst cavity so that a high dose of radiation can be delivered to the surrounding secretory epithelial layer. From a review by Blackburn et al. (1999), 121 of 149 cysts treated in 127 patients reduced in size or were obliterated in the follow-up period of 0.2 to 13 years. However, the distinction between recurrence of a cyst versus recollection of the initial lesion varied among

Table 7.2. Outcomes for craniopharyngiomas treated with Gamma Knife radiosurgery

Series	Year	Number of patients	Follow-up time (months)	Percent (%) tumor progression
Chung et al.	2000	31	36 (mean)	13
Yu et al.	2000	46	6 to 24	10 for solid tumors
				14 for mixed tumors[a]
Mokry	1999	23	28 (mean)	26

[a] intracavitary irradiation with ^{32}P was used for cystic portion of tumor

the different studies (Blackburn et al. 1999). In a study of 30 patients treated with ^{32}P where cyst regression was defined as more than 50% reduction in volume, 88% were found to have cyst regression with response occurring within 3 months of surgery and continued decrease in cyst size for up to 2 years after surgery (Pollock et al. 1995). Overall survival rate was 55% at 5 years and 45% at 10 years with a mean survival of 9 years (Voges et al. 1997). The impact of intracavitary irradiation on vision varied widely among studies ranging from 100% deterioration to 100% improvement, with improvement in 53% of patients over all studies considered (Voges et al. 1997; Blackburn et al. 1999). The effect on endocrine function was equally varied. Because of these confusing results and difficulties handling radioactive compounds, this technique has not been widely adopted.

7.7.4 Chemotherapy

The use of chemotherapeutic agents in the treatment of craniopharyngiomas is still under investigation. The most familiar technique is intracavitary instillation with bleomycin, an antibiotic with antineoplastic actions based on the inhibition of DNA, RNA, and protein synthesis. Intracavitary therapy involves initial placement of an Ommaya type catheter into the cyst cavity followed by a delayed radionuclide scan to ensure that there is no leak from the catheter or cyst. Multiple instillations of drug are also often required. Takahashi et al. (1985) first reported the administration of bleomycin in seven children with craniopharyngiomas. Of this group, four underwent partial excision and three biopsy of the tumor. Bleomycin was administered 2 weeks postoperatively via an Ommaya reservoir at a dose of 1 to 5 mg every other day. Injection of bleomycin was stopped when the cyst fluid changed from a machine-oil-like fluid to an almost colorless fluid. If necessary, hormone therapy was started in parallel with bleomycin therapy. All patients with cystic tumors were alive at 2 to 7 years follow up. Those with mixed or solid tumors did poorly and died within 2 years of treatment. Cavalheiro et al. (1996) reported the administration of bleomycin in a 16-year-old patient with decreased vi-

sual acuity, irregular menstrual cycle, and low TSH, thyroxin, cortisol, and FSH. Daily injections of 10 mg bleomycin were given via an Ommaya reservoir for 8 days. At the 1-year follow-up exam, the patient was asymptomatic endocrinologically. Her hormone levels had returned to normal and improvement in visual function was reported. More recently, Hoffman et al. (1999) reported 21 cases of pediatric cystic craniopharyngiomas that were treated with the administration of bleomycin into the cyst cavity 7 days after placement of an Ommaya reservoir. Daily doses from 2 to 10 mg were given. Fifty-seven percent had reduction in cyst size. One complication occurred from the action of bleomycin on the hypothalamus leading to seizures. Similar results were recently reported by Hader et al. (2000) who found greater than 50% reduction in cyst size at a mean follow-up period of 3 years in 57% of children treated with bleomycin.

The benefits of intracavitary bleomycin include prevention of cyst reaccumulation and thickening of the cyst wall, which may aid subsequent tumor resection. In addition, it avoids direct injury to the hypothalamus and pituitary gland, which occurs more frequently following surgery and radiation therapy. The main disadvantage is that while it is useful for tumors which are entirely cystic, radical surgery for these tumors is less likely to result in hypothalamic or pituitary injury (Hayward 1999). Other complications include headaches, hypopituitarism, and peritumoral edema (Hader et al. 2000).

Another experimental agent under investigation is interferon alpha (IFN-α), which is effective for the treatment of squamous cell carcinoma. The rationale for its use with craniopharyngiomas is that the two neoplasms share a similar epithelial origin. A phase II trial of IFN-α for progressive, recurrent, or unresectable craniopharyngiomas in children under 21 years of age has been reported by Jakacki et al. (2000) Treatment consisted of an induction phase of 8,000,000 U/m^2 daily for 16 weeks. Patients without progressive disease at 16 weeks then continued at the same dose three times a week for 32 weeks. Time to progression after discontinuation of IFN-α was 6 to 23 months. IFN-α toxicity occurred in 60% of cases during the first 8 weeks of treatment but resolved with discontinuation or dose reduction. Toxicities include hypoadrenal crisis with fever, neutropenia, transaminitis, fatigue, rash, insomnia, and seizures (Jakacki et al. 2000).

7.8 Outcome

On the basis of postoperative imaging, gross total resection varies widely in various series ranging from 29 to 77% of cases (Sanford 1994; Villani et al. 1997; Einhaus and Sanford 1999; Fahlbusch et al. 1999; Duff et al. 2000; van Effenterre and Boch 2002). Reflecting the heterogeneity of patient groups, recurrence has been reported to occur in 8 to 100% of patients after initial gross total resection. The mean duration of follow-up in these studies ranges from 5 to 10 years (Table 7.3; Hetelekidis et al. 1993; Villani et al. 1997; Fahlbusch et al. 1999; Duff et al. 2000; Kalapurakal et al. 2000). Recurrence following gross total resection can be assumed to occur because of unrecognized deposits of tumor capsule. Even high-quality imaging will miss small rests of epithelium that may eventually develop into recurrent tumors. Although most groups would not offer radiation following a gross total resection, adjunctive therapy following gross total resection has not been satisfactorily explored.

In many cases, only a portion of the tumor can be removed. The main reasons for incomplete tumor removal are adhesions to vessels and vital structures such as the optic nerve and chiasm, and major calcifications (Samii and Tatagiba 1997; Fahlbusch et al. 1999). In patients undergoing subtotal resection without radiation therapy, the recurrence rate is 43 to 75% with mean follow-up of 5 to 7 years (Villani et al. 1997; Fahlbusch et al. 1999; Khoo et al. 2001). For partial resection followed by radiotherapy the recurrence rate was 43 to 54% during a mean follow-up period of 65 to 84 months, comparable to the rate for gross total resection (Villani et al. 1997; Fahlbusch et al. 1999). The management of recurrent tumors is often fraught with difficulties. If a focal recurrence is present on imaging studies, repeat surgical exploration may be warranted. Not surprisingly, recurrent tumors are more difficult to resect and have a gross total resection rate of 13 to 50% via the transcranial approach (Villani et al. 1997; Fahlbusch et al. 1999; Duff et al. 2000) and 53% through the transsphenoidal route (Fahlbusch et al. 1999). The transsphenoidal group probably includes more intrasellar tumors which are physically confined within the bony limits of the sella and are more amenable for repeat surgery. Overall, 81% of patients who underwent surgery (intracranial or transsphenoidal) for recurrent tumor were independent on follow-up at 65 months (Fahlbusch et al. 1999).

Table 7.3. Outcomes of primary surgery, gross total resection, for craniopharyngiomas

Series	Year	Number of patients	Percent (%) recurrence-free survival at indicated time (years)	Percent (%) survival at indicated time (years)
Duff et al.	2000	121	77 at 5	88 at 10
				74 at 15
Kalapurakal et al.	2000	14	92 at 5	100 at 5
			60 at 10	86 at 10
			60 at 10	86 at 10
Fahlbusch et al.	1999	73	87 at 5	93 at 10 [a]
			81 at 10	
Villani et al.	1997	17	82 at 7	94 at 7
Hetelekidis et al.	1993	5	0 at 10	100 at 10

[a] For gross total and subtotal resections

Table 7.4. Outcomes for subtotal resection combined with radiotherapy for patients treated for primary and recurrent disease

Series	Year	Primary disease vs. recurrence	Number of patients	Percent (%) recurrence-free survival at indicated time (years)	Percent (%) survival at indicated time (years)
UCSF	2002	primary	72	89 at 5	88 at 5
				83 at 10	80 at 10
				79 at 15	77 at 15
		recurrence	36	91 at 5	87 at 5
				82 at 10	82 at 10
Habrand et al.	1999	primary and recurrent	37	78 at 5	91 at 5
				57 at 10	65 at 10
Gurkaynak	1994	primary	23	74 at 5	N/A
				62 at 10	
Hetelekidis et al.	1993	primary	37	86 at 10	86 at 10

N/A = not available

Survival of patients with craniopharyngiomas treated with radiation therapy for initial or recurrent disease is comparable to those treated with other modalities (Table 7.4). Overall survival for two recent series of patients treated in a variety of ways at 5, 10, and 15 years was 100%, 68 to 86%, and 59 to 86%, respectively (Bulow et al. 1998; Kalapurakal et al. 2000). At UCSF, the overall survival for patients treated for initial disease with surgery followed by radiation therapy at 5, 10, and, 15 years was 88%, 80%, and 77%, while disease-specific survival probabilities at 5, 10, and 15 years were 97%, 92%, and 92%. Overall survival for patients with recurrent tumors treated with radiation therapy at 5 and 10 years was similar at 87% and 82%, and disease-specific survival at 5 and 10 years was 97% and 91%. These results provide some ammunition for those who argue that radical resection should not be the primary goal for all tumors.

Radiation therapy has been shown to be an effective adjuvant treatment to subtotal surgical resection for initial disease as well as for recurrent disease compared with treatment with surgery alone. In patients treated with primary surgery, recurrence occurred in a median time of 19 months (Duff et al. 2000). In those treated with radiation combined with surgery at UCSF, recurrences occurred from 3 to 125 months, with a median of 41 months. The recurrence rate did not differ between those with radiation therapy for initial and recurrent disease. Overall freedom from progression in patients with initial disease was 89%, 83%, and 79% at 5, 10, and 15 years. Relapse-free survival at 5, 10, and 15 years was 91 to 100% for initial disease, 82 to 83%, and 83% in recurrent tumors treated with surgery and radiation therapy, and 67%, 0%, and 0% for recurrent tumors treated with surgery alone (Kalapurakal et al. 2000). For recurrent tumors, surgery combined with radiotherapy can achieve a much better result than surgery alone. However, Bulow et al. (1998) found that when patients who died within 6 months of therapy are excluded, the advantage of radiation therapy no longer becomes statistically significant. There was also no difference in rate of recurrence with respect to age or extent of surgery (Bulow et al. 1998).

Outcome did not differ between adults and pediatric patients, between papillary and adamantinomatous tumors, or between transsphenoidal and transcranial approaches. Recurrence rate also did not correlate with preoperative radiologic findings (Duff et al. 2000).

7.9 Complications

7.9.1 Complications of Surgery

The surgical resection of craniopharyngiomas is associated with significant risks to endocrine function and vision (Table 7.5). The most common postoperative complication is diabetes insipidus. Diabetes insipidus occurred in 59 to 93% following surgery (Yasargil et al. 1990; Hoffman et al. 1992; Tomita and McLone 1993; Sanford 1994; Fahlbusch et al. 1999; Hoffman et al. 1999; Rilliet et al. 1999). Fahlbusch et al. (1999) noted that normal preoperative anterior pituitary function was maintained in over 50% of patients after surgery, and the incidence of hypogonadism increased only from 77% to 80% . However, other series report that panhypopituitarism occurs in 75 to 100% patients who underwent surgical resection (de Vile et al. 1996a,b; Kalapurakal et al. 2000). Hypothalamic obesity occured in about 40% of patients postoperatively. Weight gains of 12 to 20 kg/yr persist without plateau, and often become the most debilitating aspect of the postoperative course. This phenomenon has been shown to occur due to ventromedial hypothalamus (VMH) damage, which leads to disinhibition of the vagus nerve with resultant insulin hypersecretion. Suppression of insulin secretion has been shown to be effective in preventing or reversing this complication (Lustig et al. 1999). Visual deterioration occurred in 2 to 45% of patients who underwent surgical resection (Pierre-Kahn et al. 1994; Fahlbusch et al. 1999). Minor surgical trauma to the hypothalamus can also cause sleep disorders, memory problems, apathy, and appetite changes (Samii and Tatagiba 1997).

In addition to neurological and endocrinological complications, psychological and social functions are important factors to determine whether a particular therapy is debilitating. Neuropsychological and behavioral disturbances were found in 36 to 60% of children who underwent radical resection (Anderson et al. 1997; Villani et al. 1997; Riva et al. 1998; Kalapurakal et al. 2000). Many of these children are affected by their body images as a result of obesity, which occurred in 36% of children (Kalapurakal et al. 2000). There were no changes in the long-term or short-term memory (Riva et al. 1998; Kalapurakal et al. 2000). A decrease in school performance and an increase in learning disability occurred in 0 to 36% of children (Zuccaro et al. 1996; Villani et al. 1997; Riva et al. 1998). Merchant et al. (2002) found a drop in IQ

Table 7.5. Complications for patients treated with surgery

Series	Year	Number of patients	Diabetes insipidus (%)	Panhypopi- tuitarism (%)	Visual loss (%)
Merchant et al.	2002	15	73	N/A	33 (decreased visual acuity) 40 (decreased visual field)
Kalapurakal et al.	2000	14	100	100	N/A
Duff et al.	2000	31	21	N/A	N/A
Honegger	1999	92	66 (16 at presentation)	N/A	N/A
Rilliet et al.	1999	31	74	74	22
Fahlbusch et al.	1999	89	N/A	N/A	13
Villani et al.	1997	24	81	N/A	19
Hetelekidis et al.	1993	13	79 (14 at presentation)	77	N/A
Yasargil et al.	1990	141	79 (23 at presentation)	N/A	13

N/A = not available

scores by 9.8 points in 15 pediatric patients. While neuropsychological outcome is most often studied in children, adults can have neuropsychological sequelae as well. Donnet et al. (1999) found in a study of 22 adults that 2 (9%) had severe memory and intellectual defects and 3 (14%) had moderate learning defects. In a study of 122 patients, van Effenterre and Boch (2002) found that the rate of normal neuropsychological function was 91% as assessed by patients and their families. Honegger et al. (1998) found that cognitive function in adults remained the same or improved postoperatively.

Complications from the transsphenoidal approach are similar to other surgical approaches except regarding behavioral and visual disturbance. Behavioral disturbance occurred in 9% of children, while only 0 to 1% of adults and children had visual deterioration (Laws 1994; Norris et al. 1998; Fahlbusch et al. 1999; Rilliet et al. 1999). This low complication rate can be attributed to the types of tumors for which the transsphenoidal approach is best suited, namely, intrasellar and cystic tumors, which do not generally affect the hypothalamus.

7.9.2 Complications of Radiotherapy

Radiation therapy results in endocrine dysfunction and visual defects similar to those observed following surgery; however, the severity of these complications, particularly with respect to diabetes insipidus, appears to be reduced (Table 7.6). Duff et al. (2000) found an overall good outcome rate of 60% in a retrospective study of 121 patients with a mean follow-up of 10 years. In a retrospective study of 72 patients at UCSF from 1972 to 1999 treated for initial disease, 32% had visual deficits after subtotal resection followed by radiation, although 81% of these had visual deficits prior to treatment, and 72% retained the same functional status. For 36 patients treated for recurrent disease, only 53% retained the same functional status with no difference associated with extent of surgical resection, while 78% had permanent deficits. A majority of patients had impaired endocrine function. Sixty-four percent required thyroid hormone replacement, 56% required cortisol, 44%

required sex hormones, 17% had diabetes insipidus, and 1% had elevated prolactin levels. The endocrinologic sequelae of radiotherapy compares with other series which report 6 to 38% incidence of diabetes insipidus after radiation therapy, much lower than that of patients who have undergone total resection (Einhaus and Sanford 1999). In a series by Regine et al. (1993), the incidence of endocrinologic sequelae is correlated with both age and maximum dose of radiation, being 80% in children and 26% in adults for doses greater than 61 Gy, and 36% in children and 13% in adults for doses less than 61 Gy .

The consequences of partial- or whole-brain radiation on intellectual function are much greater in younger children (Weiss et al. 1989). In children less than 3 years of age treated with either partial- or whole-brain radiation for various brain tumors not including craniopharyngiomas, 60% were mentally retarded with IQ less than 69. The incidence of mental retardation/dementia and vascular complications of radiation therapy for craniopharyngioma is highly correlated with the maximum dose, being 40% in children and 45% in adults for doses greater than 61 Gy versus 0% in children and adults at doses less than 61 Gy (Regine et al. 1993). In children who had received radiotherapy, 32 to 33% had poor school performance or required special schooling due to moderate to severe learning disability after treatment (Zuccaro et al. 1996; Habrand et al. 1999). Merchant et al. found a drop in IQ scores of 1.25 points in 15 children treated with limited surgery and radiation compared with 9.8 points in the surgery-only group (Merchant et al. 2002). Although the results of the damaging effects of radiation on the intellectual function of young children less than 3 years of age was not studied particularly in craniopharyngiomas, we do not recommend radiation therapy as an adjuvant therapy in children under 3 years of age who have undergone a subtotal resection unless they become symptomatic.

Other complications of radiation therapy seen in our series at UCSF and other series include radiation-induced neoplasms (glioblastoma, sarcoma, meningioma), radiation necrosis, vascular occlusion, radiation vasculitis, optic neuritis, dementia, calcification of basal ganglia, hypothalamic–pituitary dysfunc-

Table 7.6. Complications in patients treated with surgery and radiotherapy

Series	Year	Number of patients	Diabetes insipidus (%)	Panhypopituitarism (%)	Visual loss (%)
UCSF	2002	72 (primary disease)	17	N/A	0
		36 (recurrent disease)	72		0
Merchant et al.	2002	14	33	N/A	33 decreased visual acuity
					60 decreased visual field
Habrand et al.	1999	37	66 (22 % at presentation)	97 (22 at presentation)	0
Hetelekidis et al.	1993	34	38 (25 % at presentation)	53	N/A

N/A = not available, not reported

tion, hypothalamic obesity, and decreased intellect in children (Einhaus and Sanford 1999; Moore and Couldwell 2000; B. Fisch 2002, personal communication; Lustig et al. 2003).

7.10 Conclusion

Despite recent advances in treatment options, craniopharyngiomas remain a challenging disease. The data and experience reported in the literature do not allow a definitive recommendation to be made. In general, for tumors that do not appear to invade the hypothalamus, an attempt at gross total resection should be attempted. Attempts at gross total resection in the face of hypothalamic involvement should be avoided given the unacceptable long-term functional sequelae. Subtotal resection and treatment with external beam radiation remains an acceptable option, the aim of which is tumor control rather than removal of all neoplastic tissue. Other therapies such as intracavitary bleomycin and systemic chemotherapy either remain restricted to specific tumor subtypes or are still experimental in nature. More data are needed to understand the long-term psychological and social consequences of treatment.

References

Anderson CA, Wilkening GN et al (1997) Neurobehavioral outcome in pediatric craniopharyngioma. Pediatr Neurosurg 26:255–260

Barbosa M, Rios O et al (2001) Acetylcholinesterase and butyrylcholinesterase histochemical activities and tumor cell growth in several brain tumors. Surg Neurol 55:106–112

Barloon TJ, Yuh WT et al (1988) Frontal lobe implantation of craniopharyngioma by repeated needle aspirations. AJNR Am J Neuroradiol 9:406–407

Blackburn TP, Doughty D et al (1999) Stereotactic intracavitary therapy of recurrent cystic craniopharyngioma by instillation of 90yttrium. Br J Neurosurg 13:359–365

Bulow B, Attewell R et al (1998) Postoperative prognosis in craniopharyngioma with respect to cardiovascular mortality, survival, and tumor recurrence. J Clin Endocrinol Metab 83:3897–3904

Bunin GR, Surawicz TS et al (1998) The descriptive epidemiology of craniopharyngioma. J Neurosurg 89:547–551

Cavalheiro S, Sparapani FV et al (1996) Use of bleomycin in intratumoral chemotherapy for cystic craniopharyngioma. Case report. J Neurosurg 84:124–126

Chiou SM, Lunsford LD et al (2001) Stereotactic radiosurgery of residual or recurrent craniopharyngioma, after surgery, with or without radiation therapy. Neurooncology 3:159–166

Chung WY, Pan DH et al (2000) Gamma knife radiosurgery for craniopharyngiomas. J Neurosurg 93 [Suppl 3]:47–56

De Divitiis E, Cappabianca P et al (2000) The role of the endoscopic transsphenoidal approach in pediatric neurosurgery. Childs Nerv Syst 16:692–696

De Vile CJ, Grant DB et al (1996a) Growth and endocrine sequelae of craniopharyngioma. Arch Dis Child 75:108–114

De Vile CJ, Grant DB et al (1996b) Management of childhood craniopharyngioma: can the morbidity of radical surgery be predicted? J Neurosurg 85:73–81

Donnet A, Schmitt A et al (1999) Neuropsychological follow-up of twenty two adult patients after surgery for craniopharyngioma. Acta Neurochir (Wien) 141:1049–1054

Donovan JL, Nesbit GM (1996) Distinction of masses involving the sella and suprasellar space: specificity of imaging features. AJR Am J Roentgenol 167:597–603

Duff JM, Meyer FB et al (2000) Long-term outcomes for surgically resected craniopharyngiomas. Neurosurgery 46:291–305

Einhaus SL, Sanford RA (1999) Craniopharyngiomas. In: Albright L, Pollack I, Adelson D (eds) Principles and practice of pediatric neurosurgery. Thieme, New York

Fahlbusch R, Honneger J et al (1999) Surgical treatment of craniopharyngiomas. J Neurosurg 90:237–250

Fischbein NJ, Dillon WP et al (2000) Teaching atlas of brain imaging. Thieme, New York

Fisher PG, Jenab J et al (1998) Outcomes and failure patterns in childhood craniopharyngiomas. Childs Nerv Syst 14:558–563

Gupta K, Kuhn MJ et al (1999) Metastatic craniopharyngioma. AJNR Am J Neuroradiol 20:1059–1060

Habrand JL, Ganry O et al (1999) The role of radiation therapy in the management of craniopharyngioma: a 25-year experience and review of the literature. Int J Radiat Oncol Biol Phys 44:255–263

Hader WJ, Steinbok P et al (2000) Intratumoral therapy with bleomycin for cystic craniopharyngiomas in children. Pediatr Neurosurg 33:211–218

Harwood-Nash DC (1994) Neuroimaging of childhood craniopharyngioma. Pediatr Neurosurg 21 [Suppl 1]:2–10

Hayward R (1999) The present and future management of childhood craniopharyngioma. Childs Nerv Syst 15:764–769

Hetelekidis S, Barnes PD et al (1993) 20-year experience in childhood craniopharyngioma. Int J Radiat Oncol Biol Phys 27:189–195

Hoffman HJ, de Silva M et al (1992) Aggressive surgical management of craniopharyngiomas in children. J Neurosurg 76:47–52

Hoffman HJ, Drake JM et al (1999) Craniopharyngiomas and pituitary tumors. In: Choux M, di Rocco C, Hockley AD, Walker ML (eds) Pediatric neurosurgery. Churchill Livingstone, New York

Honegger J, Barocka A et al (1998) Neuropsychological results of craniopharyngioma surgery in adults: a prospective study. Surg Neurol 50:19–28

Israel ZH, Pomeranz S (1995) Intracranial craniopharyngioma seeding following radical resection. Pediatr Neurosurg 22:210–213

Ito M, Jamshidi J et al (2001) Does craniopharyngioma metastasize? Case report and review of the literature. Neurosurgery 48:933–935; discussion 935–936

Jakacki RI, Cohen B. H et al (2000) Phase II evaluation of interferon-alpha-2a for progressive or recurrent craniopharyngiomas. J Neurosurg 92:255–260

Kalapurakal JA, Goldman S et al (2000) Clinical outcome in children with recurrent craniopharyngioma after primary surgery. Cancer J 6:388–393

Kernohan JW (1971) Tumors of congenital origin. In: Minckler J (ed) Pathology of central nervous system. McGraw-Hill, New York, pp 1927–1937

Khoo LT, Flagel J et al (2001) Craniopharyngiomas: surgical management. In: Petrovich P, Brady LW, Apuzzo ML, Bamberg M (eds) Combined modality therapy of central nervous system tumors. Springer, Berlin Heidelberg New York, pp 187–214

Kobayashi T, Tanaka T et al (1994) Stereotactic gamma radiosurgery of craniopharyngiomas. Pediatr Neurosurg 21 [Suppl 1]:69–74

Kristopaitis T, Thomas C et al (2000) Malignant craniopharyngioma. Arch Pathol Lab Med 124:1356–1360

Laws ER Jr (1994) Transsphenoidal removal of craniopharyngioma. Pediatr Neurosurg 21 [Suppl 1]:57–63

Lee JH, Kim CY et al (1999) Postoperative ectopic seeding of craniopharyngioma. Case illustration. J Neurosurg 90:796

Leksell L, Liden K (1952) A therapeutic trial with radioactive isotope in cystic brain tumor: radioisotope techniques I. Med Physiol Appl 1:1–4

Lunsford LD, Pollock BE et al (1994) Stereotactic options in the management of craniopharyngioma. Pediatr Neurosurg 21 [Suppl 1]: 90–97

Lustig RH (2002) Hypothalamic obesity: the sixth cranial endocrinopathy. Endocrinologist 12:210–217

Lustig RH, Post SR et al (2003) Risk factors for obesity in children surviving brain tumors. J Clin Endocrinol Metab 88:611–616

Lustig RH, Rose SR et al (1999) Hypothalamic obesity caused by cranial insult in children: altered glucose and insulin dynamics and reversal by a somatostatin agonist. J Pediatr 135:162–168

Malik JM, Cosgrove GR et al (1992) Remote recurrence of craniopharyngioma in the epidural space. Case report. J Neurosurg 77:804–807

Matsuo M, Yonemitsu N et al (2001) Expression of prostaglandin H synthetase-2 in human brain tumors. Acta Neuropathol (Wien) 102:181–187

Merchant TE, Kiehna EN et al (2002) Craniopharyngioma: the St Jude Children's Research Hospital experience 1984–2001. Int J Radiat Oncol Biol Phys 53:533–542

Miller DC (1994) Pathology of craniopharyngiomas: clinical import of pathological findings. Pediatr Neurosurg 21 [Suppl 1]:11–17

Mokry M (1999) Craniopharyngiomas: a six year experience with Gamma Knife radiosurgery. Stereotact Funct Neurosurg 72 [Suppl 1]:140–149

Moore K, Couldwell WT (2000) Craniopharyngioma. In: Bernstein M, Berger MS (eds) Neuro-oncology: the essentials. Thieme, New York

Moore K, Persaud TVN (1993) The developing human: clinically oriented embryology. Saunders, Philadelphia

Nakamizo A, Inamura T et al (2001) Neuroendoscopic treatment of cystic craniopharyngioma in the third ventricle. Minim Invasive Neurosurg 44:85–87

Norris JS, Pavaresh M et al (1998) Primary transsphenoidal microsurgery in the treatment of craniopharyngiomas. Br J Neurosurg 12:305–312

Nozaki M, Tada M et al (1998) Rare occurrence of inactivating *p53* gene mutations in primary non-astrocytic tumors of the central nervous system: reappraisal by yeast functional assay. Acta Neuropathol (Berl) 95:291–296

Pierre-Kahn A, Sainte-Rose C et al (1994) Surgical approach to children with craniopharyngiomas and severely impaired vision: special considerations. Pediatr Neurosurg 21 [Suppl 1]:50–56

Pollock BE, Lunsford LD et al (1995) Phosphorus-32 intracavitary irradiation of cystic craniopharyngiomas: current technique and long-term results. Int J Radiat Oncol Biol Phys 33:437–446

Raghavan R, Dickey WT Jr et al (2000) Proliferative activity in craniopharyngiomas: clinicopathological correlations in adults and children. Surg Neurol 54:241–247

Ragoowansi AT, Piepgras DG (1991) Postoperative ectopic craniopharyngioma. Case report. J Neurosurg 74:653–655

Regine WF, Mohiuddin M et al (1993) Long-term results of pediatric and adult craniopharyngiomas treated with combined surgery and radiation. Radiother Oncol 27:13–21

Rilliet B, de Paul Djientcheu V et al (1999) Craniopharyngiomas, results in children and adolescents operated through a transsphenoidal approach compared with an intracranial approach. Front Radiat Ther Oncol 33:114–122

Riva D, Pantaleoni C et al (1998) Late neuropsychological and behavioural outcome of children surgically treated for craniopharyngioma. Childs Nerv Syst 14:179–184

Samii M, Tatagiba M (1997) Surgical management of craniopharyngiomas: a review. Neurol Med Chir (Tokyo) 37:141–149

Sanford RA (1994) Craniopharyngioma: results of survey of the American Society of Pediatric Neurosurgery. Pediatr Neurosurg 21 [Suppl 1]:39–43

Sanford RA, Muhlbauer MS (1991) Craniopharyngioma in children. Neurol Clin 9:453–465

Sarubi JC, Bei H, et al (2001) Clonal composition of human adamantinomatous craniopharyngiomas and somatic mutation analyses of the patched (PTCH), Gsalpha und Gi2alpha genes. Neurosci Lett 310:5–8

Sheline GE, Wara WM et al (1980) Therapeutic irradiation and brain injury. Int J Radiat Oncol Biol Phys 6:1215–1228

Sidawy MK, Jannotta FS (1997) Intraoperative cytologic diagnosis of lesions of the central nervous system. Am J Clin Pathol 108 [4 Suppl 1]:S56–S66

Takahashi H, Nakazawa S et al (1985) Evaluation of postoperative intratumoral injection of bleomycin for craniopharyngioma in children. J Neurosurg 62:120–127

Tarbell NJ, Barnes P et al (1994) Advances in radiation therapy for craniopharyngiomas. Pediatr Neurosurg 21 [Suppl 1]: 101–107

Thapar K, Stefaneanu L et al (1994) Estrogen receptor gene expression in craniopharyngiomas: an in situ hybridization study. Neurosurgery 35:1012–1017

Tomita T, McLone DG (1993) Radical resections of childhood craniopharyngiomas. Pediatr Neurosurg 19:6–14

Van Effenterre R, Boch A (2002) Craniopharyngioma in adults and children: a study of 122 surgical cases. J Neurosurg 97:3–11

Vidal S, Kovacs K et al (2002) Angiogenesis in patients with craniopharyngiomas: correlation with treatment and outcome. Cancer 94:738–745

Villani RM, Tomei G et al (1997) Long-term results of treatment for craniopharyngioma in children. Childs Nerv Syst 13: 397–405

Voges J, Sturm V et al (1997) Cystic craniopharyngioma: long-term results after intracavitary irradiation with stereotactically applied colloidal beta-emitting radioactive sources. Neurosurgery 40:263–269

Weiner HL, Wisoff JH et al (1994) Craniopharyngiomas: a clinicopathological analysis of factors predictive of recurrence and functional outcome. Neurosurgery 35:1001–1010

Weiss M, Sutton L et al (1989) The role of radiation therapy in the management of childhood craniopharyngioma. Int J Radiat Oncol Biol Phys 17:1313–1321

Wilson JD, Foster DW et al (1998) Williams textbook of endocrinology. Saunders, Philadelphia

Yasargil MG, Curcic M et al (1990) Total removal of craniopharyngiomas. Approaches and long-term results in 144 patients. J Neurosurg 73:3–11

Yu X, Liu Z et al (2000) Combined treatment with stereotactic intracavitary irradiation and gamma knife surgery for craniopharyngiomas. Stereotact Funct Neurosurg 75:117–122

Zuccaro G, Jaimovich R et al (1996) Complications in paediatric craniopharyngioma treatment. Childs Nerv Syst 12:385–390

Neuronal Tumors

C. S. von Koch · M. H. Schmidt · V. Perry

8.1 Ganglioglioma and Gangliocytoma

Gangliocytoma and ganglioglioma represent a family of rare, slow-growing, neuronal tumors. The term "ganglioglioma" was first introduced by Courville in 1930 to describe the mixed neuronal and glial elements typically seen in this tumor (Courville 1930).

8.1.1 Epidemiology

Gangliogliomas and gangliocytomas are rare, only accounting for 0.4% of all CNS tumors and 1.3% of all brain tumors (Zulch 1986; Kalyan and Olivero 1987). A somewhat higher percentage of 7.6% was described in one series of pediatric brain tumors (Johannsson et al. 1981). The male: female ratio varies among different series from 1.1:1 to 1.9:1, but supports a slight male predominance (Hirose et al. 1997; Lang et al. 1993; Prayson et al. 1995; Wolf et al. 1988). The mean age at diagnosis in a series of 99 children was 9.5 years and the male: female ratio was 1:1 (Johnson et al. 1997).

8.1.2 Pathology

Gangliogliomas are slow-growing tumors that can occur throughout the CNS. They occur mostly in the supratentorial region, primarily the temporal lobe, but the frontal lobes and the floor of the third ventricle are also common locations. Less frequently, they have been seen in the cerebellum, brain stem, spinal cord, pituitary, and pineal regions (Hirose et al. 1997; Lang et al. 1993; Prayson et al. 1995; Wolf et al. 1988; Kalyan and Olivero 1987).

8.1.2.1 Gross Appearance

These tumors can be either solid or cystic. Cystic masses are often associated with a mural nodule (defined as a solid tumor component eccentrically located at the margin of the cyst). Some tumors contain varying degrees of calcification. Mass effect, hemorrhage, and necrosis are rare.

8.1.2.2 Histopathology

Gangliocytomas consist of groups of large, multipolar neurons with dysplastic features. The surrounding stroma contains non-neoplastic glial elements and a network of reticulin fibers (Fig. 8.1b). Gangliocytomas are typically classified as WHO grade I tumors. Gangliogliomas, in contrast to gangliocytomas, contain neoplastic glial cells, usually astrocytes, and can be classified as either WHO grade I or II. Necrosis is absent unless the glial component undergoes malignant transformation. Tumors with evidence of malignant transformation are anaplastic gangliogliomas. Typically, tumors are well circumscribed and mitoses are rare. Perivascular lymphocytic infiltration is common, but not specific.

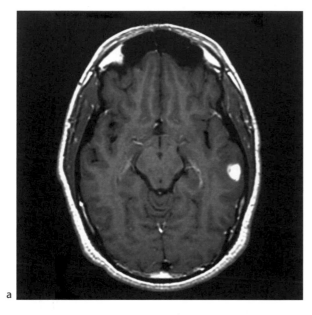

a

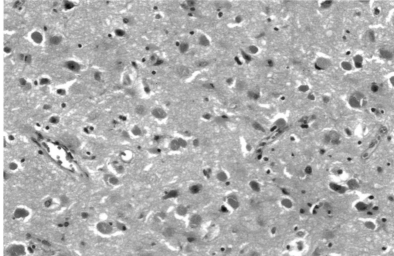

b

Figure 8.1 a,b

Ganglioglioma. **a** T1-weighted axial MRI with gadolinium of a ganglioglioma in the left temporal lobe. Nodular enhancement is seen **b** Hematoxylin and eosin staining reveals large, dysplastic neurons and a neoplastic glial component. Necrosis is not seen

8.1.2.3 Immunohistochemistry and Electron Microscopy

Immunohistochemical staining techniques are crucial for identifying neuronal and astrocytic features within these tumors. Positive staining for synaptophysin, neuropeptides, and biogenic amines are typically associated with a neuronal phenotype. Similarly, positive staining for glial fibrillary acid protein (GFAP) marks the astrocytic component of ganglioglioma. Electron microscopy can also be helpful in identifying additional neuronal features. Frequent findings include dense core granules and synaptic junctions (Hirose et al. 1997; Lantos et al. 1996; Miller et al. 1993).

8.1.2.4 Cytogenetics

In a few cases, abnormal karyotypes have been observed. Specific cytogenetic abnormalities include a ring chromosome 1, trisomy of chromosomes 5 to 7, and deletion of chromosome 6 (Neumann et al. 1993). Analysis for microsatellite marker instability in tumor DNA from 6 gangliogliomas found no abnormalities (Zhu et al. 1996). One series of ganglioglioma patients reported a comparatively high frequency of splice-site-associated single nucleotide polymorphism in the tuberous sclerosis 2 gene (*TSC2*). This may suggest an underlying genetic susceptibility (Platten et al. 1997) for sporadic ganglioglioma, although the underlying biologic mechanism remains undefined.

8.1.3 Clinical Features

Seizure is the most common presenting symptom of supratentorial tumors. The seizure history is often longstanding, with a mean duration prior to diagnosis ranging from 6 to 25 years in different series (Lang et al. 1993; Prayson et al. 1995; Wolf et al. 1988). In one series of patients examined, temporal lobe gangliogliomas represent 40% of all tumors causing chronic temporal-lobe epilepsy (Blumcke et al. 1999). The mean duration of symptoms prior to diagnosis for tumors of the brain stem or spinal cord is approximately one year (Lang et al. 1993). Patients with brainstem lesions commonly present with involvement of the motor tracts: weakness, spasticity, and gait disturbance. Gangliogliomas of the spinal cord may involve the entire spinal cord and typically produce scoliosis, gait disturbance, and progressive weakness (Park et al. 1993; Hamburger et al. 1997). These symptoms can be very longstanding. Patients with midline tumors develop symptoms and signs of hydrocephalus, such as headache, papilledema, alterations in the level of consciousness, and nausea or vomiting (Haddad et al. 1992).

8.1.4 Natural History

Gangliogliomas are indolent, slow-growing tumors. Without resection, patients often have prolonged courses of disease, depending on the location of the primary mass. Anaplastic glial changes in ganglioglioma, as well as high MIB-1 labeling indices, may be markers for more aggressive tumor behavior (Hirose et al. 1997; Kalyan and Olivero 1987; Prayson et al. 1995). Malignant transformation is rare, although one report notes that this occurs in up to 3% of gangliogliomas (Sasaki et al. 1996; Hakim et al. 1997).

8.1.5 Diagnosis and Neuroimaging

Initial diagnostic evaluation begins with detailed neuroimaging. No specific laboratory tests are available to allow a diagnosis. CT, performed as a screening test, usually reveals an iso- to hypodense solid or cystic mass. Cysts may be associated with a mural nodule, and both cyst and nodule are well circumscribed (Dorne et al. 1986). Calcifications may be present and contrast enhancement is usually seen, but occasionally can be minimal or absent. Scalloping of the overlying calvarium, presumably longstanding, has also been described.

MRI is required to adequately delineate the mass. Tumors are usually hypointense on T1-weighted images and hyperintense on T2-weighted images. Mass effect and edema are minimal. Contrast enhance-

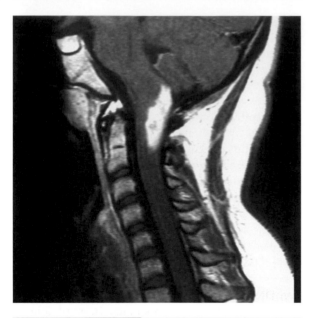

Figure 8.2

An unusual case of a ganglioglioma of the upper cervical spinal cord. The patient is a fourteen year old girl who presented with paresthesias over the left side of the neck. The sagittal T1-weighted post-contrast MRI shows a well demarcated mass arising in the dorsal portion of the spinal cord

ment varies in intensity and may be nodular, rim-like, or entirely solid (Figs. 8.1a, 8.2; Grossman and Yousem 1994; Osborne 1994). Syringobulbia or syringomyelia can be seen with spinal cord gangliogliomas (Park et al. 1993; Hamburger et al. 1997). MR spectroscopy is usually of limited value due to the indolent nature of these tumors. Angiography, rarely necessary, shows an avascular mass.

8.1.6 Treatment

Complete surgical resection is the treatment of choice, and when achievable is usually curative (Sutton et al. 1983, 1987; Ventureyra et al. 1986). The neoplasm itself contains no functioning nervous tissue. Postoperative MRI is useful for assessing the extent of resection, and follow-up surveillance neuroimaging can be done to evaluate for recurrence. Radiation therapy should be considered for tumor recurrence when further resection is not feasible. Tumors with malignant features (anaplastic features, high MIB labeling index) may require radiation as an adjuvant therapy, regardless of the extent of resection (Selch et al. 1998; Wolf et al. 1994; Hakim et al. 1997; Lang et al. 1993; Johannsson et al. 1981). The impact of radiotherapy on progression-free survival for incompletely resected benign tumors remains uncertain (Lang et al. 1993; Haddad et al. 1992). As the role of radiation therapy in the setting of a low-grade, indolent, subtotally resected tumor is unclear, it is important to weigh the risks of radiotherapy in pediatric patients against the benefits.

8.1.7 Outcome

Patients who undergo gross total resection enjoy an excellent prognosis (Khajavi et al. 1995; Sutton et al. 1983, 1987; Ventureyra et al. 1986). Tumor location is a significant predictor of outcome, most likely as a marker of resectability. Ninety-five percent of patients with hemispheric gangliogliomas remained disease free at 5 years, whereas only 53% of patients with brainstem gangliogliomas remained disease free at 3 years (Lang et al. 1993). Patients who undergo subtotal excisions, most commonly seen in patients with midline tumors, are at higher risk of tumor progression or recurrence (Haddad et al. 1992). The importance of anaplasia as a prognostic feature is unclear, with different series demonstrating conflicting results (Kalyan et al. 1987; Lang et al. 1993; Hall et al. 1986; Ventureyra et al. 1986). Retrospective analysis of one series of 34 patients, however, did demonstrate a correlation between improved survival and degree of resection as well as tumor grade (Selch et al. 1998). For patients with tumor-associated epilepsy, seizure control improves significantly after tumor resection (Haddad et al. 1992; Ventureyra et al. 1986).

8.2 Dysembryoplastic Neuroepithelial Tumor (DNET)

Dysembryoplastic neuroepithelial tumor was first described by Daumas-Duport and Scheithauer in 1988 (Daumas-Duport et al. 1988). The initial series described 39 children with a morphologically dis-

tinct brain tumor and intractable partial seizures. DNET is a benign glial–neuronal neoplasm that most commonly occurs in the supratentorial compartment.

8.2.1 Epidemiology

DNET mostly affects children and young adults in the second and third decade of life. The age at onset of seizures ranged from 2 to 18 years with a mean of 9 years (Daumas-Duport et al. 1988). True population incidence of DNET is difficult to characterize. In two different series of patients with epilepsy, the incidence of DNET ranged from 0.8 % (Wolf and Wiestler 1995) to 5 % (Morris et al. 1993). In a retrospective review of all neuroepithelial tumors at a single institution, DNETs were found in 0.6 % of patients including all ages, in 1.2 % of patients under 20 years, and in 0.2 % of patients over 20 years of age (Rosemberg and Vieira 1998). Males are more frequently affected than females (Daumas-Duport et al. 2000).

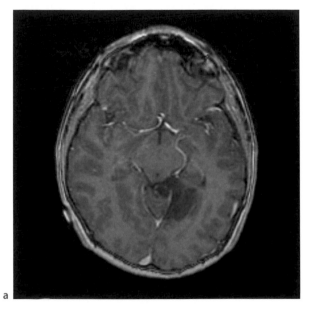

a

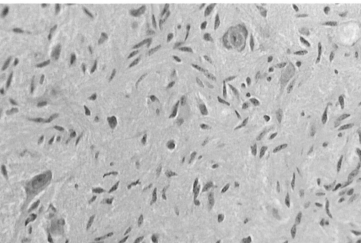

b

Figure 8.3 a,b

Dysembryoplastic neuroepithelial tumor (DNET). a T1-weighted axial MRI with gadolinium of a DNET in the mesial left temporal lobe. No enhancement or peritumoral edema is seen. b Hematoxylin and eosin staining in a complex form of DNET shows nuclear atypia of glioneuronal elements. Astrocytic, oligodendrocytic, and neuronal components are present to varying degrees

8.2.2 Pathology

8.2.2.1 Gross Appearance

The tumor expands the cortex predominantly, however, underlying white matter may be involved, especially in the temporal lobes (Daumas-Duport 1993). Distended cortical ribbons consisting of gelatinous glioneuronal elements and smaller, firmer glial nodules are seen.

8.2.2.2 Histopathology

The pathologically distinct feature is the glioneuronal element, which consists of columns of axon bundles lined with small S100 positive and GFAP negative oligodendroglia-like cells (Fig. 8.3b). Oligodendroglia-like cells have minimal cytoplasm and are rich in mucopolysaccharides. Mature neuronal cells are found interspersed within the tumor and adjacent cortical dysplasia can be found. Smaller glial nodules are found along the tumor borders of the complex variant of DNETs. In contrast to gangliogliomas, atypical neurons resembling ganglion cells and perivascular lymphocytes are not found with DNETs (Armstrong 1993; Daumas-Duport et al. 1988; Daumas-Duport 1993; Hirose et al. 1994; Raymond et al. 1994). DNETs are usually designated as WHO grade I.

8.2.2.3 Immunohistochemistry and Molecular Genetics

Neuronal elements stain positive for synaptophysin and neuronal nuclear antigen (NeuN; Wolf et al. 1997). Glial nodules stain positive for GFAP (glial fibrillary acidic protein). Proliferation potential is very low and MIB-1 labeling indices vary from 0% to 8% (Daumas-Duport 1993; Prayson and Estes 1992; Taratuto et al. 1995). Specific cytogenetic or molecular findings have not been reported for DNETs. They have been reported in patients with neurofibromatosis type I, although the overall incidence is unknown. The molecular changes within the DNETs in these patients have not been characterized (Lellouch et al. 1995).

8.2.3 Clinical Features

DNETs are associated with chronic, intractable partial seizures and account for 25% of all lesions resected for medically refractory epilepsy (Wolf et al. 1993, 1995; Raymond et al. 1995; Pasquier et al. 1996). Most DNETs are located in the supratentorial region, especially the temporal lobe; however, various locations corresponding to the topography of the secondary germinal layers have been described, including basal ganglia, thalamus, cerebellum, and pons (Cervera-Pierot et al. 1997; Kuchelmeister et al. 1995; Leung et al. 1994). Multifocal locations have been described, including temporal lobe, third ventricle, and basal ganglia in one case, and temporal lobe, thalami, cerebellum, and pons in a separate case (Leung et al. 1994).

8.2.4 Natural History

Without resection, medically intractable seizures are likely to persist. Tumor progression is rare with partially resected DNETs (Daumas-Duport et al. 1988; Daumas-Duport 1993; Raymond et al. 1994; Taratuto et al. 1995). Subtotally resected lesions can remain quiescent for extended periods of time.

8.2.5 Diagnosis and Neuroimaging

Appearance on unenhanced CT ranges from iso- to hypodense, often with calcifications and occasionally with true cyst formation. One-third of tumors show contrast enhancement, and the overlying calvarium may be remodeled, consistent with the chronic nature of the tumor (Daumas-Duport 1993; Kuroiwa et al. 1995). DNETs are cortically based and may appear as macrogyri. Usually, the lesion involves the thickness of the normal cortex. With MRI, the tumor is hypointense on T1-weighted and hyperintense on T2-weighted images (Fig. 8.3a). No peritumoral edema or mass effect is seen. Enhancement is seen in one-third of tumors (Daumas-Duport 1993; Kuroiwa et al. 1995; Koeller and Dillon 1992).

A definitive diagnosis of DNET is difficult to obtain with neuroimaging alone. However, the combination of partial seizures before age 20 years, lack of progressive neurologic deficit, cortical involvement on MRI, and absence of mass effect or edema on CT or MRI is highly suggestive of DNET (Daumas-Duport 1995). Differentiation must be made from low-grade gliomas, especially oligodendrogliomas, as management strategies differ significantly.

8.2.6 Treatment

Surgical resection is curative. Recurrence has not been reported, therefore radiation or chemotherapy are not indicated (Raymond et al. 1995). Again, it is important to differentiate DNET from oligodendroglioma to avoid unnecessarily aggressive therapy.

8.2.7 Outcome

DNETs are benign lesions. A high MIB-1 labeling index does not impact prognosis (Daumas-Duport 1993). Neither clinical nor radiographic tumor progression was seen in patients that underwent gross total or even subtotal resections (Daumas-Duport et al. 1988; Daumas-Duport 1993; Raymond et al. 1994; Taratuto et al. 1995). Resection results in high rate of seizure control.

8.3 Central Neurocytoma

8.3.1 Epidemiology

Despite their increased recognition, central neurocytomas remain rare neoplasms of the central nervous system. Central neurocytomas account for only 0.25 to 0.5% of brain tumors and are primarily tumors of adolescents and young adults (Hassoun et al. 1993). In an analysis of 207 cases, the mean age of presentation was 29 years, with a range from 8 days to 67 years (Hassoun et al. 1993; Figarella-Branger et al. 2000). Most patients (72%) present between the ages of 20 to 40 years. The incidence is similar in males and females with a ratio of 1.02:1 (Hassoun et al. 1993; Figarella-Branger et al. 2000).

8.3.2 Pathology

In 1993 Hassoun et al. reviewed the literature of 127 published cases and summarized the clinical and histological features.

8.3.2.1 Gross Appearance

These tumors are lobulated, well-circumscribed masses that are gray in color, similar to normal cortex. They typically occur in close proximity to the foramen of Monro and may be attached to the septum pellucidum. Necrosis and cyst formation are frequently seen, and some neurocytomas are very vascular. Intra-tumoral hemorrhage is unusual.

8.3.2.2 Histopathology

The histopathologic appearance of a central neurocytoma can be similar to that of an oligodendroglioma (von Deimling et al. 1990). Both neoplasms have small uniform cells with rounded nuclei and scant cytoplasm resembling perinuclear halos (the so-called "fried egg" appearance) and many intraventricular tumors previously diagnosed as oligodendrogliomas may actually have been central neurocytomas (von Deimling et al. 1990). The cytoplasm is ill defined and the nuclei are round to slightly lobulated (Fig. 8.4b). The tumor cells are dense in some areas and alternate with anuclear, less dense tumor parts. The anuclear areas in particular may have a fine fibrillary matrix. Delicate vasculature forms a branching network in a pattern similar to that found in oligodendrogliomas. Focal calcification can be seen. Mitotic figures are absent or infrequent and endothelial proliferation and necrosis are uncommon.

8.3.2.3 Immunohistochemistry and Electron Microscopy

Immunostaining for neuron-specific enolase (NSE) and synaptophysin confirm the neuronal nature of the neoplasm (von Deimling et al. 1991). GFAP staining may represent neoplastic or reactive astrocytes. It has been suggested that central neurocytomas origi-nate from bipotential (neuronal and astrocytic) pro-genitor cells in the periventricular region that persist into adulthood (von Deimling et al. 1991). An ultra-structural feature that distinguishes central neurocy-tomas from oligodendroglioma is the high degree of neuronal maturation. Electron microscopy demon-strates clear and dense core vesicles, microtubules, and synapse formation.

8.3.2.4 Cytogenetics and Molecular Genetics

Comparative genomic hybridization (CGH) analysis was used to identify losses and gains in DNA se-quences in 10 histologically confirmed central neuro-cytomas (Yin et al. 2000). Genomic alterations were found in 6 tumors. Gain in genetic material was found for chromosomes 2p and 10q in 4 tumors, chromosome 18q in 3 tumors, and chromosome 13q in two tumors. Gains in chromosome 7 were reported in 3 out 7 central neurocytomas using fluorescence in situ hybridization (FISH; Taruscio et al. 1997). No specific gene alterations have been described in cen-tral neurocytoma. The *p53* tumor suppressor gene was screened for mutations in central neurocytoma, but none were found (Ohgaki et al. 1993).

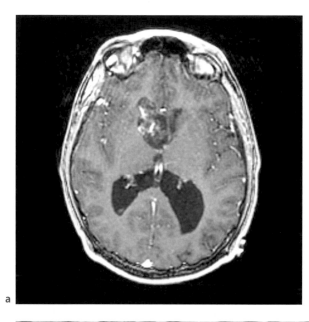

a

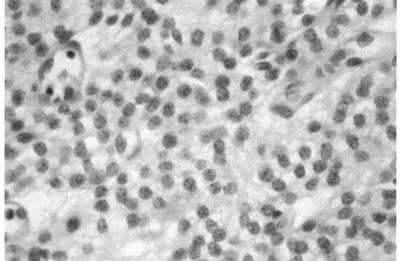

b

Figure 8.4 a,b

Central neurocytoma. a T1-weighted axial MRI with gado-linium of a typical central neuro-cytoma arising in the frontal horn of the right lateral ventri-cle. A heterogeneous pattern of enhancement is seen. b Hema-toxylin and eosin staining dem-onstrates cells with uniform round to oval nuclei with speck-led chromatin and an occasional nucleolus. Anaplastic features are not seen

8.3.3 Clinical Features

Patients present with symptoms attributable to raised intracranial pressure. As expected, these consist of headaches and visual changes; the duration of clinical symptoms and signs is typically less than 6 months. Ninety-three percent of patients complained of headaches, 37% had visual changes, and 30% experienced nausea and vomiting at presentation. Less commonly, patients complained of paresthesias (19%), lethargy (11%), balance problems (11%), and tinnitus (7%) (Schild et al. 1997). Most of these symptoms can be attributed to increased intracranial pressure secondary to obstructive hydrocephalus. The most common presenting signs were papilledema and ataxia.

8.3.4 Natural History

While most central neurocytomas have benign histology, they have been observed to recur, and can even disseminate along the CSF pathways (Eng et al. 1997; Yasargil et al. 1992). Although anaplasia has been demonstrated in central neurocytomas, the influence of this feature on prognosis is uncertain (Chang et al. 1993; von Deimling et al. 1990, 1991; Yasargil et al. 1992). An increase in GFAP positivity and vascular proliferation might suggest a more malignant course (Elek et al. 1999).

Most reports indicate that central neurocytomas have limited growth potential (Sharma et al. 1998; Söylemezoglu et al. 1997). Markers of proliferation have been studied in order to clarify the biological behavior of neurocytomas. A study with 36 central neurocytomas suggested that an MIB-1 labeling index (LI) of 2% might be predictive for recurrence (Söylemezoglu et al. 1997). Patients with an MIB-1 LI under 2% had a 22% relapse compared to relapse rate of 63% when the MIB-1 LI was over 2% for the observation period of 150 months (Söylemezoglu et al. 1997). Interestingly, an MIB-1 LI above 2% correlated with microvascular proliferation (Söylemezoglu et al. 1997). In another study comparing histological atypia, proliferation, and clinical outcome, an elevated MIB-1 LI index was felt to be indicative of biological activity (Mackenzie 1999). With longer follow-up it is possible that some of the tumors with a low MIB-1 LI might relapse. This is illustrated in a recent case report of a patient with a recurrent central neurocytoma that had a 4-fold increase in MIB-1 LI after a 9-year disease-free interval (Christov et al. 1999).

8.3.5 Diagnosis and Neuroimaging

CT scans demonstrate an iso- or slightly hyperdense mass within the body of the lateral ventricles near the foramen of Monro. Areas of hypodensity represent cystic degeneration. About half of central neurocytomas demonstrate calcification on CT imaging (Hassoun et al. 1993). These tumors are thought to arise from septal nuclei, therefore are midline, and have broad-based attachments to the superior and lateral walls of the ventricle. Obstruction of the interventricular foramen of Monro by tumor mass usually results in hydrocephalus. Contrast enhancement is mild to moderate for most central neurocytomas.

MRI reveals an isointense mass on T1-weighted images (Chang et al. 1993; Wichmann et al. 1991). Of 13 central neurocytomas, 85% contained cysts, 69% contained calcification, and 62% had flow voids from tumor vessels resulting in a heterogeneous imaging appearance (Chang et al. 1993). On T2-weighted images most central neurocytomas are isointense. Moderate gadolinium enhancement is seen (Fig. 8.4a) (Wichmann et al. 1991). Angiography is rarely performed for central neurocytomas, but if obtained shows a homogeneous vascular blush. On occasion, tumors can be avascular (Ashkan et al. 2000; Goergen et al. 1992; Hassoun et al. 1993). Arterial supply is from the posterior and anterior choroidal, pericallosal, and lenticulo striate vessels.

Central neurocytoma in the lateral ventricle of young adults must be distinguished from oligodendroglioma, subependymal giant cell astrocytoma, ependymoma, and low grade or pilocytic astrocytoma. The typical central neurocytoma is located in the supratentorial ventricular system, in the anterior half of the lateral ventricle. Some series report that the left lateral ventricle is more frequently involved (Hassoun et al. 1993).

8.3.6 Treatment

8.3.6.1 Surgery

Complete surgical resection is the treatment of choice and also re-establishes CSF pathways in patients with hydrocephalus. Clinical reports indicate that gross total resection confers long-term control for most central neurocytomas (Maiuri et al. 1995; Schild et al. 1997; Yasargil et al. 1992). In a series of 32 patients with central neurocytoma, 5-year local control and survival rates of 100% and 80%, respectively, were seen after gross total resection without adjuvant therapy (Schild et al. 1997). However, tumor recurrence after gross total resection has been reported in 3/9 patients 3 to 6 years post surgery (Yasargil et al. 1992).

Preoperative CSF shunting is rarely indicated, but if the patient continues to have hydrocephalus postoperatively a permanent shunt is required. A third ventriculostomy can be useful in patients with noncommunicating hydrocephalus and was successful in 86% of patients with intraventricular tumors (Buxton et al. 2001). After completion of tumor resection, CSF should be drained via an external ventricular drain until returns are nearly clear.

8.3.6.2 Radiation Therapy and Radiosurgery

The role of postoperative radiotherapy has been investigated in several case reports and clinical series (Kim et al. 1997; Nakagawa et al. 1993; Schild et al. 1997). Radiotherapy after gross total resection does not seem indicated since such surgery gives most patients long-term tumor control. The use of radiation for residual tumor after subtotal resection is controversial. In a retrospective analysis of 15 patients with central neurocytoma, radiation appeared to have an effect on tumor control (Kim et al. 1997). Five patients with subtotal resection received fractionated radiation. Tumor shrinkage was observed in three and the residual tumor disappeared in two. One patient experienced delayed radiation toxicity. The authors cautioned that radiation in subtotal resected tumors can result in delayed radiation toxicity, and noted that the three patients with residual tumor who did not receive radiation remained stable (Kim et al. 1997). Schild et al. (1997) demonstrated a 5-year local control rate for residual central neurocytoma of 100% with radiation compared to 50% without radiation. A case report of a child treated with surgical decompression followed by radiation at age 7 years showed the patient free of tumor progression 38 years later (Tacconi et al. 2000).

More recently the use of radiosurgery for the treatment of central neurocytomas has been reported in four cases (Cobery et al. 2001). Three patients had subtotal resections and one patient had a recurrent tumor. The patients received 9 to 13 Gy to the 30 to 50% peripheral isodose line. Marked decrease of tumor volume was detected in all patients, measuring 48%, 72%, 81%, and 77%. In another series, four patients with recurrent central neurocytomas (9 to 25 months after complete radiographic resection) were treated with radiosurgery (Anderson et al. 2001). All patients had reduction of tumor size 12 to 28 months after radiosurgery. There were no complications. Even with limited follow-up it appears that for small, residual, or recurrent tumors, radiosurgery is a reasonable treatment option.

8.3.6.3 Chemotherapy

The experience with chemotherapy for central neurocytoma is more limited. A variety of agents have been used and responses to chemotherapy have not been well documented (Brandes et al. 2000; Dodds et al. 1997; Schild et al. 1997; Sgouros et al. 1998; von Koch et al. 2001). In the series of Schild et al. (1997) four patients received chemotherapy after radiation, and all four experienced no tumor progression. Various combinations of carmustine, lomustine, prednisone, vincristine, and cisplatin were used. A case report described a 15 year old with a large central neurocytoma underwent a subtotal resection followed by four cycles of carboplatin, etoposide, and ifosfamide (Dodds et al. 1997). The tumor had a significant response but eventually the patient required reoperation and radiation therapy. A more recent study used chemotherapy in the treatment of recurrent/progressive central neurocytoma in three patients (Brandes et al. 2000). Stabilization was observed in two of them and the other had a complete remission. Follow-up was limited to 15, 18, and 36 months but the responses were maintained. At UCSF we recently treated a 20 year old woman with recurrent central neurocytoma after four subtotal resections. She refused radiation and was treated with six cycles of procarbazine, CCNU, and vincristine chemotherapy. After 2 to 3 cycles of chemotherapy the tumor reduced in size and remained stable for at least 16 months after completion of chemotherapy (von Koch et al. 2003).

8.3.7 Outcome

Overall, central neurocytomas have a favorable prognosis, but in some cases the clinical course can be more aggressive. Histological features of anaplasia do not predict biologic behavior; proliferation markers might be more useful in predicting relapse. The most important therapeutic modality remains surgery. A safe maximal resection confers the best long-term outcome. In cases of a subtotal resection standard external beam radiation can be added, or radiation can be delayed until tumor progression occurs. Smaller residual tumors or recurrences can be treated with focused radiosurgery. Reoperation for recurrence should be considered if the procedure can be performed safely. Chemotherapy may be useful for recurrent central neurocytomas that cannot be resected and have been radiated, although long-term responses have not been reported for chemotherapy.

8.4 Conclusion

Neuronal tumors are rare and usually carry a good prognosis. Gangliocytomas, gangliogliomas, and DNETs present in late childhood or early adulthood and are commonly accompanied by intractable epilepsy. This is not unexpected, given their predominance in the temporal lobe. Complete surgical resection is curative and results in improved seizure control. It is important to distinguish these tumors from low-grade astrocytomas. However, malignant transformation of the glial component of ganglioglioma has been reported.

Central neurocytomas are seen in early adulthood and present with hydrocephalus due to ventricular outflow obstruction. Although rare, tumor recurrence and progression is seen and adjuvant therapy such as chemotherapy, radiation therapy, or gamma knife radiosurgery may be necessary in addition to surgical resection.

Acknowledgements. We would like to thank Dr. Jane Uyehara-Lock for assistance with obtaining and interpreting the pathology images. Dr. Meic H. Schmidt was supported by the NIH training grant T32 CA09291.

References

Anderson RC, Elder JB, Parsa AT (2001) Radiosurgery for the treatment of recurrent central neurocytomas. Neurosurgery 48:1231–1238

Armstrong DD (1993) The neuropathology of temporal lobe epilepsy. J Neuropathol Exp Neurol 52:433–443

Ashkan K, Casey AT, D'Arrigo C (2000) Benign central neurocytoma. Cancer 89:1111–1120

Blumcke I, Lobach M, Wolf HK, Wiestler OD (1999) Evidence for developmental precursor lesions in epilepsy-associated glioneuronal tumors. Micros Res Techn 46:53–58

Brandes AA, Amista P, Gardiman M (2000) Chemotherapy in patients with recurrent and progressive central neurocytoma. Cancer 88:169–174

Buxton N, Ho KJ, Macarthur D (2001) Neuroendoscopic third ventriculostomy for hydrocephalus in adults: report of a single unit's experience with 63 cases. Surg Neurol 55:74–78

Cervera-Pierot P, Varlet P, Chodkiewicz JP, Daumas D (1997) Dysembryoplastic neuroepithelial tumors in the caudate nucleus area. Neurosurgery 40:1065–1069

Chang KH, Han MH, Kim DG (1993) MR appearance of central neurocytoma. Acta Radiol 34:520–526

Christov C, Adle-Biassette H, Le Guerinel C (1999) Recurrent central neurocytoma with marked increase in MIB-1 labelling index. Br J Neurosurg 13:496–499

Cobery ST, Noren G, Friehs GM (2001) Gamma knife surgery for treatment of central neurocytoma. J Neurosurg 94:327–330

Courville CB (1930) Ganglioglioma: tumor of the central nervous system. Review of the literature and report of two cases. Arch Neurol Psychiatry 24:438–491

Daumas-Duport C (1993) Dysembryoplastic neuroepithelial tumours. Brain Pathol 3:283–295

Daumas-Duport C (1995) Dysembryoplastic neuroepithelial tumors in epilepsy surgery. In: Guerrini R (ed) Dysplasia of cerebral cortex and epilepsy. Raven, New York, pp 125–147

Daumas-Duport C, Scheithauer BW, Chodkiewicz JP (1988) Dysembryoplastic neuroepithelial tumor (DNT): a surgically curable tumor of young subjects with intractable partial seizures: report of 39 cases. Neurosurgery 23:545–556

Daumas-Duport C, Pietsch T, Lantos PL (2000) Dysembryoplastic neuroepithelial tumour. In: Kleihaus P, Cavenee WK (eds) Pathology and genetic of tumours of the nervous system. IARC Press, Lyon, pp 103–106

Dodds D, Nonis J, Mehta M et al (1997) Central neurocytoma: a clinical study of response to chemotherapy. J Neurooncol 34:279–283

Dorne HL, O'Gorman AM, Melanson D (1986) Computed tomography of intracranial gangliogliomas. AJNR 7:281–285

Elek G, Slowik F, Eross L (1999) Central neurocytoma with malignant course. Neuronal and glial differentiation and craniospinal dissemination. Pathol Oncol Res 5:155–159

Eng DY, DeMonte F, Ginsberg L et al (1997) Craniospinal dissemination of central neurocytoma. Report of two cases. J Neurosurg 86:547–552

Figarella-Branger D, Söylemezoglu F, Kleihues P, Hassoun J (2000) Central neurocytoma. In: Kleihues P, Cavenee WK (eds) Pathology and genetics of tumours of the nervous system. IARC, Lyon, pp 107–109

Goergen SK, Gonzales MF, McLean CA (1992) Interventricular neurocytoma: radiologic features and review of the literature. Radiology 182:787–792

Grossman RI, Yousem DM (1994) Neuroradiology. The requisites. Mosby-Yearbook, St Louis

Haddad SF, Moore SA, Menezes AH (1992) Ganglioglioma: 13 years of experience. Neurosurgery 31:171–178

Hall WA, Yunis EJ, Albright AL (1986) Anaplastic ganglioglioma in an infant: case report and review of the literature. Neurosurgery 19:1016–1020

Hakim R, Loeffler JS, Anthony DC, Black PM (1997) Gangliomas in adults. Cancer 79:127–131

Hamburger C, Buttner A, Weis S (1997) Ganglioglioma of the spinal cord: report of two rare cases and review of the literature. Neurosurgery 41:1410–1415

Hassoun J, Söylemezoglu F, Gambarelli D (1993) Central neurocytoma: a synopsis of clinical and histological features. Brain Pathol 3:297–306

Hirose T, Scheithauer BW, Lopes MB, van den Berg SR (1994) Dysembryoplastic neuroepithelial tumor (DNT): an immunohistochemical and ultrastructural study. J Neuropathol Exp Neurol 53:184–195

Hirose T, Scheithauer BW, Lopes MBS, Gerber HA, Altermatt HJ, van den Berg SR (1997) Ganglioglioma: an ultrastructural and immunohistochemical study. Cancer 79:989–1003

Johannsson JH, Rekate HL, Roessmann U (1981) Gangliogliomas: pathological and clinical correlation. J Neurosurg 54:58–63

Johnson JHJ, Hariharan S, Berman J, Sutton LN, Rorke LB, Molloy P, Phillips PC (1997) Clinical outcome of pediatric gangliogliomas: ninety-nine cases over 20 years. Pediatr Neurosurg 27:203–207

Kalyan R, Olivero WC (1987) Ganglioglioma: a correlative clinicopathological and radiological study of ten surgically treated cases with follow-up. Neurosurgery 20:428–433

Khajavi K, Comair YG, Prayson RA, Wyllie E, Palmer J, Estes ML, Hahn JF (1995) Childhood ganglioglioma and medically intractable epilepsy. A clinicopathological study of 15 patients and a review of the literature. Pediatr Neurosurg 22:181–188

Kim DG, Paek SH, Kim IH (1997) Central neurocytoma: the role of radiation therapy and long term outcome. Cancer 79:1995–2002

Koeller KK, Dillon WP (1992) Dysembryoplastic neuroepithelial tumors: MR appearance. AJNR 13:1319–1325

Kuchelmeister K, Demirel T, Schlorer E, Bergmann M, Gullotta F (1995) Dysembryoplastic neurepithelial tumour of the cerebellum. Acta Neuropathol (Berl) 89:385–390

Kuroiwa T, Bergey GK, Rothman MI, Zoarski GH, Wolf A, Zagardo MT, Kristt DA, Hudson LP, Krumholz A, Barry E (1995) Radiologic appearance of the dysembryoplastic neuroepithelial tumor. Radiology 197:233–238

Lang FF, Epstein FJ, Ransohoff J, Allen JC, Wisoff J, Abbott IR, Miller DC (1993) Central nervous system gangliogliomas, part 2. Clinical outcome. J Neurosurg 79:867–873

Lantos PL, van den Berg SR, Kleihues P (1996) Tumours of the nervous system. In: Graham DI, Lantos PL (eds) Greenfield's neuropathology, 6th edn. London, Arnold, pp 583–879

Lellouch T, Bourgeois M, Vekemans M, Robain O (1995) Dysembryoplastic neuroepithelial tumors in two children with neurofibromatosis type I. Acta Neuropathol (Berl) 90:319–322

Leung SY, Gwi E, Ng HK, Fung CF, Yam KY (1994) Dysembryoplastic neuroepithelial tumor. A tumor with small neuronal cells resembling oligodendroglioma. Am J Surg Pathol 18: 604–614

Mackenzie IR (1999) Central neurocytoma: histologic atypia, proliferation potential, and clinical outcome. Cancer 85:1606–1610

Maiuri F, Spaziante R, de Caro ML (1995) Central neurocytoma: clinico-pathological study of 5 cases and review of the literature. Clin Neurol Neurosurg 97:219–228

Miller DC, Lang FF, Epstein FJ (1993) Central nervous system gangliogliomas, part I. Pathology. J Neurosurg 79:859–866

Morris HH, Estes ML, Gilmore R, van Ness PC, Barnett GH, Turnbull J (1993) Chronic intractable epilepsy as the only symptom of primary brain tumor. Epilepsia 34:1038–1043

Nakagawa K, Aoki Y, Sakata K et al (1993) Radiation therapy of well-differentiated neuroblastoma and central neurocytoma. Cancer 72:1350–1355

Newmann E, Kalousek DK, Norman MG, Steinbok P, Cockrane DD, Goddard K (1993) Cytogenetic analysis of 109 pediatric central nervous system tumors. Cancer Genet Cytogenet 71:40–49

Ohgaki H, Eibl RH, Schwab M (1993) Mutations of the p53 tumor suppressor gene in neoplasms of the human nervous system. Mol Carcinogen 8:74–80

Osborne AG (1994) Diagnostic neuroradiology. Mosby, St Louis

Park SH, Chi JG, Cho BK, Wang KC (1993) Spinal cord ganglioglioma in childhood. Pathol Res Pract 189:189–196

Pasquier B, Bost F, Peoc'h M, Barnoud R, Pasquier D (1996) Neuropathologic data in drug-resistant partial epilepsy. Report of a series of 195 cases. Ann Pathol 16:174–181

Platten M, Meyer-Puttlitz B, Waha A, Wolf HK, Nothen MM, Louis DN, Sampson JR, von Deimling A (1997) A novel splice site-associated polymorphism in the tuberous sclerosis gene may predispose to the development of sporadic gangliogliomas. Neuropathology 56:806–810

Prayson RA, Estes ML (1992) Dysembryoplastic neuroepithelial tumor. Am J Clin Pathol 97:398–401

Prayson RA, Khajavi K, Comair YG (1995) Cortical architectural abnormalities and MIB1 immunoreactivity in gangliogliomas: a study of 60 patients with intracranial tumors. J Neuropathol Exp Neurol 54:513–520

Raymond AA, Halpin SF, Alsanjari N, Cook MJ, Kitchen ND, Fish DR, Stevens JM, Harding BN, Scaravilli F, Kendall B (1994) Dysembryoplastic neuroepithelial tumor. Features in 16 patients. Brain 117:461–475

Raymond AA, Fish DR, Sisodia SM, Alsanjari N, Stevens JM, Shorvon SD (1995) Abnormalities of gyration, heterotopias, tuberous sclerosis, focal cortical dysplasia, microdysgenesis, dysembryoplastic neuroepithelial tumour and dysgenesis of the archicortex in epilepsy. Clinical, EEG and neuroimaging features in 100 adult patients. Brain 118:629–660

Rosemberg S, Vieira GS (1998) Dysembryoplastic neuroepithelial tumor. An epidemiological study from a single institution (in Portuguese). Arq Neuropsiquatr 56:232–236

Sasaki A, Hirato J, Nakazato Y, Tamura M, Kadowaki H (1996) Recurrent anaplastic ganglioma: pathological characterization of tumor cells. Case report. J Neurosurg 84:1055–1059

Schild SE, Scheithauer BW, Haddock MG (1997) Central neurocytomas. Cancer 79:790–795

Selch MT, Goy BW, Lee SP, El-Sadin S, Kincaid P, Park SH, Withers HR (1998) Gangliogliomas: experience of 34 patients and review of the literature. Am J Clin Oncol 21:557–564

Sgouros S, Carey M, Aluwihare N (1998) Central neurocytoma: a correlative clinicopathologic and radiologic analysis. Surg Neurol 49:197–204

Sharma MC, Rathore A, Karak AK (1998) A study of proliferative markers in central neurocytoma. Pathology 30:355–359

Söylemezoglu F, Scheithauer BW, Esteve J (1997) Atypical central neurocytoma. J Neuropathol Exp Neurol 56:551–556

Sutton LN, Packer RJ, Rorke LB (1983) Cerebral gangliogliomas during childhood. Neurosurgery 13:124–128

Sutton LN, Packer RJ, Zimmerman RA (1987) Cerebral gangliogliomas of childhood. Prog Exp Tumor Res 30:239–246

Tacconi L, Rossi M, Foy P (2000) Central neurocytoma: longterm follow-up of a paediatric case. J Clin Neurosci 7:542–560

Taratuto AL, Pomata H, Sevlever G, Gallo G, Monges J (1995) Dysembryoplastic neuroepithelial tumor: morphological, immunohistochemical, and deoxyribonucleic acid analyses in a pediatric series. Neurosurgery 36:474–481

Taruscio D, Danesi R, Montaldi A (1997) Nonrandom gain of chromosome 7 in central neurocytoma: a chromosomal analysis and fluorescence in situ hybridization study. Virchows Arch 430:47–51

Ventureyra E, Herder S, Mallya BK (1986) Temporal lobe gangliogliomas in children. Childs Nerv Syst 2:63–66

Von Deimling A, Janzer R, Kleihues P (1990) Patterns of differentiation in central neurocytoma. An immunohistochemical study of eleven biopsies. Acta Neuropathol (Berl) 79:473–479

Von Deimling A, Kleihues P, Saremaslani P (1991) Histogenesis and differentiation potential of central neurocytomas. Lab Invest 64:585–591

von Koch CS, Schmidt MH, Uyehara-Lock JH, Berger MS, Chang SM (2003) The role of PCV chemotherapy in the treatment of central neurocytoma: illustration of a case and review of the literature. Surg Neurol 60(6):560–565

Wichmann W, Schubiger O, von Deimling A (1991) Neuroradiology of central neurocytoma. Neuroradiology 33:143–148

Wolf HK, Wiestler OD (1995) Surgical pathology of chronic epileptic seizure disorders. Brain Pathol 3:371–380

Wolf HK, Muller MB, Spanle M, Zentner J, Schramm J, Wiestler OD (1988) Ganglioglioma: a detailed histopathological and immunohistochemical analysis of 61 cases. Acta Neuropathol (Berl) 88:166–173

Wolf HK, Campos MG, Zentner J, Hufnagel A, Schramm J, Elger CE, Wiestler OD (1993) Surgical pathology of temporal lobe epilepsy. Experience of 216 cases. J Neuropathol Exp Neurol 52:499–506

Wolf HK, Mueller MB, Spaenle M, Zentner J, Schramm J, Wiestler OD (1994) Ganglioglioma: a detailed histopathological and immunohistochemical analysis of 61 cases. Acta Neuropathol (Berl) 88:166–173

Wolf HK, Wellmer J, Mueller MB, Wistler OD, Hufnagel A, Pietsch T (1995) Glioneuronal malformative lesions and dysembryoplastic neuroepithelial tumors in patients with chronic pharmacoresistant epilepsy. J Neuropathol Exp Neurol 5:245–254

Wolf HK, Buslei R, Blumcke I, Wiestler OD, Pietsch T (1997) Neural antigens in oligodendrogliomas and dysembryoplastic neuroepithelial tumors. Acta Neuropathol (Berl) 94:436–443

Yasargil MG, von Ammon K, von Deimling A (1992) Central neurocytoma: histopathological variants and therapeutic approaches. J Neurosurgery 76:32–37

Yin XL, Pang JC, Hui AB (2000) Detection of chromosomal imbalances in central neurocytomas by using comparative genomic hybridization. J Neurosurg 93:77–81

Zhu J, Guy SZ, Beggs AH, Maruyama T, Santarius T, Dashner K, Olsen N, Wu JK, Black P (1996) Microsatellite instability analysis of primary human brain tumors. Oncogene 12: 1417–1423

Zulch KJ (1986) Brain tumors. Their biology and pathology, 3rd edn. Springer, Berlin Heidelberg New York

Choroid Plexus Tumors

N. Gupta

Contents

9.1 Introduction

The choroid plexus has the highly specific function of producing cerebrospinal fluid (CSF). It is anatomically localized to the parenchymal/ventricular junction in all four ventricles. The choroid plexus is derived from the specialization of ventricular epithelium along certain segments of the neural tube, and there is a common ontogeny between choroid epithelium and cells of glial origin. This can and does lead to diagnostic confusion in certain cases. Tumors arising from the choroid plexus can display a benign or malignant phenotype with conversion to a malignant phenotype being exceedingly rare (Chow et al. 1999a). Guerard was the first to describe a choroid plexus tumor in 1833. The first surgical resection was reported by Bielschowsky and Unger in 1906. Thereafter both Cushing and Dandy reported their experiences with this unusual tumor (Davis and Cushing 1925; Dandy 1922).

9.2 Epidemiology

Choroid plexus papilloma (CPP) and carcinoma (CPC), are uncommon, accounting for only 0.5% to 0.6% of all brain tumors. Although found in all age groups, choroid plexus neoplasms are primarily a tumor of childhood. Laurence in his review of all published cases prior to 1974 reported that 45% presented in the first year of life while 74% presented in the first decade (Lawrence 1974). As expected, reviews from pediatric centers report that a higher percentage (1.8% to 2.9%) of their cases are choroid plexus tumors (Sarkar et al. 1999; Asai et al. 1989; Ellenbogen et al. 1989). Two reviews of tumors in the first year of life, by Haddad and Galassi, found that choroid plexus tumors accounted for 14% and 12.8% of all cases (Galassi et al. 1989; Haddad et al. 1991). The majority of series noted above have not reported any predilection for right or left ventricle or sex. Laurence did note that 50% of cases reviewed were situated in the lateral ventricles, 37% in the fourth ventricle, 9% in the third ventricle, and the remainder in other locations. Other series have confirmed this geographic distribution. CPCs, while rare, account for 29% to 39% of all choroid neoplasms (Ellenbogen et al. 1989; Johnson 1989; St. Clair et al. 1991).

9.3 Pathology

9.3.1 Gross Appearance

CPP is frequently described as "cauliflower-like." Indeed, they are similar to the soft fronds of normal choroid as found in the ventricles. The shape is roughly globular with an irregular surface and intervening encapsulated areas. Old hemorrhage is sometimes apparent. Since papillomas are benign they tend to expand the ventricle rather than invade adjacent brain. Nevertheless, the proximity of these tumors to deep-seated structures such as the internal cerebral veins and limbic structures can make their removal difficult.

9.3.2 Histopathology

The microscopic appearance of papilloma recapitulates the normal choroid plexus. There are many papillae covered with a simple cuboidal or columnar epithelia. The stroma of these fibrovascular structures is composed of connective tissue and small blood vessels. The presence of the connective tissue stroma is notable mainly since it allows one to distinguish between CPP and papillary forms of ependymoma (whose stroma is composed of fibrillary neuroglia). In addition, choroid epithelial cells do not contain cilia or blepharoplasts as do ependymal cells. Mitotic figures are rare.

Villous hypertrophy of the choroid plexus is a poorly defined entity. Characteristically the choroid plexus of both lateral ventricles is enlarged and is associated with hydrocephalus from birth. Russell and Rubinstein comment that the hydrocephalus is related to hyperactivity of the choroid although the cytological appearance of the tissue is normal. Other authors have used villous hypertrophy synonymously with bilateral CPP, but this is not accurate in the strictest sense if histological evidence of neoplastic growth is not present and expansion of the choroid plexus occurs diffusely (Hirano 1994).

CPCs are diagnosed on the basis of their microscopic appearance. Two major features accompany malignancy. First is the presence of brain invasion by the tumor. This usually involves transgression of the ependymal lining and extension into the paraventricular parenchyma. Second, cytological criteria of malignancy — nuclear atypia, increased nuclear to cytoplasmic ratio, and prominent mitotic figures — are present in association with a loss of normal papillary architecture. Rarely, if a tumor demonstrates some atypical features without evidence of invasion, it can be designated as an atypical papilloma. The epithelial nature of the frank malignancy can create confusion since other tumors such as metastatic adenocarcinoma and medulloepithelioma are histologically similar. If the tumor arises in a young patient then chances of the tumor being metastatic are extremely low. Electron microscopy can reveal details such as cilia, which are not normally present in choroid plexus tumors. Grossly these tumors tend to be softer and more friable than papillomas. While carcinomas rarely metastasize from the intracranial or intraspinal compartment, they can disseminate throughout the CSF pathways (McComb and Burger 1983).

9.3.3 Immunohistochemistry

Only a few immunohistochemical stains have been found to be helpful. The calcium binding protein S-100 is positive in the vast majority of choroid tumors (Ho et al. 1991; Paulus and Janisch 1990). This is of limited value since glial tissues and normal choroid express S-100 in a parallel fashion with glial fibrillary acid protein (GFAP). Other markers such as vimentin, GFAP, and cytokeratins can be positive but also lack specificity (Cruz-Sanchez et al. 1989; Mannoji and Becker 1988). Pre-albumin or transthyretin (TTR) was initially believed to be a specific marker, but another report noted that 20% of choroid tumors were TTR negative (Herbert et al. 1990; Paulus and Janisch 1990). These investigators did find that prognostic information could be gleaned from immunohistochemical data. A poor prognosis was found in those tumors with less than 50% of the cells in a given tumor heavily stained for S-100. In addition, absence of TTR-positive cells correlated with a poor prognosis. Cellular proliferation, as measured by Ki67/MIB1 labeling, is low with papillomas and significantly higher for carcinomas (Vajtai et al. 1996).

9.3.4 Genetics

The cause of choroid plexus tumors is unknown. One report has mentioned two cases occurring in one family, but a hereditary basis has not been observed for most cases (Zwetsloot et al. 1991). There is some evidence linking SV40, a primate DNA virus, with choroid plexus tumor etiology. Large T antigen, the major regulator of late viral gene products of the SV40 virus, when expressed in mice induces the formation of choroid plexus neoplasms (Brinster et al. 1984). The large T antigen is expressed only in the choroid plexus and appears to interact with the product of the *p53* gene (Marks et al. 1989). T antigen interferes with the function of both p53 and RB tumor suppressors. This function is likely required for viral replication and growth, but may also have the effect of increasing tumor formation. Using PCR, SV40 DNA sequences were demonstrated in 50% of choroid plexus tumors and the majority of ependymomas (Bergsagel et al. 1992). Active T antigen and *p53* complexes have also been demonstrated in brain tumors (Zhen et al. 1999). More recently the expression of transgenes of the viral oncoproteins E6 and E7 from human papilloma virus have also been shown to produce tumors in 71% of offspring of which 26% of the

tumors were choroid plexus tumors (Arbeit et al. 1993).

A subset of central primitive neuroectodermal tumors (PNETs), CPCs, and medulloblastomas were recently shown to have frequent mutations in the *hSNF2/INI1* gene, which encodes for a component of the ATP-dependent chromatin-remodeling complex (Sevenet et al. 1999a). The same authors have proposed that constitutional mutations in this gene lead to a greater incidence of renal and extrarenal malignant rhabdoid tumors, CPCs, central PNETs, and medulloblastomas: a complex they have coined as the "rhabdoid predisposition syndrome" (Sevenet et al. 1999b). The penetrance of the disease is high, with many probands developing malignant tumors before 3 years of age. Some pathologic data also suggests a connection between malignant rhabdoid tumors and choroid plexus carcinomas (Wyatt-Ashmead et al. 2001).

A number of chromosomal abnormalities have been identified in both CPP and CPC (Rickert et al. 2002). Surprisingly, even benign CPP (32 of 34 cases) demonstrated chromosomal aberration. The patterns of aberrations in CPP differ from those observed in CPC.

9.4 Clinical Features: Signs and Symptoms

Hydrocephalus is the presenting symptom in the vast majority of choroid plexus tumors. It is caused by both overproduction of CSF and, in certain cases, the obstruction of CSF pathways, although it appears that overproduction is the major factor (Eisenberg et al. 1974). Resolution of hydrocephalus has been reported after complete tumor removal, suggesting that CSF hypersecretion was responsible for ventriculomegaly (Wilkins and Rutledge 1961; Matson and Crofton 1960; Gudeman et al. 1979). Variations are likely to exist, since a normal rate of CSF production has been reported in a patient harboring a papilloma (Sahar et al. 1980).

The most common presentation of choroid plexus neoplasms is related to increased intracranial pressure secondary to obstructive hydrocephalus and/or CSF overproduction (Laurence 1974; Ellenbogen et al. 1989; Humphreys et al. 1987). Since the majority of cases occur in infants and young children there are characteristic features of raised ICP; Ellenbogen described the usual presenting signs and symptoms (Ellenbogen et al. 1989). The most common symptoms described were nausea/vomiting, irritability, headache, visual difficulty, and seizure. As expected, the most common signs were craniomegaly, papilledema, and decreased level of consciousness. The duration of symptoms reported in this series varied from two months in those patients younger than two years of age to six months on average in those patients older than two years. Although choroid neoplasms are viewed as slow-growing tumors, the presence of stupor or coma as the presenting sign in 25% of children suggests a more acute clinical course in some patients. Rapid decompensation can occur either from massive hydrocephalus or from tumoral hemorrhage. Of 21 patients who had CSF examined, 2 were found to have grossly bloody fluid. Lateralizing signs are found in a minority of patients and are usually related to asymmetrical ventricular dilatation. Hydrocephalus was present in 78% of cases at the Hospital for Sick Children and 95% of cases at the Children's Hospital in Boston (Ellenbogen et al. 1989; Humphreys et al. 1987).

9.5 Diagnosis and Neuroimaging

Since most patients present with hydrocephalus and increased intracranial pressure, there is no role for sampling CSF at diagnosis. There is little information that can be gained from CSF sampling and history documents disastrous outcomes in some patients after lumbar puncture (Laurence 1974). No specific laboratory tests are available to diagnose these tumors.

9.5.1 Computed Tomography

The CT-scan appearance of CPP is often characteristic for this tumor. The mass is well demarcated from the brain, lobulated, and often has punctate calcification. These tumors enhance homogeneously after

contrast, reflecting a luxuriant blood supply (Hopper et al. 1987). Since they arise from the choroid plexus, their location is almost always intraventricular. An enlarged choroidal artery leading into the tumor mass can sometimes be seen in post-contrast images. At times, the massive size of these lesions may obscure the site of origin. Some carcinomas display a diffuse border between tumor and normal brain that may reflect areas of brain invasion. On the basis of CT, certain features distinguish a suspected choroid tumor from other possibilities. Cerebellar astrocytomas tend to stain less homogeneously and often have cystic areas. Medulloblastomas are characterized by a more heterogeneous appearance, although they also stain vividly with contrast and may cause confusion with a fourth ventricle choroid papilloma. Finally, ependymomas arise physically in similar locations but tend to enhance inhomogeneously.

9.5.2 Magnetic Resonance Imaging

Papillomas are isodense to brain on T1-weighted images (Fig. 9.1a). Areas of high signal indicate hemorrhage necrosis. Following gadolinium administration, the tumor enhances brightly (Fig. 9.1b, c), although this can be patchy in nature, reflecting areas of high flow. T2-weighted images demonstrate an intermediate to high signal intensity with areas of heterogeneous internal signal (Coates et al. 1989). MR spectroscopy of CPP and CPC is characterized by a prominent choline peak and absence of N-acetyl aspartate (Horska et al. 2001). As with CT, an enlarged choroidal artery is often noted, especially with larger tumors. The vascularity of these tumors is easily demonstrated with specific perfusion sequences (Fig. 9.2). With CPC, the boundary between the tumor and surrounding brain can be indistinct in areas, but this is not a universal finding.

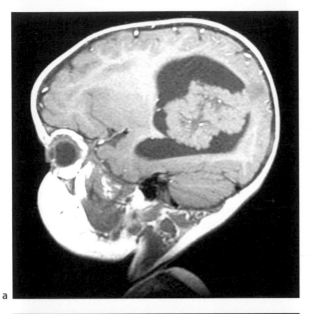

a

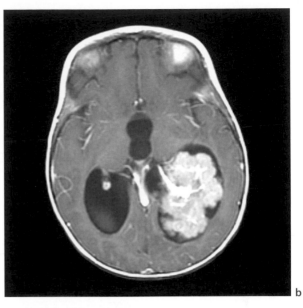

b

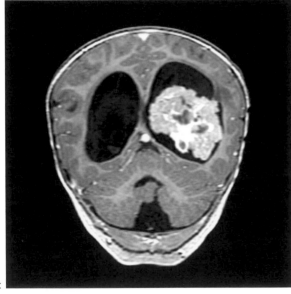

c

Figure 9.1 a–c

A large choroid plexus papilloma. **a** A sagittal pre-contrast T1-weighted MRI demonstrates a large lobulated mass within the lateral ventricle with associated enlargement of the ventricle. **b** and **c** Following contrast, the mass enhances brightly. Note that the papilloma is well demarcated from the ventricular wall

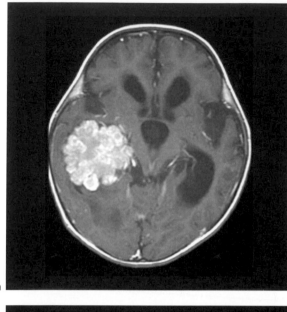

a

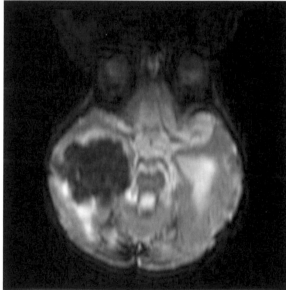

b

Figure 9.2 a,b

a An axial T1-weighted post-contrast image shows a large choroid plexus papilloma within the temporal horn of the lateral ventricle. **b** The perfusion sequence results in a "negative" image with increased vascularity depicted as a dark area. The mass is considerably darker than the adjacent brain tissue

9.6 Treatment

9.6.1 Pre-operative Planning

Since most patients present with symptoms of intracranial hypertension, the order and type of treatment is directed at relieving hydrocephalus, determining the diagnosis, and removing the tumor. Unless the patient is rapidly deteriorating urgent CSF drainage is not necessary. At the time of surgery a ventricular drain is placed in order to reduce brain tension and allow sufficient retraction. An external ventricular drain may be left in place after surgery in order to monitor ICP and to determine if shunting is required in the early postoperative period. Matson (1960) and others have reported that the successful removal of a tumor obviates the need for shunting. However, it is likely that other factors such as ventricular bleeding, postoperative changes, or meningitis can also render the patient shunt dependent. Ellenbogen's series noted that 37% of surviving patients required shunting (Ellenbogen et al. 1989). Two other series reported much higher rates of shunt dependency, ranging from 57% to 78% of cases reported (Humphrey et al. 1987; Lena et al. 1990). Raimondi and Gutierrez have recommended that third and fourth ventricle tumors require immediate shunt placement followed by a delay of 7 to 14 days prior to surgery (Raimondi and Gutierrez 1975). This method, while acceptable, can be substituted by performance of both procedures at the same time if permitted by the condition of the patient.

Angiography demonstrates that papillomas are supplied by normal choroidal vessels, which often enlarge as the tumor grows. Tumors of the lateral ventricle or third ventricle are generally supplied by branches of the anterior or posterior choroidal arteries. Mass effect tends to displace the internal occipital artery and the basal vein of Rosenthal in an inferior direction. A fourth-ventricle tumor receives its blood supply from medullary or vermian branches of the posterior inferior cerebellar artery. Conventional catheter angiography is not required for diagnosis. Rather, in combination with selective embolization it can be used as a preoperative adjunct to reduce tumor vascularity.

9.6.2 Operative Treatment

The goal of surgery is gross total resection (GTR) as measured by post-operative MR imaging. As with most intracranial tumors, the exact approach is determined by avoiding eloquent tissue (e.g. primary motor or sensory cortex, speech centers, and visual cortex). The two features of choroid plexus tumors that can make resection exceedingly difficult are: (1) profuse vascularity, and (2) large size. The tumor's arterial vessels arborize rapidly, and so control of hemorrhage within the tumor requires slow and tedious dissection. The most effective strategy focuses on initial exposure of the feeding artery and its ligation. In general, en bloc excision is recommended (Raimondi and Gutierrez 1975). For lateral ventricle papillomas, a direct cerebrotomy posterior to the angular gyrus will allow access to the entire trigone and permit the pedicle of the tumor to be identified and coagulated (Fig. 9.3). For more anteriorly located tumors, an incision can be made in the frontal convolutions and the lateral ventricle approached from an anterolateral direction. Lateral ventricle tumors can also be approached through a cerebrotomy through the superior or middle temporal gyrus.

Third ventricle tumors are rare and are approached via a midline transcallosal route. The anterior aspect of the ventricle is entered through a generous opening in the corpus callosum extending from the rostrum to the supraoptic recess. In this way the tumor can be separated from the choroid of the tela choroidea where it is usually attached and the accompanying bridging vessels can be identified and divided.

Fourth ventricle tumors almost always produce triventricular obstructive hydrocephalus and may require preoperative shunting and stabilization as noted above. Tumors in this location arise from the caudal part of the roof of the fourth ventricle and may extend into the lateral recesses or through the foramen of Magendie. The approach is via a standard midline posterior fossa craniectomy or craniotomy exposing the vermis and tonsils. The blood supply from branches of the PICA are visualized from a medial vantage.

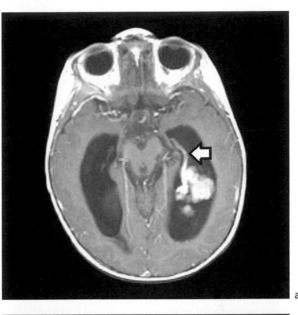

a

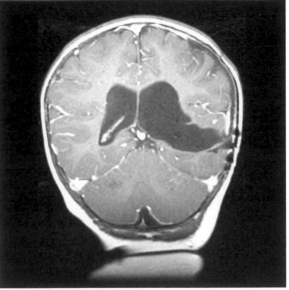

b

Figure 9.3 a,b

The same case as shown in Fig. 9.1. **a** The axial T1-weighted image clearly shows an enlarged choroidal artery leading into the tumor. **b** The postoperative coronal MRI image shows the route through the temporal lobe used to access initially the feeding artery and then the tumor itself. Once the blood supply was interrupted, the tumor removal proceeded uneventfully

9.6.3 Choroid Plexus Carcinomas

Overall, reported results in the literature appear to confirm that GTR has a favorable impact upon survival for carcinomas (see Outcome below). For this reason, aggressive surgical treatment with GTR should be the primary objective. Nevertheless, GTR with carcinoma is achieved in less than 50% of cases. Combined with adjunctive therapy, either radiation or chemotherapy, survival following GTR ranges from 67 to 91% (Fitzpatrick et al. 2002). Technical considerations with choroid plexus carcinoma include the expected increased tumor vascularity as well as additional difficulties relating to the lack of a well developed plane between the brain and tumor and excessive friability of the tumor tissue. The rate of recurrence associated with GTR alone suggests that adjunctive therapy is useful, although definitive guidelines are not available (Fitzpatrick et al. 2002).

Most chemotherapy regimens rely upon cyclophosphamide, etoposide, vincristine, and a platinum agent (St. Clair et al. 1991; Packer et al. 1992; Berger et al. 1998). Wolff et al. (2002) noted that only 8 of 22 carcinomas responded to chemotherapy, a disappointing observation. Use of combination chemotherapy (ifosfamide, carboplatinum, and etoposide) after an initial surgical procedure was found to reduce tumor volume and allow a more complete resection during a second-stage operation (St. Clair et al. 1991; Razzaq and Cohen 1997). Importantly, the vascularity of the tumor appeared to be greatly reduced, as measured blood loss during the second procedure was on average 15% of blood volume compared to an average of 64% of blood volume during the first procedure.

Postoperative radiation is usually recommended if the child is over three years of age, although this therapy has not been subjected to a clinical trial. Radiation is also used in the presence of leptomeningeal dissemination, subtotal resection (STR), and drop metastases. In one series, ten patients with choroid plexus carcinoma were treated with either chemotherapy and/or craniospinal radiation (Chow et al. 1999a). Some of these patients demonstrated no evidence of disease following chemotherapy alone, but others required radiation to achieve disease control.

The authors do suggest that radiation can be used as salvage therapy but whether radiation for all patients with carcinoma would reduce the relapse rate remains unclear. Fitzpatrick et al. (2002) noted that following STR, radiation therapy, either alone or in combination with chemotherapy, offered a survival advantage. The question of whether to use adjunctive therapy following GTR remains unclear, although the presence of relapse despite chemotherapy and radiation in a small group of patients suggests that surgery alone is not sufficient for CPC. Wolff et al. (1999) support this view and state that GTR alone is insufficient for carcinoma and should be supplemented with radiation. The role of conformal radiation and radiosurgery is unknown, as is the role of intrathecal chemotherapy. The experience reported by Packer suggests that disease relapse confers a poor prognosis (Packer et al. 1992).

9.7 Outcome

The vast majority of patients with CPP can expect excellent long-term survival. The survival for CPC, however, is much worse. In a recent meta-analysis, the one, five, and ten year survival for papilloma was 90, 81, and 77%, compared to only 71, 41, and 35% for carcinoma (Wolff et al. 2002). The extent of surgery is the most important treatment variable impacting long-term survival for both papilloma and carcinoma (Ellenbogen et al. 1989; Packer et al. 1992; Wolff et al. 2002). The overall crude survival rate in Ellenbogen's series was 88% for patients with papillomas and 50% for carcinomas (Ellenbogen et al. 1989).

Packer et al. (1992) reported that GTR for carcinoma without adjunctive therapy offers the highest likelihood of success. Four of five patients with GTR remained disease free at a median of 45 months after diagnosis. Five of six patients who had a STR relapsed (Packer et al. 1992). While the authors of this study were pessimistic regarding the value of adjunctive therapy, the timing of this therapy may prove to be important with regard to survival after multi-modality treatment. Two other reports noted that 5-year survival following GTR of carcinomas ranged from 26 to 40% (Berger et al. 1998; Pencalet et al. 1998).

Berger et al. (1998) also noted that surgery was the most important prognostic factor for choroid plexus carcinoma. The role of radiation also remains unclear. A brief report recently noted that the five-year survival for patients with carcinoma and GTR followed by radiation was 68% compared to 16% for those not irradiated (Wolff et al. 1999). The two groups were not exactly comparable but the clear suggestion is that surgery alone is insufficient to prevent recurrence for carcinomas.

Although papillomas are histologically benign and potentially curable, morbidity and mortality are significant concerns. With respect to operative mortality, modern series provide figures of 8% to 9.5% (Humphrey et al. 1987; Lena et al. 1990). In the series from the Hospital for Sick Children the cumulative mortality was 36%, the majority of which (6 of 8) occurred in patients below 12 months of age. Morbidity remains an important problem. In one series 33% of patients with papillomas have persisting motor sequelae and psychomotor retardation (Lena et al. 1990). In another series 26% of patients were classified as having a fair or poor recovery (Ellenbogen et al. 1989).

As noted above, the treatment of hydrocephalus goes hand-in-hand with the treatment of choroid neoplasms. Associated complications also occur. One of note is the presence of large subdural collections that may develop following tumor resection through a transcortical approach. The cause is believed to be a persistent ventriculosubdural fistula. Boyd and Steinbok (1987) appear to have dealt with this problem by applying pial sutures at the conclusion of the procedure. The role of preoperative shunting in the causation of this entity is unclear.

9.8 Conclusion

Choroid plexus tumors represent a well-defined subset of brain tumors that occur mainly in young children. Surgical resection for papilloma is usually curative while adjunctive therapy for carcinoma should include chemotherapy and/or radiation. The long-term survival for carcinoma remains poor.

References

Arbeit JM, Munger K, Howley PM, Hanahan D (1993) Neuroepithelial carcinomas in mice transgenic with human papillomavirus type 16 E6/E7 ORFs. Am J Pathol 142:1187–1197

Asai A, Hoffman HJ, Hendrick EB, Humphreys RP, Becker LE (1989) Primary intracranial neoplasms in the first year of life. Childs Nerv Syst 5:230–233

Berger C, Thiesse P, Lellouch-Tubiana A, Kalifa C, Pierre-Kahn A, Bouffet E (1998) Choroid plexus carcinomas in childhood: clinical features and prognostic factors. Neurosurgery, 42:470–475

Bergsagel DJ, Finegold MJ, Butel JS, Kupsky WJ, Garcea RL (1992) DNA sequences similar to those of simian virus 40 in ependymomas and choroid plexus tumors of childhood. N Engl J Med 326:988–993

Boyd MC, Steinbok P (1987) Choroid plexus tumors: problems in diagnosis and management. J Neurosurg 66:800–805

Brinster RL, Chen HY, Messing A, van Dyke T, Levine AJ, Palmiter RD (1984) Transgenic mice harboring SV40 T-antigen genes develop characteristic brain tumors. Cell 37:367–379

Chow E, Jenkins JJ, Burger PC, Reardon DA, Langston JW, Sanford RA, Heideman RL, Kun LE, Merchant TE (1999a) Malignant evolution of choroid plexus papilloma. Pediatr Neurosurg 31:127–130

Chow E, Reardon DA, Shah AB, Jenkins JJ, Langston J, Heideman RL, Sanford RA, Kun LE, Merchant TE (1999b) Pediatric choroid plexus neoplasms. Int J Radiat Oncol Biol Phys 44:249–254

Coates TL, Hinshaw DB Jr, Peckman N, Thompson JR, Hasso AN, Holshouser BA, Knierim DS (1989) Pediatric choroid plexus neoplasms: MR, CT, and pathologic correlation. Radiology 173:81–88

Cruz-Sanchez FF, Rossi ML, Hughes JT, Coakham HB, Figols J, Eynaud PM (1989) Choroid plexus papillomas: an immunohistological study of 16 cases. Histopathology 15:61–69

Dandy W (1922) Diagnosis, localization, and removal of tumours of the third ventricle. Bull Johns Hopkins Hosp 33:188

Davis LE, Cushing H (1925) Papillomas of the choroid plexus with a report of six cases. Arch Neurol Psychiatry 13:681

Eisenberg HM, McComb JG, Lorenzo AV (1974) Cerebrospinal fluid overproduction and hydrocephalus associated with choroid plexus papilloma. J Neurosurg 40:381–385

Ellenbogen RG, Winston KR, Kupsky WJ (1989) Tumors of the choroid plexus in children. Neurosurgery, 25:327–335

Fitzpatrick LK, Aronson LJ, Cohen KJ (2002) Is there a requirement for adjuvant therapy for choroid plexus carcinoma that has been completely resected? J Neurooncol 57:123–126

Galassi E, Godano U, Cavallo M, Donati R, Nasi MT (1989) Intracranial tumors during the 1st year of life. Childs Nerv Syst 5:288–298

Gudeman SK, Sullivan HG, Rosner MJ, Becker DP (1979) Surgical removal of bilateral papillomas of the choroid plexus of the lateral ventricles with resolution of hydrocephalus. Case report. J Neurosurg 50:677–681

Haddad SF, Menezes AH, Bell WE, Godersky JC, Afifi AK, Bale JF (1991) Brain tumors occurring before 1 year of age: a retrospective reviews of 22 cases in an 11-year period (1977–1987). Neurosurgery 29:8–13

Herbert J, Cavallaro T, Dwork AJ (1990) A marker for primary choroid plexus neoplasms. Am J Pathol 136:1317–1325

Hirano H, Hirahara K, Asakura T, Shimozuru T, Kadota K, Kasamo S, Shimohonji M, Kimotsuki K, Goto M (1994) Hydrocephalus due to villous hypertrophy of the choroid plexus in the lateral ventricles. J Neurosurg, 80:321–323

Ho DM, Wong TT, Liu HC (1991) Choroid plexus tumors in childhood. Histopathologic study and clinico-pathological correlation. Childs Nerv Syst 7:437–441

Hopper KD, Foley LC, Nieves NL, Smirniotopoulos JG (1987) The interventricular extension of choroid plexus papillomas. AJNR Am J Neuroradiol 8:469–472

Horska A, Ulug AM, Melhem ER, Filippi CG, Burger PC, Edgar MA, Souweidane MM, Carson BS, Barker PB (2001) Proton magnetic resonance spectroscopy of choroid plexus tumors in children. J Magn Reson Imaging 14:78–82

Humphreys RP, Nemoto S, Hendrick EB, Hoffman HJ (1987) Childhood choroid plexus tumors. Conc Pediatr Neurosurg 7:1–18

Johnson DL (1989) Management of choroid plexus tumors in children. Pediatr Neurosci 15:195–206

Laurence KM (1974) The biology of choroid plexus papilloma and carcinoma of the lateral ventricle. In: Vinken PJ, Bruyn GW (eds) Handbook of clinical neurology. Elsevier, New York, pp 555–595

Lena G, Genitori L, Molina J, Legatte JR, Choux M (1990) Choroid plexus tumours in children. Review of 24 cases. Acta Neurochir (Wien) 106:68–72

Mannoji H, Becker LE (1988) Ependymal and choroid plexus tumors. Cytokeratin and GFAP expression. Cancer 61:1377–1385

Marks JR, Lin J, Hinds P, Miller D, Levine AJ (1989) Cellular gene expression in papillomas of the choroid plexus from transgenic mice that express the simian virus 40 large T antigen. J Virol 63:790–797

Matson DD, Crofton FD (1960) Papilloma of choroid plexus in childhood. J Neurosurg 17:1002

McComb RD, Burger PC (1983) Choroid plexus carcinoma. Report of a case with immunohistochemical and ultrastructural observations. Cancer 51:470–475

Packer RJ, Perilongo G, Johnson D, Sutton LN, Vezina G, Zimmerman RA, Ryan J, Reaman G, Schut L (1992) Choroid plexus carcinoma of childhood. Cancer 69:580–585

Paulus W, Janisch W (1990) Clinicopathologic correlations in epithelial choroid plexus neoplasms: a study of 52 cases. Acta Neuropathol (Berl) 80:635–641

Pencalet P, Sainte-Rose C, Lellouch-Tubiana A, Kalifa C, Brunelle F, Sgouros S, Meyer P, Cinalli G, Zerah M, Pierre-Kahn A, Renier D (1998) Papillomas and carcinomas of the choroid plexus in children. J Neurosurg 88:521–528

Raimondi AJ, Gutierrez FA (1975) Diagnosis and surgical treatment of choroid plexus papillomas. Childs Brain 1:81–115

Razzaq AA, Cohen AR (1997) Neoadjuvant chemotherapy for hypervascular malignant brain tumors of childhood. Pediatr Neurosurg 27:296–303

Rickert CH, Wiestler OD, Paulus W (2002) Chromosomal imbalances in choroid plexus tumors. Am J Pathol 160:1105–1113

Sahar A, Feinsod M, Beller AJ (1980) Choroid plexus papilloma: hydrocephalus and cerebrospinal fluid dynamics. Surg Neurol 13:476–478

Sarkar C, Sharma MC, Gaikwad S, Sharma C, Singh VP (1999) Choroid plexus papilloma: a clinicopathological study of 23 cases. Surg Neurol 52:37–39

Sevenet N, Lellouch-Tubiana A, Schofield D, Hoang-Xuan K, Gessler M, Birnbaum D, Jeanpierre C, Jouvet A, Delattre O (1999a) Spectrum of hSNF5/INI1 somatic mutations in human cancer and genotype-phenotype correlations. Hum Mol Genet 8:2359–2368

Sevenet N, Sheridan E, Amram D, Schneider P, Handgretinger R, Delattre O (1999b) Constitutional mutations of the hSNF5/INI1 gene predispose to a variety of cancers. Am J Hum Genet 65:1342–1348

St Clair SK, Humphreys RP, Pillay PK, Hoffman HJ, Blaser SI, Becker LE (1991) Current management of choroid plexus carcinoma in children. Pediatr Neurosurg 17:225–233

Vajtai I, Varga Z, Aguzzi A (1996) MIB-1 immunoreactivity reveals different labelling in low grade and in malignant epithelial neoplasms of the choroid plexus. Histopathology 29:147–151

Wilkins RH, Rutledge BJ (1961) Papillomas of the choroid plexus. J Neurosurg 18:14

Wolff JE, Sajedi M, Brant R, Coppes MJ, Egeler RM (2002) Choroid plexus tumours. Br J Cancer 87:1086–1091

Wolff JE, Sajedi M, Coppes MJ, Anderson RA, Egeler RM (1999) Radiation therapy and survival in choroid plexus carcinoma. Lancet, 353:2126

Wyatt-Ashmead J, Kleinschmidt-DeMasters B, Mierau GW, Malkin D, Orsini E, McGavran L, Foreman NK (2001) Choroid plexus carcinomas and rhabdoid tumors: phenotypic and genotypic overlap. Pediatr Dev Pathol 4:545–549

Zhen HN, Zhang X, Bu XY, Zhang ZW, Huang WJ, Zhang P, Liang JW, Wang XL (1999) Expression of the simian virus 40 large tumor antigen (Tag) and formation of Tag-p53 and Tag-pRb complexes in human brain tumors. Cancer 86:2124–2132

Zwetsloot CP, Kros JM, Paz y Gueze HD (1991) Familial occurrence of tumours of the choroid plexus. J Med Genet 28:492–494

Intramedullary Spinal Cord Tumors

A. Quinones-Hinojosa · M. Gulati
M. H. Schmidt

Contents

10.1 Introduction

Intramedullary spinal cord tumors (IMSCTs) are rare and account for only 4 to 6% of all pediatric central nervous system tumors (DeSousa et al. 1979). Approximately 100 to 200 cases are diagnosed each year in the US (Constantini and Epstein 1995), representing an incidence of less than 1 in 100,000. Pediatric IMSCTs are usually located in the cervical or thoracic spine (90 to 95%) and occur infrequently in the lumbar spine (Epstein and Ragheb 1994; Goh et al. 2000). There is an equal male and female distribution in the reported pediatric series (Brotchi et al. 1992; Goh et al. 1997; Zileli et al. 1996).

Initially, the presenting symptoms are minimal, often leading to delay in recognition. The parents usually report that mild symptoms have been present for months to years prior to diagnosis. Signs and symptoms include pain, weakness, paresthesias, spinal deformity, sphincter disturbance, and cervicomedullary symptoms (Goh et al. 2000). Slow deterioration of neurological function can also occur (Constantini et al. 1996). The primary treatment for primary IMSCTs is surgical resection; however, resection may leave a patient with severe neurological deficits. Effective treatment requires an interdisciplinary approach incorporating specialists in pediatric neurosurgery, neurooncology, child neurology, pediatrics, and nursing.

10.2 Ependymoma

10.2.1 Epidemiology and Etiology

Ependymomas can either arise from the cranial ventricular system or within the spinal cord. Those originating in the spinal cord presumably arise from the remnants of the central canal and can be seen both in children and in young adults. Ependymomas are found most commonly in the cervical region in children, and have a lower incidence than astrocytomas (Brotchi et al. 1991; Fine et al. 1995). In a study by Miller (2000) ependymomas were found in 16 out of 117 pediatric patients (16%) with intramedullary spinal cord tumors . Ependymomas tend to increase in incidence with age. A recent study by Constantini and colleagues reported no ependymomas in a series of intramedullary spinal cord tumors in patients under three years of age (Constantini et al. 1996).

Ependymomas (WHO grade II) have been found to contain SV40 virus large-T-antigen-related DNA sequences. This finding has received a great deal of attention since widespread use of SV40-contaminated polio vaccines may have occurred between 1955 to 1962 (Huang et al. 1999). However, these findings have not been corroborated by other investigators and the role of SV40 in the pathogenesis of ependymomas still remains to be established (Salewski et al. 1999). Intramedullary spinal cord ependymomas are associated with neurofibromatosis type 2 (NF2) (Egelhoff et al. 1992), a genetic syndrome inherited in an autosomal dominant pattern (see Chap. II). In fact, one recent study showed mutations of the NF2 transcript occur in a majority of sporadic intramedullary spinal cord ependymomas (Birch et al. 1996). In this study, five of seven intramedullary spinal cord ependymomas had mutations that resulted in truncation of the predicted protein product, probably rendering the protein product inactive (Birch et al. 1996).

10.2.2 Pathology

10.2.2.1 Grading

Eighty-nine percent of IMSCTs in children are low-grade tumors (Constantini et al. 1996). Four different entities are delineated according to the most recent WHO classification of tumors (Kleihues et al. 2000). The subependymoma (WHO grade I) is a benign, slowly growing intraventricular tumor that is often detected incidentally and carries a very good prognosis. These tumors have histological features of both subependymomas and ependymomas. The myxopapillary type (WHO grade I) arises in the filum terminale or conus medullaris almost exclusively and carries a good long-term prognosis. Classic ependymoma (WHO grade II) is a common intramedullary neoplasm found in the spinal cord in children. Anaplastic ependymoma (WHO grade III) is thought to arise from a malignant transformation of low-grade ependymoma (Kleihues et al. 2000).

10.2.2.2 Histopathology

The myxopapillary ependymoma has a pseudopapillary architecture and abundant mucin production. This variety of ependymoma is characterized by GFAP-expressing tumor cells with a cuboidal or elongated morphology arranged radially in a papillary manner around vascularized stromal cores. Mitotic activity is almost absent and a mucoid matrix material accumulates between tumor cells and blood vessels. Subependymomas are rarely mitotically active, and are characterized by clusters of isomorphic nuclei embedded in a dense fibrillary matrix of glial cell processes, often with small cysts.

Ependymomas are highly cellular tumors regardless of their grade. Their characteristic features include pseudorosettes and perivascular grouping. Since ependymomas are highly cellular, neuropathologists may on occasion disagree on the grade of a given specimen (McLaughlin et al. 1998). In particular, there is a tendency to attribute a higher grade to low-grade tumors.

Figure 10.1

Histological features of ependymoma. This image illustrates the ependymal rosettes that are formed from columnar cells arranged around a central lumen. Also in the top right hand corner, a pseudorosette, cells arranged radially around a blood vessels, can be appreciated

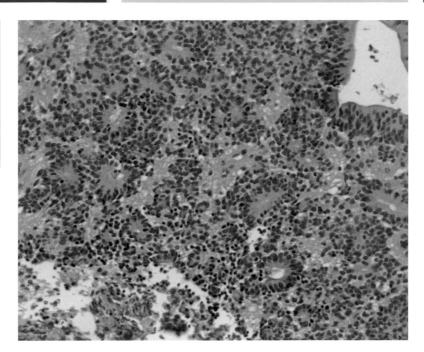

Classic ependymomas contain perivascular pseudorosettes which are immunoreactive for glial fibrillary acidic protein (GFAP) and, uncommonly, true epithelial-lined ependymal rosettes (Fig. 10.1). The perivascular pseudorosettes originate from tumor cells arranged radially around blood vessels and occur in the great majority of these tumors. True rosettes appear as a number of nuclei forming a ring from which neurofibrils, which can be demonstrated by silver staining, extend to interlace in the center. These tumors are well delineated and mitotic figures are rare. An occasional non-palisading focus of necrosis is sometimes observed and is compatible with lower-grade histology. Unusual variants such as the clear-cell ependymoma and the tanycytic ependymoma can mimic oligodendroglioma and astrocytoma, respectively (Goh et al. 2000). Other histopathological variants include cellular and papillary ependymoma. The differential diagnosis can be aided by the presence of epithelial differentiation demonstrated using immunohistochemistry or electron microscopy.

The anaplastic ependymoma differs from the classic ependymoma. While the cells of the classic ependymoma are morphologically similar to normal ependymal cells, those of the anaplastic ependymoma have clear histologic features of malignancy. More specifically, the anaplastic ependymoma is characterized by aggressive mitotic activity and increased cellularity often associated with microvascular proliferation and pseudopalisading necrosis. Anaplastic ependymomas can be very invasive and are often poorly differentiated.

10.2.2.3 Molecular Biology and Cytogenetics

A study by von Haken et al. (1996) reported a 50% incidence of allelic losses on the short arm of chromosome 17 in 18 pediatric ependymomas. The tumor-suppressor gene *p53* was excluded, and therefore a candidate gene has yet to be identified. Recognizing the increased incidence of ependymomas in patients with NF2, some investigators have reported evidence for mutations of the *NF2* gene located on chromosome 22q12. One group analyzed 62 ependymal tumors for loss of heterozygosity (LOH) 22q, LOH 10q, and for mutations of the *NF2* tumor-suppressor gene. Six of the tumors revealed mutations of NF2, all of which came from patients with IMSCTs (Ebert et al. 1999). This may suggest that spinal intramedullary ependymomas constitute a distinct phenotypic variant of an altered *NF2* gene. Additional cytogenetic changes have been found in a significant number of ependymomas. In a series of 22 childhood ependymomas, loss of chromosome 22 was found in 2 cases, deletion of chromosome 17 in 2 cases and rearrangements or deletions of chromosome 6 in 5 cases (Kramer et al. 1998). In anaplastic ependymoma, the

genetic alterations remain largely undefined. A recent study of 23 anaplastic ependymomas revealed LOH 10q in 4 cases, but the significance of this finding is unknown (Ebert et al. 1999).

10.2.3 Clinical Features

Intramedullary spinal cord tumors occur commonly in the cervical region. Children most often present with pain, reported in 42% of cases. Motor regression with weakness is present in 36%, gait abnormality or deterioration in 27%, torticollis in 27%, and progressive kyphoscoliosis in 24% of cases (Constantini et al. 1996). Hydrocephalus occurs with greater frequency than in adult patients and may require treatment with a CSF shunt (Houten and Weiner 2000) (Table 10.1).

10.2.4 Diagnostic Imaging

Magnetic resonance imaging (MRI) has greatly improved the preoperative evaluation of spinal cord tumors. The exact histologic diagnosis of these tumors, however, cannot be made by MRI features and patterns of enhancement (Table 10.2). Tumor tissue is still required in virtually all cases to establish a definitive diagnosis. Since ependymomas originate from the ependymal walls, they tend to be more central in location as compared with astrocytomas. On average,

Table 10.1. Presenting symptoms of intramedullary spinal cord tumors in children

Pain
Motor regression
Weakness
Gait abnormality/deterioration
Torticollis
Progressive kyphoscoliosis
Hydrocephalus
Sphincter disturbance
Reflex changes
Sensory impairment

Table 10.2. Magnetic resonance imaging features of intramedullary spinal cord tumors

	Ependymomas	Astrocytomas
Location	centrally located; mostly in the cervical spine but in children also present in the conus	Eccentrically located; usually widens the spinal cord; 75% of astrocytomas in the cervical-thoracic regions; 20% in the distal cord; 5% in the filum terminale
T1-weighted image	Isointense/hypointense	Isointense/hypointense
T1-weighted image with contrast	axial view; cord symmetrically expanded; enhances with contrast but less than astrocytomas	Ill-defined borders Axial view; cord asymmetrical, "lumpy"; heterogeneous, moderate, partial contrast enhancement

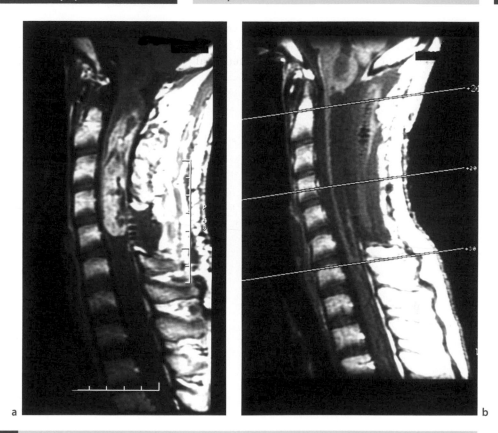

a   b

Figure 10.2 a,b

A 17-year-old male presented with left-arm numbness and tingling. **a** The preoperative MRI scan reveals an intramedullary cervical cord mass in the sagittal T1-weighted image with contrast. Gross total resection was achieved, and pathology was consistent with a grade II ependymoma. **b** A postoperative MRI showed resection of the mass with no evidence of residual tumor as demonstrated in the sagittal T1-weighted image with contrast

ependymomas span three to four vertebral bodies (Baleriaux 1999). The pattern of enhancement is homogeneous, usually with well-defined borders (Fig. 10.2). A "cap sign" is often seen, which corresponds to a low-signal-intensity area on either side of the tumor mass itself. The caps represent hemosiderin deposits secondary to chronic hemorrhage (Baleriaux 1999). These tumors can on occasion present with subarachnoid hemorrhage. Ependymomas are also often associated with large intramedullary satellite cysts. These can extend many segments above or below the solid component of the tumor.

Miyasawa and colleagues reported that the typical MRI characteristics of ependymoma include an enhancing border, sharply defined margins, and a central location in the spinal cord (Miyazawa et al. 2000). Axial post-contrast sequences demonstrate symmetric expansion of the spinal cord, unlike astrocytoma, in which the pattern of expansion is often asymmetric or nodular. The study also concluded that hemorrhage within the tumor, hemosiderin deposits, or calcifications are more frequent in ependymomas, which may be attributed the presence of a highly vascular connective tissue stroma.

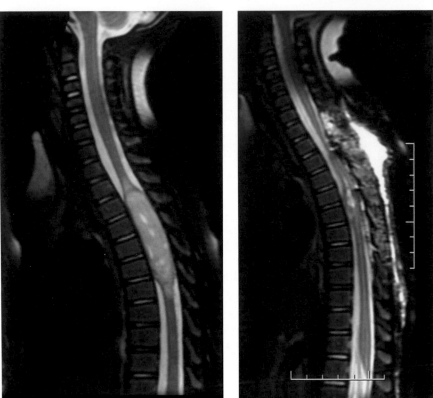

a

b

Figure 10.3 a,b

A three-year-old girl presented with six months of intermittent, worsening back pain. a The sagittal T2-weighted MRI revealed a large intramedullary mass extending from T3–T7. Histology was consistent with a juvenile pilocytic astrocytoma. b The postoperative MRI scan demonstrates removal of the centrally located tumor, nodular enhancement in the area of the surgery, shown in a sagittal T2-weighted image (bB). Although nodular enhancement was present in the first postoperative imaging study, subsequent MRIs showed complete resolution of the abnormality

10.3 Astrocytoma

Astrocytomas are the largest group (about 60%) of pediatric IMSCTs (Epstein and Ragheb 1994; Reimer and Onofrio 1985; Rossitch et al. 1990). They are typically large and mostly located in the thoracic region. A cystic component may be present, commonly intratumoral. Satellite cysts and secondary hydromyelia may also be observed (Baleriaux 1999). The histology in all age groups is usually low grade; high-grade tumors occur in only 10 to 15% of cases (Allen et al. 1998; DeSousa et al. 1979). In children, the most common IMSCT is the pilocytic astrocytoma (Figs. 10.3, 10.4). Pilocytic astrocytomas are well circumscribed, slowly growing, often cystic tumors that are characterized histologically by a biphasic pattern with varying proportions of compacted bipolar cells with Rosenthal fibers.

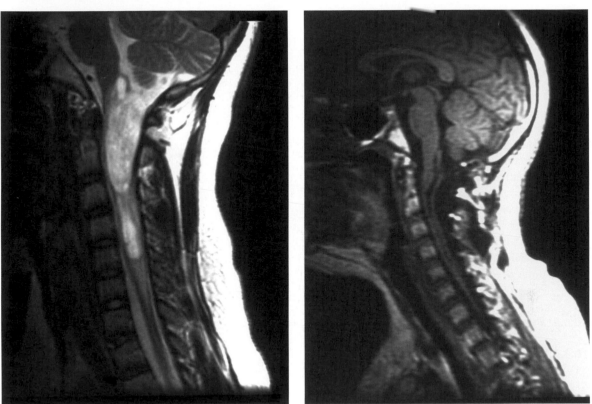

a   b

Figure 10.4 a,b

A twelve-year-old girl presented with a three-month history of progressive right arm weakness and clumsiness. **a** The preoperative MRI scan revealed an intramedullary spinal cord tumor extending from the cervicomedullary junction to C4, as shown in a sagittal T2-weighted image. Histology was consistent with a juvenile pilocytic astrocytoma. **b** The postoperative MRI demonstrates that the enhancing mass has been resected, as shown in the sagittal T1-weighted image

10.3.1 Epidemiology and Etiology

Low-grade astrocytomas such as pilocytic astrocytoma most often present in the first two decades of life with no clear gender predilection. In adults, they are mostly encountered in younger patients (mean age 29 years) with a predominance in males (63%) (Baleriaux 1999). Previous irradiation is known to play a causative role in the formation of CNS gliomas. Nevertheless, very few case reports of radiation-induced intramedullary astrocytomas exist in the literature. Grabb and colleagues (1996) reported a case of a ra-

diation-induced spinal cord glioma in a 20-year-old woman who presented with neck pain and new significant neurological deficits 17 years after resection of a posterior fossa medullomyoblastoma and craniospinal irradiation. She was found to have a cervical intramedullary tumor consistent with anaplastic astrocytoma.

Familial clustering of astrocytomas is frequently described. These tumors are associated with inherited syndromes such as Li-Fraumeni syndrome, Turcot's syndrome, tuberous sclerosis, multiple enchondromatosis (Maffucci/Ollier disease), and neurofibromatosis (NF) (Frappaz et al. 1999; Mellon et al. 1988; van Nielen and de Jong 1999). The typical picture of spinal involvement with NF is the presence of multiple, extramedullary, spinal nerve root neurofibromas. These tumors can cause spinal cord compression but are anatomically outside the spinal cord itself. Lee and colleagues (1996) have reported a series of nine patients with NF that had developed IMSCTs (ages ranged from 4 to 31 years). Three patients had neurofibromatosis type1 (NF1), five patients had NF2, and one patient had an undefined variety. The pathology of the tumors was also variable, with five ependymomas, three astrocytomas, and one intramedullary schwannoma reported (Lee et al. 1996). Based on limited data it is unclear whether IMSCTs are a subgroup of NF-associated neoplasms, or simply represent the higher tumor predisposition in these patients.

10.3.2 Pathology

10.3.2.1 Grading

Grading is based on areas with the highest degree of anaplasia. The WHO classification of astrocytomas consists of four grades: grade I (pilocytic astrocytoma), grade II (diffuse astrocytoma), grade III (anaplastic astrocytoma) (Fig. 10.5), and grade IV (glioblastoma multiforme).

10.3.2.2 Histopathology

The pilocytic astrocytoma is characterized by elongated "hair" cells with coarse cytoplasmic process. Intracytoplasmic Rosenthal fibers and eosinophilic granular bodies are characteristic but not specific features. Cellular pleomorphism, vascular proliferation, infiltration of the meninges, and occasional mitoses can also be present but have no prognostic value and do not represent malignant features.

The diffuse fibrillary astrocytoma is an infiltrative tumor that produces fusiform enlargement of the cord. The typical features include hypercellularity, nuclear atypia and an infiltrative growth pattern. The dominant cell types are well differentiated fibrillary

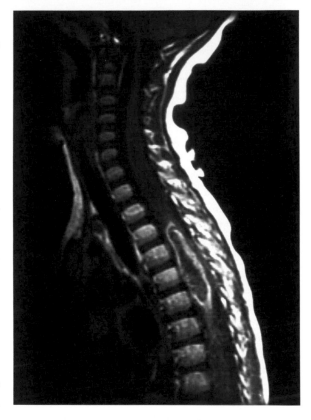

Figure 10.5

A two-year-old boy presented with several weeks of slowly progressive disuse of his lower extremities. The preoperative MRI demonstrated a six centimeter intramedullary thoracic cord mass from T3 to T7 with marked edema spanning the entire length of the spinal cord. Histopathology showed the tumor to be a grade III oligoastrocytoma. The patient's tumor progressed despite treatment

or gemistocytic neoplastic astrocytes in a background of a loosely structured, often microcystic matrix. Mitotic activity is mostly absent. Three major variants can be distinguished based upon the appearance of the astrocytes: fibrillary (fibrillary neoplastic astrocytes), gemistocytic (a conspicuous though variable fraction of gemistocytic astrocytes), and protoplasmic (small cell body with few, flaccid processes with a low content of glial filaments and scant

GFAP expression). Higher-grade tumors, anaplastic astrocytoma and glioblastoma multiforme, have increased cellularity, anaplasia, and marked mitotic activity. A tumor is classified as a glioblastoma multiforme when endothelial proliferation and necrosis are also present.

10.3.2.3 Molecular Biology and Cytogenetics

Some astrocytomas are known to lose chromosome 17q, which includes the region encoding the *NF1* gene (van Deimling et al. 1993). Screening of *NF1*-coding sequences such as the GRD (GAP related domain) region, the only functional region of the *NF1* mRNA transcript identified to date, has failed to detect any mutations. Current evidence has failed to support a role for the tumor-suppressor gene *NF1* in the oncogenesis of pilocytic astrocytomas (Kleihues and Cavenee 2000).

Cytogenetic studies of pilocytic astrocytomas have revealed a variety of aberrations but no specific pattern suggestive of a specific tumor-suppressor gene has been reported (Ransom et al. 1992). Ransom and colleagues attempted to locate tumor-suppressor genes on chromosome 10 by correlating cytogenetic studies and LOH analysis in human astrocytomas and mixed oligoastrocytomas. Of 53 specimens, 45 were diffuse astrocytomas, 1 was an astroblastoma, and 7 were mixed oligoastrocytomas. By cytogenetic analyses the most common numeric chromosome abnormalities were +7, -10, -13, -14, -17, +19, -22, and -Y. The most common structural abnormalities involved chromosome arms 1p, 1q, 5p, and 9p. By LOH and dosage analysis the most common molecular genetic abnormalities were of chromosome arms 5p, 6p, 7q, 9p, 10p, 10q, 13q, 14q, 17p, and 19p. When the results of all methods were combined, the most commonly abnormal chromosomes were, in descending frequency, 10, Y, 17, 7, 13, and 9. In 80 percent of cases the cytogenetic and molecular genetic studies were concordant. The authors concluded that, based on the genetic analyses of these tumors, there may be 2 regions on chromosome 10 that contain tumor-suppressor genes (Ransom et al. 1992).

10.3.3 Clinical Features

The clinical features of intramedullary astrocytomas are similar to the symptoms of intramedullary ependymomas (Table 10.1). Gait disturbance, pain, and sphincter disturbance are the most common presenting symptoms, while reflex changes, paralysis, and sensory impairment are the most frequent physical findings (DeSousa et al. 1979). Spinal deformity can be present in up to 30% of patients (Steinbok et al. 1992). Epstein and colleagues, in a series of 152 spinal cord astrocytomas, reported that scoliosis was the most common early sign in 34 cases of thoracic tumors while torticollis was present in 21 cases of cervical spine astrocytomas (Epstein 1986). Tumors involving the cervicomedullary junction can present with unusual symptoms. If the medulla is involved, children can develop: (1) failure to thrive due to nausea, vomiting, choking, and dysphagia; (2) frequent respiratory tract infections from chronic aspiration; (3) dysphonia and dysarthria; and (4) sleep apnea from respiratory center involvement. If the tumor mainly arises from the cervical cord then children can present with long-standing neck pain and torticollis, slowly evolving motor deficits in the limbs, sometimes with associated muscle atrophy, sensory dyesthesias, hyperreflexia, and occasionally hydrocephalus (Abbott 1993; Robertson et al. 1994) (Fig. 10.4).

10.3.4 Diagnostic Imaging

As with all spinal cord tumors, MRI is the diagnostic tool of choice. Astrocytomas are commonly located eccentrically within the spinal cord (Table 10.2). On MRI, there is heterogeneous, moderate, and partial contrast enhancement following gadolinium administration, with ill-defined borders (Baleriaux 1999) (Figs. 10.3 to 10.5). Approximately 75% of astrocytomas occur in the cervico–thoracic region, 20% in the distal spinal cord, and 5% in the filum terminale (Osborn 1994). Whereas the mean extent of an ependymoma corresponds to three to four vertebral bodies, astrocytomas are in general much more extensive, with one series reporting a mean span of 5.6 vertebral bodies (minimum 2, maximum 19) (Baleriaux 1999).

10.4 Treatment

The treatment of choice for intramedullary tumors, both ependymomas and astrocytomas, is surgical resection. The resection is aided by motor and sensory evoked-potential monitoring. Gross total resection can be achieved in the majority of ependymomas and will very likely result in cure (Houten and Weiner 2000). Astrocytomas, on the other hand, are infiltrating neoplasms and gross total resection is occasionally possible only in the pediatric population. Outcome for low-grade astrocytomas is better in children than adults, but not as favorable as that for ependymomas. The role of radical resection of low-grade fibrillary astrocytomas of the spinal cord in children has not been definitively demonstrated in the literature (Houten and Weiner 2000).

10.4.1 Surgery

10.4.1.1 Surgical Approach

Bone exposure by laminectomy (removal of the vertebral lamina to unroof the spinal canal) is centered on the solid part of the tumor, as identified by preoperative MRI. Osteoplastic laminotomy (removal of the laminar roof in one piece and replacement at the end of the case) is the preferred technique in children (Houten and Weiner 2000). This preserves the posterior tension band, restores normal anatomy, and may result in bony fusion of the reapproximated lamina (Raimondi et al. 1976). There is evidence that this technique results in a reduced incidence of postoperative spinal deformity (Constantini and Epstein 1995). Intraoperative ultrasound is crucial to verify that the rostral-caudal bony exposure is sufficient to expose the entire solid component of the tumor (Brunberg et al. 1991; Raghavendra et al. 1984). More importantly, intraoperative ultrasound has been shown to reduce the extent of the laminectomy, dural opening and myelotomy needed for resection (Maiuri et al. 2000).

10.4.1.2 Technical Considerations During Tumor Removal

Conventional orthodromic somatosensory evoked potentials (SSEPs) are used to measure dorsal-column function during surgery (Goh et al. 2000). This is done by electrically stimulating the extremities and recording at higher points, including the head. Excessive traction or injury to the spinal cord will result in a reduction of these potentials. At our center, we have reported the use of antidromic-elicited SSEPs to assist placement of the myelotomy (Quinones-Hinojosa et al. 2002). This antidromic recording is performed by stimulating along the posterior surface of the spinal cord, while recording evoked responses in the extremities. In a patient whose SSEP recordings are shown (Fig. 10.6), a stimulating electrode was applied to the area of the dorsal columns and recordings of elicited antidromic SSEPs were made at the medial malleoli bilaterally. Beginning left of midline, stimulation evoked the SSEPs seen at the top of the figure. Moving towards the midline, stimulation evoked no SSEP at the area marked "septum," indicating the optimal electrical site of myelotomy.

A number of other techniques are used to reduce postoperative neurologic deficits. These include transcranial epidural and/ or transcranial muscle motor-evoked potentials (referred to as epidural and muscle Tc-MEPs). Tc-MEPs are obtained by stimulating electrodes over the patient's motor cortical regions, and recording EMG activity either epidurally or at the extremities (Kothbauer et al. 1997). Direct stimulation of the spinal cord is also possible with simultaneous recordings of extremity EMG recordings. In the patient whose EMG recording is shown (Fig. 10.7) tonic contractions of the right hand were noted during dissection of the ventral aspect of the tumor, amplitude of Tc-MEPs from the right hand dropped significantly, and direct intramedullary stimulation evoked EMG activity in the right upper extremity. This technique helped differentiate tumor from spinal cord, and prevented damage to the corticospinal tracts (Quinones-Hinojosa et al. 2002).

Ependymomas are usually encapsulated, and a dissection plane can be established, allowing for removal of the entire tumor. With astrocytomas or very

Figure 10.6

Dorsal median sulcus mapping performed by stimulation of the dorsal columns followed by recording of antidromic SSEPs in the extremities. This technique assists placement of the spinal cord myelotomy at the true electrophysiologic midline of the cord, which is often distorted by tumor growth   ▶

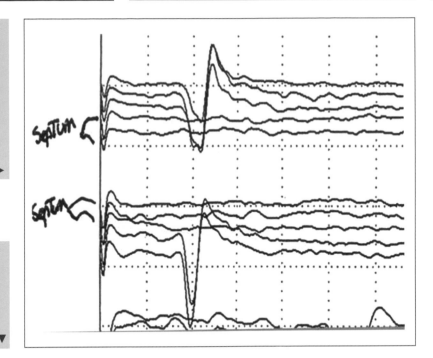

Figure 10.7

EMG recording in the extremities following direct intramedullary stimulation in the spinal cord can confirm corticospinal tract integrity during tumor resection   ▼

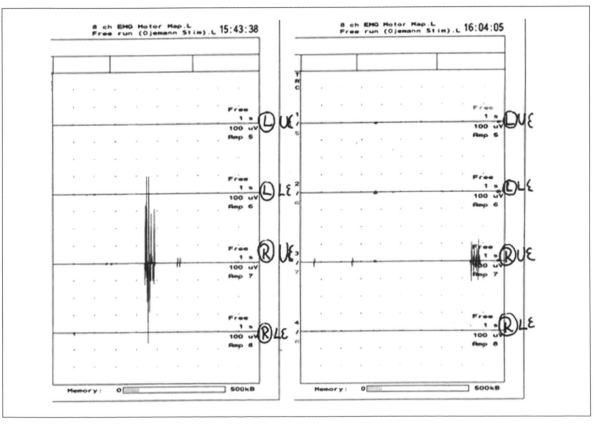

large tumors, the interface between tumor and cord tissue often cannot be identified. At the completion of surgery, the extent of resection should be reassessed by ultrasound before closing, and by postoperative MRI in the immediate postoperative period. Gross total resection is defined as more than 90% tumor removal, subtotal resection as 50 to 90%, and partial as less than 50%.

10.4.2 Radiation Therapy

Radiation therapy has played a limited role in the primary management of IMSCTs in children. The side effects associated with CNS irradiation include growth retardation, endocrine dysfunction, decreased IQ, radionecrosis, vasculopathy, and alopecia (Avizonis et al. 1992). Some investigators advocate radiotherapy only for incompletely resected tumors and high-grade astrocytomas.

In a recent review of the literature regarding radiation therapy and the management of intramedullary spinal-cord tumors, Isaacson (2000) concluded that low-grade, completely resected astrocytomas should be followed by serial imaging studies. Low-grade astrocytomas with incomplete resection appear to benefit from postoperative radiation. For high-grade astrocytomas in the spine some authors recommend aggressive surgical resection followed by radiotherapy, but these tumors can relapse early. Isaacson recommended that all high-grade astrocytomas be treated with radiation (Isaacson 2000).

Literature supporting the use of radiotherapy for intramedullary spinal cord ependymoma in children is scarce and inconclusive (Isaacson 2000). Nagib and colleagues treated three children, ages 7, 8, and 13 years, for conus medullaris myxopapillary ependymoma over a 2-year period with a 24-month follow-up. One child received radiation therapy following a recurrence. Based on this patient and a literature review including 11 other cases, the authors concluded that the gross feature of myxopapillary ependymoma that allows for complete resectability appears to be the key prognostic factor, and that radiotherapy appeared to have no proven value in completely resected conus medullaris myxopapillary

ependymoma tumors in children (Nagib and O'Fallon 1997).

Isaacson in his review of the literature concluded that patients with gross total resection of low-grade ependymomas with no evidence of disease should be observed with serial imaging studies (Isaacson 2000). High-grade and multifocal benign ependymomas should be given adjuvant radiation therapy. Complete imaging of the neuraxis and cerebrospinal fluid analysis should be obtained to assist in the decision-making process. Isaacson's specific radiation therapy guidelines are: (1) low-grade astrocytomas and low-grade ependymomas with residual disease after surgery should be prescribed a total dose of 5040 cGy in 180 cGy fractions over 28 treatment days using external beam radiation therapy (EXBRT); (2) for high-grade astrocytomas despite complete resection, the treatment recommended is the same (5040 cGy with 180 cGy fractions with EXBRT); (3) malignant ependymomas and benign multifocal ependymomas are treated with a locally delivered dose of 5040 to 5400 cGy in 28 to 30 fractions with occasional consideration of radiation to the neuraxis (Isaacson 2000).

10.4.3 Chemotherapy

Chemotherapy for the treatment of IMSCTs as an adjunct to surgery, radiotherapy, or both is not standardized. Adjuvant chemotherapy may play an important role in children younger than 3 years old, mainly in an effort to delay radiotherapy (Prados et al. 1997). Chemotherapy guidelines for IMSCTs are mainly based upon the clinical experience with intracranial low-grade gliomas. As with radiotherapy, no randomized trials have been performed, and only anecdotal reports and small series have been reported (Doireau et al. 1999; Hassall et al. 2001; Lowis et al. 1998; Merchant et al. 2000).

Lowis and colleagues described two children with astrocytomas (Lowis et al. 1998). The first child, a 19-month-old, had an anaplastic astrocytoma of the cervical spinal cord that progressed rapidly after initial partial resection. Chemotherapy was given according to the United Kingdom Children's Cancer Study Group Baby Brain Protocol (Lashford et al. 1996) with marked clinical improvement. This regimen comprised cycles of chemotherapy (carboplatin, vincristine, cyclophosphamide, methotrexate, and cisplatin) given every two weeks, regardless of count, for a period of 1 year. No evaluable disease remained at the end of treatment (Lowis et al. 1998). The second child was a 4-year-old with a recurrent low-grade astrocytoma. Chemotherapy was given for 3 months according to an International Society of Paediatric Oncology protocol for low-grade gliomas. This regimen consisted of cycles of carboplatin and vincristine administered every 3 weeks and vincristine administered weekly for the first 10 weeks, then carboplatin and vincristine administered every 4 weeks up to 1 year. Marked tumor regression was observed, accompanied by neurological recovery. The authors concluded that these patients demonstrate the potential value and low morbidity of chemotherapy in spinal cord astrocytoma (Lowis et al. 1998).

A study by Hassall and colleagues reported responses to carboplatin in three patients with progressive low-grade spinal cord gliomas (Hassall et al. 2001). The diagnoses of the tumors were juvenile pilocytic astrocytoma (Allen et al. 1998) and ganglioglioma (Abbott 1993). With a mean follow-up of 27 months, one patient had a complete response, one patient had partial response, and one patient had stable disease (Hassall et al. 2001). The potential role of chemotherapy in the management of spinal cord astrocytoma remains to be defined.

10.5 Outcome

Different studies have consistently demonstrated that there are only two significant predictors of outcome in patients with intramedullary spinal cord tumors: the histologic grade of the tumor and the preoperative neurologic status at the time of surgery (Cristante and Herrmann 1994). In general, patients with ependymoma have a more favorable outcome than those with low-grade astrocytoma (WHO grade II). In a series of 21 patients, Sandler reported a five-year survival of 57% in patients with grade I or II spinal cord astrocytoma (Sandler et al. 1992). Patients with pilocytic astrocytoma, the most common spinal cord

tumor found in children, have an even more favorable prognosis (Houten and Weiner 2000). Patients with malignant astrocytomas do very poorly, with no correlation between the extent of resection and survival. In one study of 19 patients with malignant astrocytomas of the spinal cord, median survival was only six months. At the time of publication, 15 (79%) of the 19 patients in the series had died. Although all underwent radical excision, none of the patients improved following their operations. Hydrocephalus and dissemination of disease occurred in a majority of patients (Cohen et al. 1989). Some data, however, suggest that surgery for malignant spinal astrocytomas is not always futile. In one study of 18 children with spinal astrocytomas, gross total resection was achieved in 5, including 3 with anaplastic tumors. All 5 of the patients in whom gross total resection was achieved were alive and disease free between 12 and 18 years after treatment (Przybylski et al. 1997).

The prognosis and outcome of patients with intramedullary ependymomas mainly depends on the extent of the original resection. Ependymomas are slow-growing tumors and late recurrence has been seen up to 12 years after surgery as reported at our institution (Linstadt et al. 1989). Gross total resection of benign intramedullary ependymomas more commonly results in long-term tumor control or cure than do subtotal resection and radiation therapy together (Cristante and Herrmann 1994; Epstein et al. 1993; Hoshimara et al. 1999; McCormick et al. 1990). Some authors have reported up to 100% recurrence-free survival following gross total resection (McCormick et al. 1990), whereas others have reported recurrence rates of 5 to 10% (Cooper 1989; Guidetti et al. 1981). The current consensus is that gross total resection is the most efficacious treatment and that radiation therapy is unnecessary if complete removal has been accomplished (Cooper 1989; McCormick et al. 1990; McLaughlin et al. 1998a,b; Wen et al. 1991)

10.6 Conclusion

Although spinal cord tumors are rare, early diagnosis plays an important role in the management of the lesion and it is an important factor in prognosis and outcome. In the pediatric population, low-grade astrocytomas predominate; ependymomas increase in frequency with age and are the most common IMSCT in adults. Unexplained and intractable lumbar pain in childhood should be investigated with a high-quality MRI scan. Postoperative baseline MRI and regular sequential imaging studies are essential for long-term follow-up in patients that have undergone resection of an intramedullary spinal cord tumor. The mainstay of treatment to date for IMSCTs is surgery. Electrophysiological monitoring has proven to be a useful adjunct in aiding the resection of these lesions. In the future, appropriate management of these lesions will require a more complete understanding of their molecular genetics.

References

Abbott R (1993) Tumors of the medulla. Neurosurg Clin North Am 4:519–527

Allen JC, Aviner S, Yates AJ, Boyett JM, Cherlow JM, Turski PA, Epstein F, Finlay JL (1998) Treatment of high-grade spinal cord astrocytoma of childhood with "8-in-1" chemotherapy and radiotherapy: a pilot study of CCG-945. Children's Cancer Group. J Neurosurg 88:215–220

Avizonis VN, Fuller DB, Thomson JW, Walker MJ, Nilsson DE, Menlove RL (1992) Late effects following central nervous system radiation in a pediatric population. Neuropediatrics 23:228–234

Baleriaux DL (1999) Spinal cord tumors. Eur Radiol 9:1252–1258

Birch BD, Johnson JP, Parsa A, Desai RD, Yoon JT, Lycette CA, Li YM, Bruce JN (1996) Frequent type 2 neurofibromatosis gene transcript mutations in sporadic intramedullary spinal cord ependymomas. Neurosurgery 39:135–140

Brotchi J, Dewitte O, Levivier M, Baleriaux D, Vandesteene A, Raftopoulos C, Flament-Durand J, Noterman J (1991) A survey of 65 tumors within the spinal cord: surgical results and the importance of preoperative magnetic resonance imaging. Neurosurgery 29:651–656

Brotchi J, Noterman J, Baleriaux D (1992) Surgery of intramedullary spinal cord tumours. Acta Neurochir (Wien) 116:176–178

Brunberg JA, DiPietro MA, Venes JL, Dauser RC, Muraszko KM, Berkey GS, D'Amato CJ, Rubin JM (1991) Intramedullary lesions of the pediatric spinal cord: correlation of findings from MR imaging, intraoperative sonography, surgery, and histologic study. Radiology 181:573–579

Cohen AR, Wisoff JH, Allen JC, Epstein F (1989) Malignant astrocytomas of the spinal cord. J Neurosurg 70:50–54

Constantini S, Epstein F (1995) Intraspinal tumors in children and infants. In: Youmans J (ed) Neurological surgery. Saunders, Philadelphia, pp 3132–3167

Constantini S, Houten J, Miller DC, Freed D, Ozek MM, Rorke LB, Allen JC, Epstein FJ (1996) Intramedullary spinal cord tumors in children under the age of 3 years. J Neurosurg 85:1036–1043

Cooper PR (1989) Outcome after operative treatment of intramedullary spinal cord tumors in adults: intermediate and long-term results in 51 patients. Neurosurgery 25:855–859

Cristante L, Herrmann HD (1994) Surgical management of intramedullary spinal cord tumors: functional outcome and sources of morbidity. Neurosurgery 35:69–74

DeSousa AL, Kalsbeck JE, Mealey J Jr, Campbell RL, Hockey A (1979) Intraspinal tumors in children. A review of 81 cases. J Neurosurg 51:437–445

Doireau V, Grill J, Zerah M, Lellouch-Tubiana A, Couanet D, Chastagner P, Marchal JC, Grignon Y, Chouffai Z, Kalifa C (1999) Chemotherapy for unresectable and recurrent intramedullary glial tumours in children. Brain Tumours Subcommittee of the French Society of Paediatric Oncology (SFOP). Br J Cancer 81:835–840

Ebert C, von Haken M, Meyer-Puttlitz B, Wiestler OD, Reifenberger G, Pietsch T, von Deimling A (1999) Molecular genetic analysis of ependymal tumors. NF2 mutations and chromosome 22q loss occur preferentially in intramedullary spinal ependymomas. Am J Pathol 155:627–632

Egelhoff JC, Bates DJ, Ross JS, Rothner AD, Cohen BH (1992) Spinal MR findings in neurofibromatosis types 1 and 2. AJNR Am J Neuroradiol 13:1071–1077

Epstein F (1986) Intraaxial tumor of the spinal cord and cervicomedullary junction in children. In: Hoffman HJ (ed) Advances in pediatric neurosurgery. Hanley and Belfus, Philadelphia, pp 17–34

Epstein F, Ragheb J (1994) Intramedullary tumors of the spinal cord. In: Cheek W (ed) Pediatric neurosurgery: surgery of the developing nervous system. Saunders, Philadelphia, pp 446–457

Epstein FJ, Farmer JP, Freed D (1993) Adult intramedullary spinal cord ependymomas: the result of surgery in 38 patients. J Neurosurg 79:204–209

Fine MJ, Kricheff II, Freed D, Epstein FJ (1995) Spinal cord ependymomas: MR imaging features. Radiology 197:655–658

Frappaz D, Ricci AC, Kohler R, Bret P, Mottolese C (1999) Diffuse brain stem tumor in an adolescent with multiple enchondromatosis (Ollier's disease). Childs Nerv Syst 15:222–225

Goh K, Muszynski C, Teo J, Constantini S, Epstein F (2000) Excision of spinal intramedullary tumors. In: Kaye A, Black P (eds) Operative neurosurgery, Churchill Livingstone: London, pp 1947–1959

Goh KY, Velasquez L, Epstein FJ (1997) Pediatric intramedullary spinal cord tumors: is surgery alone enough? Pediatr Neurosurg 27:34–39

Grabb PA, Kelly DR, Fulmer BB, Palmer C (1996) Radiation-induced glioma of the spinal cord. Pediatr Neurosurg 25:214–219

Guidetti B, Mercuri S, Vagnozzi R (1981) Long-term results of the surgical treatment of 129 intramedullary spinal gliomas. J Neurosurg 54:323–330

Hassall TE, Mitchell AE, Ashley DM (2001) Carboplatin chemotherapy for progressive intramedullary spinal cord low-grade gliomas in children: three case studies and a review of the literature. Neurooncology 3:251–257

Hoshimaru M, Koyama T, Hashimoto N, Kikuchi H (1999) Results of microsurgical treatment for intramedullary spinal cord ependymomas: analysis of 36 cases. Neurosurgery 44:264–269

Houten JK, Weiner HL (2000) Pediatric intramedullary spinal cord tumors: special considerations. J Neurooncol 47:225–230

Huang H, Reis R, Yonekawa Y, Lopes JM, Kleihues P, Ohgaki H (1999) Identification in human brain tumors of DNA sequences specific for SV40 large T antigen. Brain Pathol 9:33–42

Isaacson SR (2000) Radiation therapy and the management of intramedullary spinal cord tumors. J Neurooncol 47:231–238

Kleihues P, Cavenee WK (eds) (2000) Pathology and genetics of tumours of the nervous system. IARC Press, Lyon

Kothbauer K, Deletis V, Epstein FJ (1997) Intraoperative spinal cord monitoring for intramedullary surgery: an essential adjunct. Pediatr Neurosurg 26:247–254

Kramer DL, Parmiter AH, Rorke LB, Sutton LN, Biegel JA (1998) Molecular cytogenetic studies of pediatric ependymomas. J Neurooncol 37:25–33

Lashford LS, Campbell RH, Gattamaneni HR, Robinson K, Walker D, Bailey C (1996) An intensive multiagent chemotherapy regimen for brain tumours occurring in very young children. Arch Dis Child 74:219–223

Lee M, Rezai AR, Freed D, Epstein FJ (1996) Intramedullary spinal cord tumors in neurofibromatosis. Neurosurgery 38:32–37

Linstadt DE, Wara WM, Leibel SA, Gutin PH, Wilson CB, Sheline GE (1989) Postoperative radiotherapy of primary spinal cord tumors. Int J Radiat Oncol Biol Phys 16:1397–1403

Lowis SP, Pizer BL, Coakham H, Nelson RJ, Bouffet E (1998) Chemotherapy for spinal cord astrocytoma: can natural history be modified? Childs Nerv Syst 14:317–321

Maiuri F, Iaconetta G, Gallicchio B, Stella L (2000) Intraoperative sonography for spinal tumors. Correlations with MR findings and surgery. J Neurosurg Sci 44:115–122

McCormick PC, Torres R, Post KD, Stein BM (1990) Intramedullary ependymoma of the spinal cord. J Neurosurg 72:523–532

McLaughlin MP, Buatti JM, Marcus RB Jr, Maria BL, Mickle PJ, Kedar A (1998) Outcome after radiotherapy of primary spinal cord glial tumors. Radiat Oncol Invest 6:276–280

McLaughlin MP, Marcus RB Jr, Buatti JM, McCollough WM, Mickle JP, Kedar A, Maria BL, Million RR (1998) Ependymoma: results, prognostic factors and treatment recommendations. Int J Radiat Oncol Biol Phys 40:845–850

Mellon CD, Carter JE, Owen DB (1988) Ollier's disease and Maffucci's syndrome: distinct entities or a continuum. Case report: enchondromatosis complicated by an intracranial glioma. J Neurol 235:376–378

Merchant TE, Kiehna EN, Thompson SJ, Heideman R, Sanford RA, Kun LE (2000) Pediatric low-grade and ependymal spinal cord tumors. Pediatr Neurosurg 32:30–36

Miller DC (2000) Surgical pathology of intramedullary spinal cord neoplasms. J Neurooncol 47:189–194

Miyazawa N, Hida K, Iwasaki Y, Koyanagi I, Abe H (2000) MRI at 1.5 T of intramedullary ependymoma and classification of pattern of contrast enhancement. Neuroradiology 42:828–832

Nagib MG, O'Fallon MT (1997) Myxopapillary ependymoma of the conus medullaris and filum terminale in the pediatric age group. Pediatr Neurosurg 26:2–7

Osborn AG (1994) Diagnostic neuroradiology. Mosby, St Louis

Prados MD, Edwards MS, Rabbitt J, Lamborn K, Davis RL, Levin VA (1997) Treatment of pediatric low-grade gliomas with a nitrosourea-based multiagent chemotherapy regimen. J Neurooncol 32:235–241

Przybylski GJ, Albright AL, Martinez AJ (1997) Spinal cord astrocytomas: long-term results comparing treatments in children. Childs Nerv Syst 13:375–382

Quinones-Hinojosa A, Lyon R, Gulati M, Lyon R, Gupta N, Yingling C (2002) Spinal cord mapping as an adjunct for resection of intramedullary tumors: Surgical technique with case illustrations. Neurosurgery 51:1199–1206

Raghavendra BN, Epstein FJ, McCleary L (1984) Intramedullary spinal cord tumors in children: localization by intraoperative sonography. AJNR Am J Neuroradiol 5:395–397

Raimondi AJ, Gutierrez FA, di Rocco C (1976) Laminotomy and total reconstruction of the posterior spinal arch for spinal canal surgery in childhood. J Neurosurg 45:555–560

Ransom DT, Ritland SR, Kimmel DW, Moertel CA, Dahl RJ, Scheithauer BW, Kelly PJ, Jenkins RB (1992) Cytogenetic and loss of heterozygosity studies in ependymomas, pilocytic astrocytomas, and oligodendrogliomas. Genes Chromosomes Cancer 5:348–356

Ransom DT, Ritland SR, Moertel CA, Dahl RJ, O'Fallon JR, Scheithauer BW, Kimmel DW, Kelly PJ, Olopade OI, Diaz MO et al (1992) Correlation of cytogenetic analysis and loss of heterozygosity studies in human diffuse astrocytomas and mixed oligo-astrocytomas. Genes Chromosomes Cancer 5:357–374

Reimer R, Onofrio BM (1985) Astrocytomas of the spinal cord in children and adolescents. J Neurosurg 63:669–675

Robertson PL, Allen JC, Abbott IR, Miller DC, Fidel J, Epstein FJ (1994) Cervicomedullary tumors in children: a distinct subset of brainstem gliomas. Neurology 44:1798–1803

Rossitch E Jr, Zeidman SM, Burger PC, Curnes JT, Harsh C, Anscher M, Oakes WJ (1990) Clinical and pathological analysis of spinal cord astrocytomas in children. Neurosurgery 27:193–196

Salewski H, Bayer TA, Eidhoff U, Preuss U, Weggen S, Scheidtmann KH (1999) Increased oncogenicity of subclones of SV40 large T-induced neuroectodermal tumor cell lines after loss of large T expression and concomitant mutation in p53. Cancer Res 59:1980–1986

Sandler HM, Papadopoulos SM, Thornton AF Jr, Ross DA (1992) Spinal cord astrocytomas: results of therapy. Neurosurgery 30:490–493

Steinbok P, Cochrane DD, Poskitt K (1992) Intramedullary spinal cord tumors in children. Neurosurg Clin North Am 3:931–945

Van Nielen KM, de Jong BM (1999) A case of Ollier's disease associated with two intracerebral low-grade gliomas. Clin Neurol Neurosurg 101:106–110

Von Deimling A, Louis DN, Menon AG, von Ammon K, Petersen I, Ellison D, Wiestler OD, Seizinger BR (1993) Deletions on the long arm of chromosome 17 in pilocytic astrocytoma. Acta Neuropathol (Berl) 86:81–85

Von Haken MS, White EC, Daneshvar-Shyesther L, Sih S, Choi E, Kalra R, Cogen PH (1996) Molecular genetic analysis of chromosome arm 17p and chromosome arm 22q DNA sequences in sporadic pediatric ependymomas. Genes Chromosomes Cancer 17:37–44

Wen BC, Hussey DH, Hitchon PW, Schelper RL, Vigliotti AP, Doornbos JF, VanGilder JC (1991) The role of radiation therapy in the management of ependymomas of the spinal cord. Int J Radiat Oncol Biol Phys 20:781–786

Zileli M, Coskun E, Ozdamar N, Ovul I, Tuncbay E, Oner K, Oktar N (1996) Surgery of intramedullary spinal cord tumors. Eur Spine J 5:243–250

Neurocutaneous Syndromes and Associated CNS Tumors

B. S. Tseng · D. Haas-Kogan

Contents

11.1 Introduction

In the Greek language, *phakos* means spot, mole, or lentil, and "phakomatosis" suggests the presence of a congenital lesion or birthmark (Berg 1991). This term was applied historically to a group of genetic disorders that are defined by involvement of the central nervous system and skin. Over time, these disorders expanded to include over 40 entities, each with its own specific features (Chalhub 1976). This chapter will review six of the more common neurocutaneous syndromes and the current designations for these disorders, with a particular emphasis on the CNS tumors occurring in each disease: neurofibromatosis types 1 (NF1) and 2 (NF2), Tuberous sclerosis (TS), ataxia–telangiectasia (AT), von Hippel–Lindau disease (VHL), and Sturge–Weber syndrome (SWS). Other comprehensive reviews discuss each entity in detail (Chalhub 1976; Berg 1991; Roach 1992; Korf 1997; Roach et al. 1998). More up-to-date information on current molecular genetics is available through the Online Mendelian Inheritance in Man website (http://www.ncbi.nlm. nih.gov/omim/).

Dysplasia caused by specific genetic alterations within ectodermal tissue is thought to give rise to the abnormalities seen in neurocutaneous syndromes (skin and neural tissues). The same underlying molecular defects predispose affected individuals to further genetic alterations with increasing risks of developing a neoplasm. Although the responsible genes for many of these syndromes are known, the molecular mechanisms leading to variations in disease phenotype remain poorly understood. Clinical characterization of these syndromes has improved, accelerated by advances in both computed tomography (CT) and magnetic resonance imaging (MRI) (Braffman et al. 1988; Fischbein et al. 2000; Herron et al. 2000). Imaging is now essential to define major and minor criteria for diagnosis of neurocutaneous syndromes. In many patients, the neuroradiographic features often precede clinically significant findings or patient symptoms.

Most oncologists should be familiar with the neurocutaneous syndromes for several reasons. First, these patients are at increased risk for the development of CNS tumors. Second, the natural history of these tumors differ from sporadically occurring versions of the same tumors (Rosser and Packer 2002). Finally, the incidence of these inherited syndromes is relatively high. Similar to other genetic syndromes and heritable diseases, great variability exists among patients with phakomatoses due in part to mosaicism, expressivity, and genetic penetrance. Such variability exists among patients afflicted with the same neurocutaneous syndrome, even within a single family. Not surprisingly, lag times of over 8 years have been reported between symptoms or signs of neurocutaneous syndromes and clinical diagnoses (Parry et al. 1994). Further complexity is added by spontaneous mutations that result in neurocutaneous syndromes that lack a family history but incur subsequent risk for patients and their progeny.

11.2 Neurofibromatosis Type 1

11.2.1 Epidemiology

Also known as von Recklinghausen's disease, NF1 is an autosomal dominant disease with an estimated incidence of 1:3,000 to 4,000, equal sex distribution, and no apparent ethnic predisposition (Szudek et al. 2000; Korf 2002). It is one of the most common single-gene disorders, with as many as 50% of cases arising sporadically as new mutations. Most cases of NF1 can be detected in infancy based on skin abnormalities, which although subtle usually intensify with age, especially after puberty. The clinical diagnosis of NF1 is frequently delayed until the teen years. NF1

exhibits nearly 100% penetrance by adulthood (Riccardi 1987; Friedman 1999).

11.2.2 Genetics and Molecular Biology

The *NF1* gene maps to chromosome 17q11.2 and consists of 59 exons spread over 350 kb of genomic DNA. More than 100 different mutations have been observed in patients with NF1 (Rosser and Packer 2002; Viskochil 2002). The NF1 gene product, neurofibromin, has been cloned and is believed to interact with key signaling pathways regulating cell growth and division. Neurofibromin is a 2,818 amino acid cytoplasmic protein that contains a large amino acid segment exhibiting homology to the functional domain of the p21ras-GTPase-activating protein. This protein inactivates the oncogene p21ras by stimulating its GTPase activity, thus converting the active form of p21ras into its inactive form. Mutations of neurofibromin allow constitutive activation of p21ras and probably account for the many phenotypic abnormalities seen in NF1, including benign and malignant neoplasms. Although speculative, such molecular signaling abnormalities might underlie the learning disabilities described in approximately half of all patients with NF1 (Szudek et al. 2000).

11.2.3 Diagnostic Criteria and Clinical Features

The clinical features of NF1 are divided into major and minor subgroups (Table 11.1). The most recognizable clinical feature of NF1 is the café au lait spot, a smooth, non-raised, brown discoloration of the skin, which appears before adulthood in 95% of patients with NF1. Dermal neurofibromas, which arise from Schwann cells, occur in >99% of patients. These tumors appear during adolescence and increase in number and size with age. Other manifestations seen in patients with NF1 include axillary freckling, Lisch nodules (pigmented hamartomas of the iris), optic gliomas, and bone dysplasias (Szudek et al. 2000; Korf 2002). As outlined in an earlier NIH meeting (NIH Consensus Development Conference, Neurofibromatosis: Conference Statement 1988), the diagnosis of

Table 11.1. Major and minor features of NF1. NIH Consensus Development Conference, Neurofibromatosis: Conference Statement (1988)

Major features	Minor features
Café au lait spots and skin freckling	Macrocephaly
Peripheral neurofibromas	Short stature as growth hormone deficiency is found even in NF1 patients that do not have hypothalamic lesions
Lisch nodules (iris hamartomas)	Hypsarrhythmia
Plexiform neurofibromas	Intellectual difficulties (e.g. learning difficulties)
CNS tumors (optic gliomas, spinal neurofibromas)	Epilepsy
Distinctive osseous lesions (ribbon ribs, sphenoid wing dysplasia, pseudoarthroses, or thinning of long bone cortex)	Hypertension – may be due to aortic coarctation, renal artery stenosis, or pheochromocytoma

NF1 is made if a patient has met two or more of the following criteria:

1. Six or more café au lait spots (>5 mm if prepubertal, >15 mm if postpubertal)
2. Two or more neurofibromas of any type, or one or more plexiform neurofibromas
3. Freckling in the axilla or inguinal regions (Crowe's sign)
4. Two or more Lisch nodules (iris hamartomas)
5. An optic pathway tumor
6. A distinctive osseous lesion such as sphenoid wing dysplasia, or thinning of the cortex of the long bones with or without pseudoarthroses
7. First degree relative (parent, sibling, or offspring) with NF1 by the above criteria

There is an increased incidence of specific CNS neoplasms in patients with NF1 (Korf 2000; Rosser and Packer 2002). The most common NF1-associated tumors are optic gliomas, especially chiasmatic gliomas, the majority of which are diagnosed in childhood (Turgut et al. 1991; Balestri et al. 1993). Although optic gliomas are symptomatic in only 2 to 4% of patients with NF1, MRI findings of optic gliomas exist in 12 to 20% of patients. Optic gliomas rarely give rise to clinical manifestations and the typical progression is often slow. If symptomatic, these tumors may present with decreased visual acuity, visual field defects, proptosis and precocious puberty due to hy-

pothalamic compression. Although serial MRI scans are recommended every 6 to 12 months, visual field and acuity testing is a more sensitive indicator for tumor progression. One prospective study of the utility of MRI scans (Listernick et al. 1994) noted that there was no instance of tumor progression that would not have been identified clinically and concluded that screening MRI alone does not alter management for optic gliomas in NF1 patients.

In addition to optic gliomas, NF1 is associated with an increased incidence of parenchymal gliomas, particularly in the brainstem, cerebellar peduncles, globus pallidus, and midbrain. The biological behavior of brainstem gliomas in patients with NF1 differs significantly from that of lesions with similar appearance in patients without NF1 (Pollack et al. 1996; Listernick et al. 1999). With NF1, there is a higher predilection for development in girls (female:male ratio of 2:1) and location in the third ventricle, hypothalamus, cerebellum, and spinal cord. Other CNS neoplasms that occur in NF1 patients with increased incidence are ependymomas, meningiomas, and medulloblastomas. Also noted is a preponderance of paraspinal neurofibromas with an incidence of 4% of symptomatic neurofibromas and >25% of asymptomatic but radiographically evident tumors.

NF1 patients develop not only central nervous system lesions but also peripheral nervous system tumors. Neurofibromas and schwannomas arise most commonly from major peripheral nerves, particularly

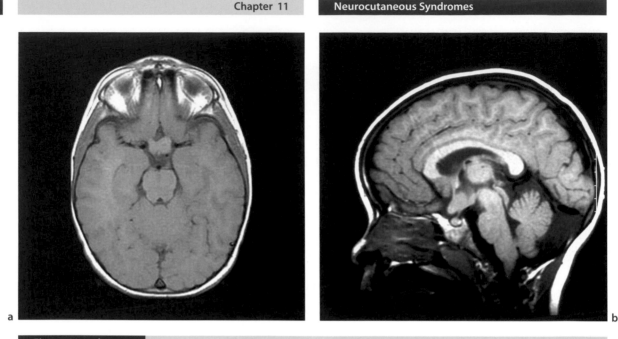

a   b

Figure 11.1 a,b

Optic pathway gliomas associated with NF1. a The T1-weighted axial images shows asymmetry of the optic chiasm with the left optic nerve being larger than the right. The mass did not enhance following gadolinium. b A sagittal T1-weighted image clearly shows the thick chiasm directly above the pituitary gland

the radial and ulnar nerves. Malignant transformation of neurofibromas into neurofibrosarcomas occurs in less than 5% of children with NF1 but more frequently in adults with NF1. The clinical signs associated with malignant transformation are rapid growth and/or pain. In this situation, the mass should be surgically resected. The other general indication for surgical resection is for removal of very large tumors that create a cosmetic problem. Patients with NF1 are also at risk for non-CNS tumors, including Wilms tumor, rhabdomyosarcoma, leukemia, melanoma, medullary thyroid carcinoma, and pheochromocytoma.

11.2.4 Natural History and Prognosis

NF1 is a progressive disease that can affect almost every organ (Rasmussen et al. 2001; Korf 2002). Sorensen noted that overall survival was reduced in patients with NF1 (Sorensen et al. 1986). The causes of death in NF1 patients include neurofibrosarcoma, CNS tumors, and systemic conditions such as hypertension (Friedman and Ricardi 1999, Zoller et al. 1995). Patients with NF1 have a 34-fold greater likelihood of having malignant connective tissue or soft tissue neoplasms compared with non-NF1 individuals (Rasmussen et al. 2001).

11.2.5 Laboratory Studies

DNA testing is limited because present techniques only detect approximately 70% of NF1 mutations (Menkes and Maria 2000). Although performed in some research laboratories, widespread genetic testing for NF1 is currently not available.

11.2.6 Imaging Studies

On CT head scans, the characteristic features of an optic glioma are fusiform enlargement of the optic nerve(s), optic tract and/or optic chiasm. Remodel-

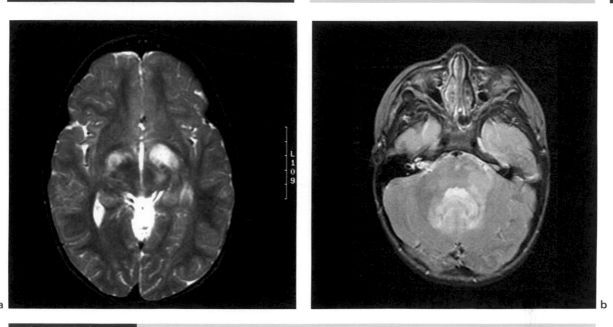

a   b

Figure 11.2 a,b

White matter lesions associated with NF1. These lesions are best seen on T2-weighted images. a In this axial image, there are bilateral (larger on the patient's left side) lesions within the basal ganglia that do not produce much mass effect. These lesions do not enhance following gadolinium. b Similar lesions can be seen in the posterior fossa. Here, the area of T2 prolongation extends from the cerebellar peduncle toward the pons

ing of the optic canal and medial sphenoid wing may also be present. Sphenoid wing dysplasia is usually associated with plexiform neurofibroma and bupthalmos (Balestri et al. 1993; Mukonoweshuro et al. 1999; Fischbein et al. 2000; Kornreich et al. 2001). With MR brain imaging, optic nerve gliomas are easily visible with enlargement of the optic nerve(s), chiasm, and/or optic tract (Fig. 11.1). Asymptomatic optic gliomas are present in up to 20% of NF1 patients. The extent of involvement is often underestimated with T1-weighted images while T2-weighted images provide better representation of the involved areas. Contrast enhancement can occur and may either be heterogeneous or homogeneous. Brainstem gliomas are relatively common (Aoki et al. 1989; Balestri et al. 1993; Mukonoweshuro et al. 1999; Fischbein et al. 2000; Kornreich et al. 2001).

Non-enhancing foci of T2 prolongation within deep gray nuclei and the white matter may represent myelin vacuolization. These are most common in the globus pallidus, followed by the cerebellum and brainstem, internal capsules, centrum semiovale, and corpus callosum and occur in up to 60% of NF1 patients (Fig. 11.2). Parenchymal tumors (usually astrocytomas) have a predilection for the thalami and basal ganglia and appear as T2-prolonging mass lesions with variable post-gadolinium enhancement.

11.2.7 Treatment

Patients with NF1 should have a thorough annual physical examination. Although the value of screening imaging studies is not proven, most patients will at some point undergo a screening MRI of the brain and spine. Even if a mass is identified, treatment focuses on symptomatic lesions (Turgut et al. 1991; Pollack et al. 1996). Most optic pathway gliomas associated with NF1 are asymptomatic and some have been

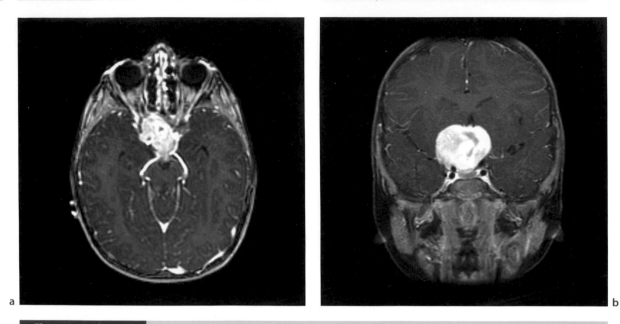

a   b

Figure 11.3 a,b

Large optic pathway glioma in a patient with NF1. This 3 year old girl presented with visual loss and was noted to have an extremely large optic glioma as seen on axial **a** and coronal **b** T1-weighted images following contrast. The optic chiasm and nerves cannot be differentiated from the tumor. Because of the degree of visual loss, the patient underwent biopsy to confirm the diagnosis and then was started on chemotherapy

noted to regress spontaneously (Parsa et al. 2001). Pathologically, these tumors are classified as pilocytic astrocytomas (WHO grade I), although their clinical course is more indolent than in non-NF1 patients. Gradual enlargement of the mass can cause compression of nearby structures and may require surgical debulking. Hydrocephalus from obstruction of the anterior third ventricle is treated by placement of a ventriculoperitoneal shunt.

Slow enlargement of optic pathway gliomas clearly demonstrated on serial imaging studies and accompanied by symptoms can be managed by systemic chemotherapy. Gururangan et al., treated 22 NF1 patients with low-grade gliomas as part of a large phase II study and found that they had better overall survival than non-NF1 patients (Gururangan et al. 2002). Patients were treated if they met one or more of the following criteria: (a) >25% increase in the size of the tumor (Fig. 11.3A, B), (b) papilledema, (c) loss of vision, (d) increase in proptosis, or (e) increase in the diameter of the optic nerve >2 mm. Usually, protocols tailored for low-grade astrocytic tumors are used (see Chapter 1). Surgery is often required for plexiform neurofibromas that have become disfiguring or painful, but new biologic-based approaches are being advocated (Packer et al. 2002).

11.3 Neurofibromatosis Type 2

11.3.1 Epidemiology

Neurofibromatosis type 2 (NF2) is inherited in an autosomal dominant manner with an incidence of 1:37,000 and has no gender predilection (Mautner et al. 1993; Parry et al. 1994). Generally NF2 patients become symptomatic at puberty or thereafter. The mean age of onset of symptoms is approximately 17 years of age, usually with acute hearing loss.

11.3.2 Molecular Biology and Cytogenetics

The NF2 gene is located on chromosome 22 between markers D22S212 and D22S28. The protein product is a 595 amino acid protein called merlin, or schwannomin, and demonstrates a high degree of homology with a family of F-actin binding proteins including talin, ezrin, radixin, and moesin (De Vitis et al. 1996a,b). Merlin localizes at the cell membrane and acts as a membrane–cytoskeletal linker. It can revert Ras-induced malignant phenotypes, indicating that the NF2 gene product is a tumor suppressor protein. The full biochemical consequences of merlin mutations and the mechanism underlying NF2 phenotypic features remain unclear. Mutations of the NF2 gene occur not only in neoplasms associated with NF2 but also in 30% of melanomas and 41% of mesotheliomas (De Vitis et al. 1996a,b). The reason why NF2 mutations predispose to the formation of bilateral vestibular schwannomas remains unclear.

11.3.3 Diagnostic Criteria and Clinical Features

Clinical criteria are used to determine the diagnosis of NF2 (Table 11.2). Bilateral vestibular schwannomas, which are characteristic lesions in patients with NF2, usually present with hearing loss (Mautner et al. 1993; Parry et al. 1994; Mautner et al. 1996). These tumors are found in 96% of NF2 patients; bilateral in 90% and unilateral in 6%. Vestibular schwannomas were formerly called "acoustic neuromas," an inaccurate term because they arise from

Schwann cells and typically involve the vestibular rather than the acoustic (cochlear) branch of the 8th cranial nerve. NF2 patients exhibit an overall predilection for tumors of meninges and Schwann cells and may also present with facial nerve, trigeminal nerve, and multiple spinal nerve schwannomas, as well as meningiomas. Symptoms at time of presentation include hearing loss, tinnitus, and disequilibrium from vestibular schwannomas. The onset of symptoms ranges from 15 to 74 years of age. It is widely believed that hemorrhage into vestibular schwannomas may trigger sudden hearing loss and acute hydrocephalus although this event is quite rare. NF2 patients under 10 years of age present most commonly with visual deficits or rapidly growing skin tumors.

NF2 patients develop other central neurofibromas including paraspinal tumors that may compress the spinal cord and present with myelopathy. These lesions, the source of major morbidity and mortality, are surprisingly common (90%) in patients with NF2. Additional lesions associated with NF2 include posterior subcapsular cataracts (63%), retinal hamartomas, optic nerve sheath meningiomas, meningiomas (meningeal), ependymomas (usually spinal cord), gliomas, and trigeminal schwannomas (Mautner et al. 1996).

11.3.4 Natural History and Prognosis

The mean age of onset of symptoms is 17 years of age while the mean age of NF2 diagnosis is 22 years. Relentless progression of vestibular schwannomas and other tumors may lead to loss of vision, paresis, and

Table 11.2. NF2 Diagnostic criteria. NIH Consensus Development Conference, Neurofibromatosis: Conference Statement (1988)

Clinical features – one of the following	Or, two of the following
Bilateral eighth cranial nerve masses (vestibular schwannomas) seen with imaging techniques	Multiple meningiomas
A first-degree relative with NF2 and unilateral vestibular schwannoma or any two of: neurofibroma, glioma, meningioma, schwannoma, juvenile posterior subcapsular lenticular opacity	Unilateral vestibular schwannoma
	Neurofibroma, glioma, schwannoma, glioma, cerebral calcification or subcapsular lens opacity

eventual death from brainstem compression (Parry et al. 1994). The prognosis for NF2 patients is variable, as a spectrum of phenotypes exists. Early detection offers distinct advantages to the patients as hearing preservation remains a challenge. The diagnosis of NF2 raises great concern for potential CNS tumors (schwannomas, meningiomas, gliomas, and neuromas) that may involved the brain, cranial nerves, or spinal cord.

11.3.5 Laboratory Studies

Laboratory diagnosis relies on the presence of DNA mutation in merlin and requires linkage studies from DNA derived from at least two affected family members.

11.3.6 Imaging Studies

Schwannomas on CT head scanning are round or ovoid extra-axial masses. They are iso to mildly hypodense on non-contrast CT scan unless cystic or hemorrhagic. Meningiomas are dural-based extra-axial masses, often with an associated dural tail. They are typically isodense to brain on non-contrast CT scans (Aoki et al. 1989; Mautner et al. 1996; Fischbein et al. 2000).

On MR imaging, schwannomas are iso to mildly hypointense compared to brain parenchyma on T1-weighted-images. They are iso to hyperintense to brain parenchyma on T2-weighted images. Intense homogeneous enhancement after contrast administration is typically seen (Fig. 11.4a), although areas of cystic change or hemorrhage may lead to heterogeneous enhancement. Large lesions may cause brainstem compression and/or hydrocephalus. Similar to schwannomas, meningiomas are isointense to gray

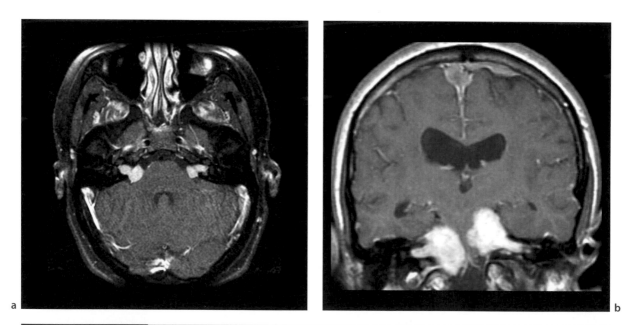

a   b

Figure 11.4 a,b

NF2 tumors. a Typical apperance of bilateral vestibular schwannomas in a teenage girl. On this fat-suppressed T1-weighted axial image, the tumors are clearly seen arising from the internal acoustic meati on either siede. b Although convexity and falcine meningiomas are visualized, the bilateral schwannomas are much larger.

matter on T1- and T2-weighted images. They usually enhance intensely and homogeneously following gadolinium administration and calcifications are common (Fig. 11.4B; Mautner et al. 1996; Fischbein et al. 2000).

11.3.7 Treatment

Schwannomas generally progress slowly, and if small and asymptomatic, patients can be followed by serial imaging studies. Surgical resection, and/or stereotactic radiosurgery may be required for symptomatic lesions (Parry et al. 1994). A recent retrospective study (Moffat et al. 2003) spanning 17 years concluded that surgery unequivocally offered superior tumor control over stereotactic radiosurgery (Gamma Knife, Elekta AB) when hearing preservation and facial nerve function were the endpoints studied. Half of the tumors in this study were treated conservatively with annual surveillance alone and did not require intervention. In another study (Samii 1995), 74 NF2 patients with bilateral tumors following surgical resections had a total rate of hearing preservation of 36%, while another group (Brackmann et al. 2001) reported 42.5% hearing preservation with early proactive surgical intervention. Others report that stereotactic radiosurgery is a safe and effective treatment for NF2 tumors and may in fact have better rates of hearing preservation, approximately 43% (Subach et al. 1999). Patients with small vestibular schwannomas can suffer deafness without imaging changes in tumor size (Walsh et al. 2000). At this time, more clinical experience is warranted to better define the most effective treatment(s) and key criteria for initiating therapy.

11.4 Tuberous Sclerosis Complex

11.4.1 Epidemiology

Tuberous sclerosis complex (TSC), previously known as Bourneville's disease, is an autosomal dominant disorder with an incidence of 1:10,000 to 1:30,000. It is the second most common neurocutaneous syndrome after NF1. There is no race or gender predilection and onset of symptoms varies from infancy to late childhood (Roach et al. 1998; Sparagana and Roach 2000).

11.4.2 Molecular Biology and Genetics

TSC is genetically heterogeneous with two implicated genes: TSC1 on chromosome 9q34 encodes hamartin, a 130 kDa protein with no significant homology to any other known vertebrate protein; and TSC2 on chromosome 16p13 encodes tuberin, a 200 kDa tumor-suppressor protein. Tuberin protein is most abundant in cerebral gray matter and increases during prenatal and postnatal development. Interestingly, hamartin and tuberin associate physically *in vitro* and inactivation of either is believed to prevent the formation of a functional protein complex. The details of how these two gene products manifest the phenotype of TSC remain unknown but are the topic of active investigation (Sparagana and Roach 2000).

In TSC, it is widely held that the disease phenotype results from deficits in cell migration, proliferation and differentiation. In the CNS, primitive cells in the germinal matrix fail to differentiate into neuronal and glial populations while other cells fail to migrate at all. Features of this aberrant CNS development in TSC include cortical tubers, also known as hamartias, constituting defects in tissue combination during development. Other examples of aberrant CNS development in TSC include subependymal nodules also known as hamartomas, which are defined as benign tumor-like nodules composed of a disorganized overgrowth of mature cells.

11.4.3 Diagnostic Criteria and Clinical Features

The classic TSC triad consists of seizures, mental retardation, and adenoma sebaceum (Hanno and Beck 1987; Curatolo 1996; Roach et al. 1998). Adenoma sebaceum growths are pathologically better characterized as facial angiofibromas. In infants, the combination of depigmented areas of skin, infantile spasms and delayed development is diagnostic of TSC. A variety of clinical criteria are used to establish the diagnosis of TSC (Table 11.3). For a definitive diagnosis of TSC, either two major features or one major feature and two minor features must be present. For a probable diagnosis of TSC, one major feature or two or more minor features must be present.

In 70% of TSC patients, seizures begin before 1 year of age (Webb et al. 1996), are often refractory to treatment, and thus present a major therapeutic challenge (Hanno and Beck 1987; Curatolo 1996; Roach et al. 1998). Signs of intellectual deterioration can be a consequence of either frequent uncontrolled seizures or increased intracranial pressure caused by obstruction of the foramen of Monro. The degree of mental retardation varies widely and many patients develop autism or pervasive developmental delay. Only one-third of TSC patients maintain normal intelligence.

Hypomelanotic lesions, ash-leaf macular depigmented nevi resembling vitiligo, may be noted at birth and can be seen in more than half of TSC patients before 2 years of age. These are best visualized with ul-

Table 11.3. Diagnostic criteria for tuberous sclerosis (Roach et al. 1998)

Major features	Minor features
Facial angiofibromas or forehead plaque	Multiple randomly distributed pits in dental enamel
Non-traumatic ungula or periungual fibroma	Hamartomatous rectal polyps – histologic confirmation is suggested
Hypomelanotic macules (≥3)	Bone cysts – radiologic confirmation is sufficient
Shagreen patch (connective tissue nevus)	Cerebral white matter radial migration lines – radiologic confirmation is sufficient (one panel member felt strongly that >3 radial migration lines should constitute a major sign)
Multiple retinal nodular hamartomas	Gingival fibromas
Cortical tuber – when cerebral cortical dysplasia and cerebral white matter migration tracts occur together, they should be counted as 1 rather than 2 features of TS	Non-renal hamartoma – histologic confirmation is suggested
Subependymal nodule	Retinal achromic patch
Subependymal giant cell astrocytoma	Confetti skin lesions
Cardiac rhabdomyoma, single or multiple	Multiple renal cysts – histologic confirmation is suggested
Lymphangiomyomatosis – when both lymphangiomyomatosis and renal angiomyolipomas are present, other features of TS should be present before a definite diagnosis is assigned	Cardiac rhabdomyomas (some neonates may present with congestive heart failure)
Renal angiomyolipoma – when both lymphangiomyomatosis and renal angiomyolipomas are present, other features of TS should be present before a definite diagnosis is assigned	Macrocephaly
	Multiple ungual fibromas: fleshy lesions arising from around or underneath the nails; more in toes than fingers and more in girls than boys; seen in 15--20% of TS patients but usually not seen before adolescence
	Retinal hamartomas
	Renal angiomyolipomas and cysts

traviolet light (Wood lamp), and are seen in up to 90 % of patients with TSC. Facial angiofibromas (adenoma sebaceum) are skin lesions consisting of vascular and connective tissue elements. They form a red papular rash that typically extends over the nose and down the nasolabial folds toward the chin, cheeks, and malar regions. Skin lesions gradually enlarge, manifesting in 12 % of affected children by 1 year of age, 40 % by 3 years of age and ultimately in as many as 80 % of TSC patients (Hanno and Beck 1987; Curatolo 1996; Roach et al. 1998).

11.4.4 Natural History and Prognosis

Major CNS manifestations of TSC include subependymal nodules (hamartias) and cortical tubers (hamartomas), white matter lesions, and giant cell astrocytomas of the foramen of Monro (Curatolo 1996; Roach et al. 1998; Sparagana and Roach 2000). Not surprisingly, involvement of the cortex can lead to neurologic deficits marked by infantile spasms and medically refractory seizures. It remains unclear if the number of cortical tubers dictates the extent of mental retardation or the severity of the seizure disorder. Additional abnormalities occur in the brain, eyes, skin, kidneys, bones, heart, and lungs. Prognosis varies with the individual manifestations of the disease. In severe cases, death occurs in the second decade of life (Curatolo 1996; Webb et al. 1996; Sparagana and Roach 2000). Major causes of death in a large TSC Scottish cohort were renal disease, followed by brain tumors, pulmonary lymphangiomyomatosis, status epilepticus, and bronchopneumonia (Shepherd and Stephenson 1992).

11.4.5 Laboratory Studies

Genetic testing of TSC has limited utility as two-thirds of all cases are considered sporadic. Thus such assays are not typically employed for prenatal diagnosis nor confirmation of a clinical diagnosis of TSC.

11.4.6 Imaging Studies

Clinical criteria are commonly used to establish the diagnosis of TSC with a head CT scan performed as a confirmatory test. Approximately 95 % of patients with clinical features of TSC have abnormalities on CT scans (Menkes and Maria 2000). Typically, there are hypodense subependymal nodules lining the ventricles (Fig. 11.5q), usually calcified after the first year of life and 50 % of affected individuals demonstrate calcified cortical hamartomas. Giant cell astrocytomas located at or near the foramen of Monro enhance brightly following contrast administration. Calcified subependymal and cortical nodules are seen in 95 % of individuals with TSC, and thus can be diagnosed by CT, obviating the need for MRI and its attendant requirement for general anesthesia in children (Braffman et al. 1990; Menor et al. 1992; Fischbein et al. 2000; Mukonoweshuro et al. 2001).

MRI brain imaging is preferable for defining the exact number and location of cerebral cortical and subcortical tubers, white matter lesions, and areas of heterotopias (Braffman et al. 1990; Menor et al. 1992; Fischbein et al. 2000; Mukonoweshuro et al. 2001). Gadolinium-enhanced MRI imaging helps distinguish subependymal giant cell astrocytomas from benign subependymal nodules. Tubers or sclerotic white patches involving the gyri or white matter occur mostly in the cerebrum, while cerebellar, brainstem, and spinal cord lesions occur less commonly. Cortical tubers/hamartomas change in appearance as the brain myelinates. They are initially hyperintense on T1-weighted-images and hypointense on T2-weighted-images, but as brain myelination progresses, this imaging pattern reverses. White matter lesions appear as hyperintense linear bands in cerebrum and cerebellum. In infants, bands are hypointense to unmyelinated white matter on T2-weighted-images becoming hyperintense to white matter in older children and adults (Fig. 11.5b). Giant cell astrocytomas at or near foramen of Monro display intense post-contrast enhancement, although the pattern can be heterogeneous (Fig. 11.5c). MR spectroscopy can be useful to distinguish them from cortical tubers.

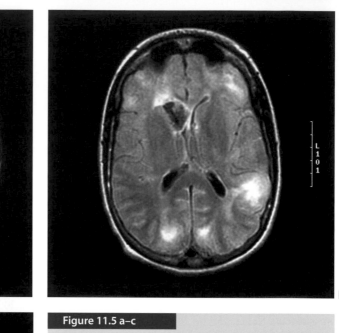

a

b

c

Figure 11.5 a–c

Tuberous sclerosis complex. **a** Axial CT image of multiple calcified subependymal nodules. Other calcifications are also seen within the cortex. **b** Bilateral cortical tubers of varying sizes and a frontal subependymal giant cell astrocytoma (SEGA) are seen on this T2-weighted image. **c** A post-contrast T1-weighted coronal image from the same patient demonstrates the proximity of the tumor to the foramen of Monro

11.4.7 Treatment

To prevent possible degeneration into higher grade tumors, complete tumor excision of giant cell astrocytomas is prudent when lesions are symptomatic and accessible. Resection of intraventricular tumors is necessary for children who develop obstructive hydrocephalus. Medical management of TSC can prove challenging, with 75 to 90% of patients displaying focal or generalized seizures, many refractory to treatment. In addition to antiepileptic agents, a surgical option for control of intractable seizures is gaining attention. In selected cases, surgical resection of dominant seizure foci that have an established concordance of neuroimaging, electrophysiologic, and clinical findings can be effective in achieving seizure control. Regular clinical surveillance every 6 to 12 months for clinical signs and symptoms such as visual field deficits or visual impairment is advisable, rather than frequent neuroimaging in the absence of clinical manifestations (Curatolo 1996; Webb et al. 1996; Miller et al. 1998; Roach et al. 1998). Potential involvement of additional tissues warrants regular screening for lesions such as cardiac myxomas and renal angiolipoma tumors.

11.5 Ataxia-Telangiectasia (AT)

11.5.1 Epidemiology

Ataxia-telangiectasia (AT) is an autosomal recessive disorder with an incidence of 1:40,000 to 80,000 and equal sex predilection. Patients with AT may present during infancy with ataxia without any cutaneous manifestations, which may become apparent after 2 years of age (Gosink et al. 1999; Lavin 1999; Lavin and Khanna 1999).

11.5.2 Molecular Biology and Genetics

The gene for AT has been mapped to the long arm of chromosome 11 (11q23.3). The Ataxia Telangiectasia Mutated (*ATM*) gene product is a member of the phosphatidylinositol 3-kinase (PI3-kinase) family. The ATM protein detects DNA double-strand breaks and activates a number of cell-cycle checkpoints (Lavin and Khanna 1999). ATM plays an important role in cellular responses to DNA damage, cell-cycle control and maintenance of telomere length. ATM is a 370 kDa phosphoprotein that contains a PI3-kinase domain, a putative leucine zipper, and a proline-rich region that has been shown to bind the non-receptor tyrosine kinase c-Abl. The ATM kinase is thought to have specificity for serine and threonine residue and can act as a tumor suppressor (Gosink et al. 1999).

Over 300 different mutations have been identified in AT patients. Database screening has revealed that most mutations are unique to a given family. Mutations are distributed anywhere within 66 exons across the full 150 kilobases (kb) of the *ATM* gene. Immunoblotting for ATM protein expression reveals absence in 85% of patients. In the remaining 15% of patients that express ATM protein, ATM kinase assays for enzymatic activity assess the function of the protein.

11.5.3 Diagnostic Criteria and Clinical Features

The hallmark findings are oculocutaneous lesions and oculomotor apraxia (Table 11.4). Progressive oculocutaneous telangiectasias represent a key feature of AT (Paller 1987; Gosink et al. 1999; Lavin et al. 1999; Kamiya et al. 2001). Bulbar conjunctivae telangiectasias first appear between 2 and 6 years of age and subsequently involve ears, eyelids, malar prominences, neck, antecubital and popliteal fossae, as well as dorsum of hands and palate. Initially they appear as bright-red, thick, symmetrical streaks that resemble atypical conjunctivitis and only later become frank telangiectasias. The AT skin lesions become more prominent with sunlight exposure and older age.

AT is the most common ataxia in infancy (Kamiya et al. 2001), although the initial manifestations of cerebellar ataxia may not be noted until early walking. AT is a common cause of progressive ataxia in children younger than 10 years of age, second only to tumors of the posterior fossa.

Table 11.4. Clinical features of ataxia telangiectasia (Menkes and Maria 2000)

Clinical features
Slowly progressive cerebellar ataxia
Choreoathetosis
Telangiectasia of skin and conjunctiva
Susceptibility to sinobronchopulmonary infections, lymphoreticular neoplasia, and other malignancies

11.5.4 Natural History and Prognosis

Neurologic deterioration is progressive and older children are eventually confined to wheelchairs with myoclonic jerks, drooling, choreoathetosis, oculomotor abnormalities, and dysarthric speech (Paller 1987). Eighty-five percent of AT patients develop choreoathetosis, apraxia of eye movements, and nystagmus. Intelligence is usually normal in young children but deteriorates with progressive disease (Menkes and Maria 2000). Facial expression is typically alert when smiling but dull and hypotonic when relaxed. Older children may have a stooped posture with mask-like facies and dystonic posturing of fingers.

Growth retardation occurs in 72% of patients with AT. Progeric changes have been noted in almost 90% of AT patients with early loss of subcutaneous fat, loss of skin elasticity, and premature graying of hair by adolescence (Paller 1987). AT patients are immunodeficient with compromised humoral immune surveillance. Specifically, AT patients have IgA deficiencies that predispose them to infectious agents that enter through exposed sites. Consequently, they tend to suffer from recurrent bacterial and viral sinopulmonary infections that can be life threatening (Paller 1987).

Children with AT have an increased incidence of cancer, primarily lymphoid tumors, due to acute sensitivity to ionizing radiation and defective cell-cycle checkpoints. AT patients are 40 to 100 times more likely to develop leukemias, lymphomas, lymphosarcomas, and Hodgkin's disease. Lymphoreticular malignancies predominate in younger patients whereas epithelial malignancies occur most frequently in adult patients (Paller 1987). Not surprisingly, death frequently occurs in late childhood or early teenage years. Mean age of death is 14 years (Kamiya et al. 2001) due to pulmonary infections and malignancy.

Some penetrance appears in AT heterozygotes leading to intermediate radiosensitivity and increased risk of cancer, particularly breast cancer. ATM heterozygotes have a 9-fold increased risk of developing breast cancer, characterized by bilateral disease and early age of onset (Lavin et al. 1999).

11.5.5 Laboratory Studies

Highly elevated serum alpha-fetoprotein is detected in nearly 95% cases, and this laboratory marker often precedes the appearance of telangiectasias by several years (Menkes and Maria 2000). Patients may display elevated levels of carcinoembryonic antigen (CEA) and low or absent total IgA or IgE. Markedly decreased serum IgA (<80 mg/L) is noted in 70 to 80%, and low IgE (<3 mg/L) in 80 to 90% of AT patients. Conversely, IgM, IgG1 and IgG3 levels tend to be high (Menkes and Maria 2000). Elevated hepatic transaminases are seen in 40 to 50% of patients and glucose intolerance is seen in 50% of patients. An unusual form of adolescent diabetes is observed in which hyperglycemia occurs with rare glycosuria, absent ketosis, insulin hypersecretion, and peripheral insulin resistance.

Chromosomal abnormalities occur 2 to 18 times more frequently in AT patients than in normal individuals, with chromosomal abnormalities observed in 80% of AT patients. Rearrangements of chromosomes 7 and 14 and especially 14:14 translocations may anticipate the development of lymphoreticular malignancies (Lavin et al. 1999). Analysis of amniotic fluid allows prenatal diagnosis using measurements of alpha-fetoprotein and high-resolution chromosomal analysis. New ATM protein and enzyme assays are in development but not yet commercially available.

11.5.6 Imaging Studies

Brain MR imaging (Fischbein et al. 2000) best visualizes posterior fossa abnormalities that include cerebellar atrophy, particularly of the anterior vermis, atrophy of the dentate and olivary nuclei, while spine MR imaging demonstrates degeneration of the posterior columns. These imaging findings correlate with well-described neuropathologic features of AT. In the cerebellum, there is a reduction in Purkinje cell number and atrophy of dentate nuclei. In addition, there is atrophy of anterior horn cells, and demyelination of gracile fasciculi in the spinal cord and nucleocytomegalic cells in the anterior pituitary.

11.5.7 Treatment

Supportive efforts include prophylactic therapy for infections. Antibiotics and plasma gamma globulin infusions have been utilized for IgA deficiencies and intercurrent sinopulmonary infections. Thymus gland and bone marrow transplantations have been reported as well. Judicious use of sunscreen is warranted to retard actinic-like skin progeric changes. Radiation therapy and radiomimetic chemotherapeutic agents should be avoided in treating lymphoreticular malignancies. Early pulmonary physiotherapy and physical therapy appropriate for neurologic dysfunction should be instituted. Many treatments employed for ataxia, including acetylcholine, gamma-aminobutyric acid, dopamine, diazepam, chlordiazepoxide, trihexyphenidyl, diphenhydramine, and haloperidol have been ineffective. A patient disabled with an extremely severe involuntary movement disorder responded well to dantrolene, a hydantoin compound. Unfortunately to date, no specific treatment prevents the neurologic progression of AT (Paller 1987; Lavin et al. 1999). Neoplastic processes that require aggressive treatment with chemotherapy or radiation present a formidable challenge given the high vulnerability to further oncologic insults in AT patients.

11.6 Von Hippel–Lindau Disease

11.6.1 Epidemiology

Von Hippel–Lindau (VHL) disease is an autosomal dominant disorder with an incidence of 1 per 40,000 (Maher and Kaelin 1997). It exhibits 90% penetrance and equal incidence in males and females. Generally, VHL does not present during childhood, but more often during the second or third decades of life (Singh et al. 2001).

11.6.2 Molecular Biology and Cytogenetics

The VHL gene has been mapped to chromosome 3p25-p26 and is a putative tumor-suppressor gene. The VHL gene product is a component of an E3 ubi-

quitin ligase that regulates the stability of the HIF (hypoxia-inducible factor) transcription factor, which in turn influences the angiogenic nature of VHL-associated neoplasms (Kondo and Kaelin 2001).

11.6.3 Diagnostic Criteria and Clinical Features

Although it is classified as a neurocutaneous syndrome, VHL is not associated with any specific cutaneous lesion (Richard et al. 2000; Sims 2001), but rather appears to be a multisystem disorder with marked phenotypic variability (Table 11.5). Cardinal features are retinal angiomas and hemangioblastomas of the cerebellum (Friedrich 2001). Diagnostic features include a positive family history of VHL with identification of a CNS hemangioblastoma or a visceral lesion (Richard et al. 2000; Sims 2001). For example, a retinal or cerebellar hemangioblastoma, renal cell carcinoma, or pheochromocytoma in an at-risk individual would be adequate for diagnosing VHL. In isolated cases with absent family histories, two or more retinal or cerebellar hemangioblastomas or a single hemangioblastoma and a visceral tumor are required for diagnosis. Multiple, frequent retinal angiomas may lead to retinal detachment, hemorrhage, and blindness if left untreated.

CNS hemangioblastomas occur most often in the superficial posterior-lateral cerebellum (75%) followed by the spinal cord (13%), medulla (5%), and rarely supratentorial brain (1.5%). Wanebo et al. re-

Table 11.5. Clinical features of von Hippel–Lindau disease (Maher and Kaelin 1997; Richard et al. 2000; Sims 2001)

Clinical Features
Cerebellar hemangioblastoma with angiomas of the spinal cord
Multiple congenital cysts of the pancreas
Kidney and renal carcinoma
Retinal hemangioma
Polycythemia

port a higher incidence of spinal cord hemangioblastomas (53%) than in other studies (Wanebo et al. 2003). These lesions are often multiple, and generally benign without metastases. Surgical excision results in excellent clinical outcome. Mean age at onset of cerebellar hemangioblastomas in VHL is considerably younger than in sporadic cases (Richard et al. 2000; Sims 2001). Cerebellar hemangioblastomas are found in approximately 75% of patients with VHL. However, only 5 to 30% of all patients with cerebellar hemangioblastomas are found to have VHL. Many patients with VHL ultimately develop multiple CNS hemangioblastomas and management of brainstem and spinal tumors can be difficult. Thus, CNS involvement remains an important cause of morbidity and mortality in VHL.

Fifty to seventy percent of VHL patients develop renal cysts, although renal impairment from them is rare. However, the lifetime risk of clear cell renal cell carcinoma (RCC) is greater than 70% and RCC is a major cause of death in VHL. Pheochromocytomas, angiomas of the liver and kidneys, papillary cystadenomas, and endolymphatic sac tumors all develop at increased rates in patients with VHL. Frequency of pheochromocytomas in patients with VHL disease varies between 7% and 20%.

11.6.4 Natural History and Prognosis

Patients with VHL usually present in adulthood. Initial symptoms are often visual and related to retinal angiomas with a mean age of onset of 25 years. Symptoms from cerebellar hemangioblastomas present later and include headache, disequilibrium, nausea, and vomiting. In a large 10-year retrospective NIH study of 160 consecutive VHL patients, many patients presented with mass effect attributable to a cyst that was far greater in size than the causative tumor (Wanebo et al. 2003). Neither tumors nor cysts spontaneously diminished in size although many untreated tumors remained the same size for several years. The tumors demonstrated a step-wise pattern of growth with enlargement followed by a plateau. Usually the mass effect caused by the cyst was responsible for symptoms.

The median age of death for patients with VHL is 49 years. Fifty-three percent of deaths are due to complications of cerebellar hemangioblastomas while 32% are due to RCCs (Singh et al. 2001). Pure solid lesions have worse prognoses than mixed (cystic and solid) hemangioblastomas.

11.6.5 Laboratory Studies

Laboratory studies are very non-specific. Urinary catecholamines, VMA and HVA, may be elevated. Hemangioblastomas may produce excess erythropoietin resulting in elevated hematocrit values. No DNA genetic testing is available to date.

11.6.6 Imaging Studies

With CT head scanning, a low density cystic mass is often present in the posterior fossa. Isodense mural nodules may enhance intensely with contrast (Fischbein et al. 2000). On MR imaging, brain cysts may be isointense to CSF or proteinaceous (hyperintense on T1-weighted sequences) with variable hyper- or hypointensity on T2 (Fig. 11.6). Prominent flow voids are seen in and adjacent to solid portions of the hemangioblastoma. Conventional catheter angiography demonstrates intense tumor blush localized to the posterior fossa. The typical blood supply is from superior cerebellar, anterior inferior cerebellar, or posterior inferior cerebellar arteries, but may also arise from branches of the internal and external carotid arteries. Angiography may assist with operative planning and, if possible, embolization may reduce the tumor vascularity allowing resection with reduced blood loss.

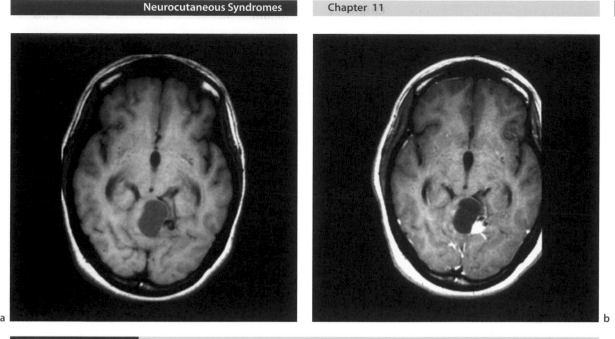

a   b

Figure 11.6 a,b

VHL syndrome. T1-weighted images, pre- and post-contrast, demonstrating a small enhancing tumor nodule adjacent to a cyst located within the cerebellar vermis. The cyst contents are slightly hyperintense to CSF

11.6.7 Treatment

To identify retinal angiomas, ophthalmologic examinations are required and, when indicated, laser therapy and cryotherapy are effective (Hes et al. 2001). Surgical removal of symptomatic lesions may also be considered. The NIH group emphasize that the pattern of growth may be variable (Wanebo et al. 2003). Some tumors remain quiescent for many years while others grow quickly over several months. As mentioned above, the growth of the cyst is often greater than the tumor itself and is responsible for the development of symptoms related to mass effect. In their series, asymptomatic patients rarely underwent surgery. Overall, surgical resection of cerebellar, and even brainstem and spinal cord tumors was associated with acceptable morbidity. External beam radiation or stereotactic radiosurgery may be helpful for multiple or inaccessible lesions.

11.7 Sturge–Weber Syndrome

11.7.1 Epidemiology

Sturge–Weber syndrome (SWS), or encephalofacial angiomatosis, occurs sporadically. It is a readily recognizable congenital disorder with no definable genetic pattern of sexual or ethnic predilection (Oakes 1992; Maria et al. 1998a; Bodensteiner and Roach 1999). Although there are rare familial cases of SWS, there is no convincing data to suggest that it is a heritable condition. Skin findings are generally noticed at birth and seizures may present in infancy. Classic manifestations include an ipsilateral facial "port-wine" stain, mental retardation, contralateral hemiparesis, contralateral hemiatrophy, and contralateral homonymous hemianopsia. Other features of the syndrome include glaucoma, dental abnormalities, and skeletal lesions.

11.7.2 Genetic and Molecular Biology

There are no known molecular biology factors or cytogenetic features (Oakes 1992; Maria et al. 1998a), but from a pathologic perspective, malformations of embryonic vascular plexus give rise to abnormalities of the skin, leptomeninges, choroids, and cortex. Interference with vascular drainage at 5 to 8 weeks of gestation affects the face, eye, leptomeninges, and brain. Resultant angiomatosis is accompanied by poor superficial cortical venous drainage with enlarged regional transmedullary veins developing as alternate pathways. It is postulated that inefficient outflow of venous blood causes chronic hypoxia that results in brain tissue loss and dystrophic calcifications.

11.7.3 Diagnostic Criteria and Clinical Features

Two essential features of SWS are facial cutaneous nevi (commonly known as "port-wine" stains) and leptomeningeal angiomas (Table 11.6; Menkes and Maria 2000). The other accepted name for "port-wine" stain is capillary vascular malformation. Although the diagnosis of SWS is seldom difficult, challenges remain in predicting functional outcome (Oakes 1992; Maria et al. 1998a). While facial nevi are the most obvious of the SWS manifestations, the ipsilateral leptomeningeal angioma is regarded as the most important component in determining prognosis. Children with widespread vascular lesions often have more seizures and greater intellectual impairment. The SWS clinical triad consists of (1) seizure disorder, (2) mental retardation, and (3) facial angiomas.

Facial nevi are relatively common malformations, occurring in approximately 3 in 1,000 births, and only 15% of infants with typical "port-wine" cutaneous lesions have SWS. In fact, up to 85% of patients with typical upper face hemifacial nevi are not associated with leptomeningeal angiomatosis found classically in SWS. Conversely, 13% of patients with cerebral manifestation of SWS do not display facial nevi. Involvement of the eyelid is associated with ipsilateral brain involvement and usually conforms to the distribution of the first division of the trigeminal nerve. The second and third divisions of the trigeminal nerve can also be involved. There is no correlation between size of facial involvement and CNS malformations (Bodensteiner and Roach 1999). Cutaneous facial nevi are usually present at birth but may become more prominent, thicker, and darker with age.

Seizures often begin in the first year of life as the initial presenting feature in 80% of patients with SWS, and are often medically refractory (Oakes 1992; Maria et al. 1998a). Seizures usually arise focally at first but may become secondarily generalized into tonic-clonic seizures. In addition, patients experience focal neurologic deficits that develop acutely in conjunction with flurries of seizures, and also experience the more readily recovering post-seizure episodes known as Todd's paralysis. Hemiparesis occurs with or without seizures and affected extremities often grow poorly, eventually resulting in hemiatrophy. Visual field defects result from involvement of one or both occipital lobes or optic tracts with leptomeningeal angiomatosis. Hydrocephalus may occur as a result of increased venous pressure from thromboses of deep venous channels or extensive arteriovenous anastomoses.

Table 11.6. Clinical features of Sturge–Weber syndrome (Bodensteiner and Roach 1999; Menkes and Maria 2000)

Major clinical features	Additional features
Congenital facial vascular nevus	Glaucoma/bupthalmos
Focal or generalized seizures	Neurologic deterioration
Brain MRI leptomeningeal enhancement after gadolinium administration plus enlarged transmedullary veins and unilateral hypertrophy of the choroid plexus	CT head parieto-occipital calcifications arranged in parallel lines ("tram tracks")

Mental retardation is common in SWS, with IQs lower than 90 in 70% of patients (Menkes and Maria 2000). Early developmental milestones may reveal delays. There is some controversy in the SWS literature regarding intellectual status. One study reports that most SWS patients without seizures are mentally normal (Sujansky and Conradi 1995). A conflicting study reports that although most infants with SWS have normal neurologic function, nearly all adults with SWS are impaired, suggesting a pervasive deterioration of function regardless of seizures (Maria et al. 1998).

Other signs and symptoms of SWS include headaches, stroke-like episodes, contralateral hemiplegia, hemisensory deficits, and contralateral homonymous hemianopsia. Ocular involvement is common (up to 40% of patients) and includes glaucoma and buphthalmos (enlarged globes). The vascular malformations of the conjunctiva, episclera, choroid, and retina predispose to abnormal intra-globe fluid dynamics.

11.7.4 Natural History and Prognosis

SWS is associated with progressive CNS disease that results in seizures as well as decreased motor, sensory, visual, and cognitive abilities. Early development of intractable seizures associated with hemiparesis and bilateral involvement are poor prognostic signs for cognitive development and general health.

11.7.5 Laboratory Studies

Neither laboratory nor genetic tests are available for the diagnosis of SWS.

11.7.6 Imaging Studies

Although facial nevi are the most obvious manifestations of SWS, leptomeningeal angiomas are clearly the most important determinants of ultimate patient prognosis. Leptomeningeal malformations typically involve posterior cerebral hemispheres, especially occipital lobes. Such malformations cause ischemia in adjacent brain resulting in gliosis, demyelination, parallel cortical calcifications, focal cerebral atrophy, and hemiatrophy. Other findings include absent superficial cortical veins adjacent to the malformation and enlarged choroid plexus of the ipsilateral deep venous system.

Head CT scans reveal gyral or "tram-track" cortical calcifications (absent in very young patients), most commonly over posterior hemispheres. There is often underlying cortical atrophy. Enlargement of the skull, diploic space, subarachnoid space, sinuses, and mastoid air cells all occur ipsilateral to port-wine stains. Contrast-enhanced scans may reveal diffuse staining of involved cerebral cortex and intense leptomeningeal enhancement if performed prior to the development of cortical calcifications (Fischbein et al. 2000).

Brain MRI scans (Fischbein et al. 2000) demonstrate ipsilateral parenchymal atrophy, compensatory skull thickening, and sinus enlargement. There is marked gadolinium enhancement in areas of leptomeningeal angiomatosis. Enlargement of the ipsilateral choroid plexus occurs secondary to angiomatosis. T2 shortening in the white matter underlies angiomatous malformations, usually seen in infants and may be due to ischemia. In later life, areas of T2 shortening are usually secondary to calcifications. Enlargement of deep venous structures occurs ipsilateral to meningeal angiomas.

11.7.7 Treatment

Unlike other neurocutaneous syndromes, SWS is not associated with heightened predisposition to CNS tumors. Treatment of facial nevi has been revolutionized by vascular-specific pulsed dye laser therapy. Ophthalmologic consultation is often required for aggressive medical and surgical management of glaucoma. If intractable seizures affect neurologic development and quality of life in young patients, there is general agreement that surgical resection (lobectomy, hemispherectomy) can significantly reduce seizure frequency and improve quality of life (Kossoff et al. 2002). This usually requires removal of the involved cortex and leptomeningeal abnormality. One author provided limited evidence that aspirin therapy at 2 to 5 mg/kg per day may be associated with two-thirds fewer stroke-like episodes but confirmatory data is lacking (Maria et al. 1998b).

11.8 Conclusion

The neurocutaneous syndromes are among the most common genetic disorders observed in humans. Furthermore, patients suffering from one or another in this unique group are at higher risk for the development of CNS neoplasms. The responsible genes have already been identified although the molecular pathophysiology remains unclear in many cases. For the clinical oncologist, the challenge is the decision to treat or observe. Generally, this decision is driven by the tempo and severity of the patient's clinical picture, although a clear understanding of the natural history of the disease is essential. Fortunately, most patients do not develop malignant tumors, but this information is tempered by the need for life-long observation and follow-up.

Internet sites regarding the phakomatoses are listed in Table 11.7.

Table 11.7. Internet sites with additional information for the phakomatoses

Neurofibromatosis	www.nf.org
Tuberous sclerosis	www.tsalliance.org
Ataxia telangiectasia	www.atsociety.org.uk
	www.atcp.org
Von Hippel–Lindau	www.vhl.org
Sturge–Weber	www.sturge-weber.com

References

Aoki S, Barkovich AJ, Nishinura K et al (1989) Neurofibromatosis types 1 and 2: cranial MR findings. Radiology 172:527–34

Balestri P, Calistri L, Vivarelli R et al (1993) Central nervous system imaging in reevaluation of patients with neurofibromatosis type 1. Childs Nerv Syst 9:448–451

Berg BO (1991) Current concepts of neurocutaneous disorders. Brain Dev 13:9–20

Bodensteiner JB, Roach ES (1999) Sturge–Weber syndrome. Sturge–Weber Foundation, Mt Freedom

Brackmann DE, Fayad JN, Slattery WH et al (2001) Early proactive management of vestibular schwannomas in neurofibromatosis type 2. Neurosurgery 49:274–280

Braffman BH, Bilaniuk LT, Zimmerman RA (1988) The central nervous system manifestations of the phakomatoses on MR. Radiol Clin North Am 26:773–800

Braffman BH, Bilaniuk LT, Zimmerman RA et al (1990) MR of central nervous system neoplasia of the phakomatoses. Semin Roentgenol 25:198–217

Chalhub EG (1976) Neurocutaneous syndromes in children. Pediatr Clin North Am 23:499–516

Curatolo P (1996) Neurological manifestations of tuberous sclerosis complex. Childs Nerv Syst 12:515–521

De Vitis LR, Tedde A, Vitelli F et al (1996a) Screening for mutations in the neurofibromatosis type 2 (NF2) gene in sporadic meningiomas. Hum Genet 97:632–637

De Vitis LR, Tedde A, Vitelli F et al (1996b) Analysis of the neurofibromatosis type 2 gene in different human tumors of neuroectodermal origin. Hum Genet 97:638–641

Fischbein NJ, Dillon WP, Barkarich AJ (2000) Teaching atlas of brain imaging. Thieme, New York

Friedman JM (1999) Epidemiology of neurofibromatosis type 1. Am J Med Genet 89:1–6

Friedman JM, Riccardi VM (1999) Neurofibromatosis: Phenotype, natural history, and pathogenesis. Johns Hopkins University Press, Baltimore

Friedrich CA (2001) Genotype-phenotype correlation in von Hippel–Lindau syndrome. Hum Mol Genet 10:763–767

Gosink EC, Chong MJ, McKinnon PJ (1999) Ataxia telangiectasia mutated deficiency affects astrocyte growth but not radiosensitivity. Cancer Res 59:5294–5298

Gururangan S, Cavazos CM, Ashley D et al (2002) Phase II study of carboplatin in children with progressive low-grade gliomas. J Clin Oncol 20:2951–2958

Hanno R, Beck R (1987) Tuberous sclerosis. Neurol Clin 5:351–360

Herron J, Darrah R, Quaghebeur G (2000) Intra-cranial manifestations of the neurocutaneous syndromes. Clin Radiol 55:82–98

Hes FJ, van der Luijt RB, Lips CJ (2001) Clinical management of Von Hippel–Lindau (VHL) disease. Nether J Med 59:225–234

Kamiya M, Yamanouchi H, Yoshida T et al (2001) Ataxia telangiectasia with vascular abnormalities in the brain parenchyma: report of an autopsy case and literature review. Pathol Int 51:271–276

Kondo K, Kaelin WG Jr (2001) The von Hippel–Lindau tumor suppressor gene. Exp Cell Res 264:117–125

Korf BR (1997) Neurocutaneous syndromes: neurofibromatosis 1, neurofibromatosis 2, and tuberous sclerosis. Curr Opin Neurol 10:131–136

Korf BR (2000) Malignancy in neurofibromatosis type 1. Oncologist 5:477–485

Korf BR (2002) Clinical features and pathobiology of neurofibromatosis 1. J Child Neurol 17:573–577; discussion 602–604, 646–651

Kornreich L, Blaser S, Schwarz M et al (2001) Optic pathway glioma: correlation of imaging findings with the presence of neurofibromatosis. AJNR Am J Neuroradiol 22:1963–1969

Kosoff EH, Buck Cm Freeman IM (2002) Outcomes of 32 hemispherecontnies for Sturge-Weber syndrome worldwide. Neurology 59:1735–1738

Lavin MF (1999) ATM: the product of the gene mutated in ataxia-telangiectasia. Int J Biochem Cell Biol 31:735–740

Lavin MF, Concannon P, Galti RA (1999) Eighth international workshop on ataxia-telangiectasia (ATW8). Cancer Res 59:3845–3849

Lavin MF, Khanna KK (1999) ATM: the protein encoded by the gene mutated in the radiosensitive syndrome ataxia-telangiectasia. Int J Radiat Biol 75:1201–1214

Listernick R, Charrow J, Greenwald M et al (1994) Natural history of optic pathway tumors in children with neurofibromatosis type 1: a longitudinal study. J Pediatr 125:63–66

Listernick R, Charrow J, Guttman DH (1999) Intracranial gliomas in neurofibromatosis type 1. Am J Med Genet 89:38–44

Maher ER, Kaelin WG Jr (1997) Von Hippel–Lindau disease. Medicine (Baltimore) 76:381–391

Maria BL, Neufeld JA, Rosainz LL et al (1998a) High prevalence of bihemispheric structural and functional defects in Sturge–Weber syndrome. J Child Neurol 13:595–605

Maria BL, Neufeld JA, Rosainz LL et al (1998b) Central nervous system structure and function in Sturge–Weber syndrome: evidence of neurologic and radiologic progression. J Child Neurol 13:606–618

Mautner VF, Tatagiba M, Gutthof R et al (1993) Neurofibromatosis 2 in the pediatric age group. Neurosurgery 33:92–96

Mautner VF, Lindenau M, Baser ME et al (1996) The neuroimaging and clinical spectrum of neurofibromatosis 2. Neurosurgery 38:880–885; discussion 885–886

Menkes JH, Maria BL (2000) Neurocutaneous syndromes. In: Menkes JH, Sarnat HB (eds) Child neurology. Lippincott Williams and Wilkins, Philadelphia

Menor F, Marti-Bonmati L, Mulas F et al (1992) Neuroimaging in tuberous sclerosis: a clinicoradiological evaluation in pediatric patients. Pediatr Radiol 22:485–489

Miller SP, Tasch T, Sylvain M et al (1998) Tuberous sclerosis complex and neonatal seizures. J Child Neurol 13:619–623

Moffat DA, Quaranta N Baquley DM (2003) Management strategies in neurofibromatosis type 2. Eur Arch Otorhinolaryngol 260:12–18

Mukonoweshuro W, Griffiths PD, Blaser S (1999) Neurofibromatosis type 1: the role of neuroradiology. Neuropediatrics 30:111–119

Mukonoweshuro W, Wilkinson ID, Griffiths PD (2001) Proton MR spectroscopy of cortical tubers in adults with tuberous sclerosis complex. AJNR Am J Neuroradiol 22:1920–1925

Neurofibromatosis. Conference statement. National Institutes of Heath Consensus Development Conference. Arch Neurol. 45:575–578

Oakes WJ (1992) The natural history of patients with the Sturge–Weber syndrome. Pediatr Neurosurg 18:287–290

Packer RJ, Gutmann DH, Rubinstein A et al (2002) Plexiform neurofibromas in NF1: toward biologic-based therapy. Neurology 58:1461–1470

Paller AS (1987) Ataxia-telangiectasia. Neurol Clin 5:447–449

Parry DM., Eldridge R, Kaiser-Kupta MI et al (1994) Neurofibromatosis 2 (NF2): clinical characteristics of 63 affected individuals and clinical evidence for heterogeneity. Am J Med Genet 52:450–461

Parsa CF, Hoyt CS, Lesser RL et al (2001) Spontaneous regression of optic gliomas: thirteen cases documented by serial neuroimaging. Arch Ophthalmol 119:516–529

Pollack IF, Shultz B, Mulrihik JJ (1996) The management of brainstem gliomas in patients with neurofibromatosis 1. Neurology 46:1652–1660

Rasmussen SA, Yang Q, Friedman JM (2001) Mortality in neurofibromatosis 1: an analysis using US death certificates. Am J Hum Genet 68:1110–1118

Riccardi VM (1987) Neurofibromatosis. Neurol Clin 5:337–349

Richard S, David P, Marsot-Dupuch K et al (2000) Central nervous system hemangioblastomas, endolymphatic sac tumors, and von Hippel–Lindau disease. Neurosurg Rev 23:1–22

Roach ES (1992) Neurocutaneous syndromes. Pediatr Clin North Am 39:591–620

Roach ES, Gomez MR, Northrap H (1998) Tuberous sclerosis complex consensus conference: revised clinical diagnostic criteria. J Child Neurol 13:624–628

Rosser T, Packer RJ (2002) Intracranial neoplasms in children with neurofibromatosis 1. J Child Neurol 17:630–637; discussion 646–651

Samii M (1995) Hearing preservation in bilateral acoustic neurinomas. Br J Neurosurg 9:413–424

Shepherd CW, Stephenson JB (1992) Seizures and intellectual disability associated with tuberous sclerosis complex in the west of Scotland. Dev Med Child Neurol 34:766–774

Sims KB (2001) Von Hippel–Lindau disease: gene to bedside. Curr Opin Neurol 14:695–703

Singh AD, Shields CL, Shields JA (2001) Von Hippel–Lindau disease. Surv Ophthalmol 46:117–142

Sorensen SA, Mulvihill JJ, Nielsen A (1986) Long-term follow-up of von Recklinghausen neurofibromatosis. Survival and malignant neoplasms. N Engl J Med 314:1010–1015

Sparagana SP, Roach ES (2000) Tuberous sclerosis complex. Curr Opin Neurol 13:115–119

Subach BR, Kondziolka D, Lunsford LD et al (1999) Stereotactic radiosurgery in the management of acoustic neuromas associated with neurofibromatosis Type 2. J Neurosurg 90:815–822

Sujansky E, Conradi S (1995) Sturge-Weber syndrome: age of onset of seizures and glaucoma and the prognosis for offerted children. J Child Neurol 10:49–58

Szudek J, Birch P, Riccardi VM et al (2000) Associations of clinical features in neurofibromatosis 1 (NF1). Genet Epidemiol 19:429–439

Turgut M, Ozcan OE, Saglam S (1991) Central neurofibromatosis. Case report and review of the literature. Eur Neurol 31:188–192

Viskochil D (2002) Genetics of neurofibromatosis 1 and the NF1 gene. J Child Neurol 17:562–570; discussion 571–572, 646–651

Walsh RM, Bath AP, Bance ML et al (2000) The natural history of un-treated vestibular schwannomas. Is there a role for conservative management? Rev Laryngol Otol Rhinol (Bord) 121:21–26

Wanebo JE, Lonser RR, Glenn GM et al (2003) The natural history of hemangioblastomas of the central nervous system in patients with von Hippel–Lindau disease. J Neurosurg 98:82–94

Webb DW, Fryer AE, Osborne JP (1996) Morbidity associated with tuberous sclerosis: a population study. Dev Med Child Neurol 38:146–155

Zoller M, Rembeck B, Akesson HO et al (1995) Life expectancy, mortality and prognostic factors in neurofibromatosis type 1. A twelve-year follow-up of an epidemiological study in Goteborg, Sweden. Acta Derm Venereol 75:136–140

Modern Neuroimaging of Pediatric CNS Tumors

S.O. Bryant · S. Cha · A.J. Barkovich

Contents

Neuroimaging has been an important tool in the diagnosis of brain tumors and the assessment of their response to therapy for more than 20 years. Pre- and post-contrast magnetic resonance (MR) imaging remains the most important tool in the assessment of CNS neoplasms. Recently, however, technical advances have allowed the development of new techniques that enable the noninvasive evaluation of physiologic aspects of brain tumors and the surrounding brain. In this chapter, the new techniques and their applications to the assessment of brain tumors are discussed.

12.1 MR Spectroscopy

12.1.1 Principles

Proton MR spectroscopy (MRS) is a powerful, sensitive technique that can be added to a standard MR scan with only a small time penalty (Hunter and Wang 2001). MRS gives information about specific metabolites that can supplement the morphologic information obtained by current MR imaging (Kim et al. 1997; Kimura et al. 2001). Data suggest that MRS may be useful to differentiate tumor from normal tissue, determine relative tumor grade, plan biopsies, distinguish treatment injury from recurrent neoplasm, and distinguish cystic infection from cystic neoplasm (Dowling et al. 2001; Horska et al. 2001; Lazareff et al. 1999; Martin et al. 2001; Nelson et al. 1997; Nelson et al. 1999; Norfray et al. 1999; Ott et al. 1993; Poptani et al. 1995; Shimizu et al. 1996; Vigneron et al. 2001; Wang et al. 1996; Yousem et al. 1992). Currently, MR imaging alone may misrepresent tumor extent in up to 40 % of cases (Ott et al. 1993).

MRS can detect peaks from functional groups of numerous neurochemicals (Salibi and Brown 1998). Several of these are important in the analysis of patients with brain tumors, including N-acetylaspartate (NAA), trimethylamines [choline (Cho) and related compounds], creatine constituents (Cr), lactate (Lac), myo-inositol (Myo), and amino acids (AA) (Birken and Oldendorf 1989; Dezortova et al. 1999; Hunter and Wang 2001; Norfray et al. 1999; Poptani et al. 1995; Tomoi et al. 1997; Urenjak et al. 1993). The first four merit a more in-depth discussion to understand how spectroscopic information is beneficial in the setting of pediatric brain tumors.

A normal NAA peak is thought to indicate a normal number of mature, normally functioning neurons (Birken and Oldendorf 1989; Hunter and Wang 2001). NAA is believed to be a key component in an acetyl-group carrier between neuronal mitochondria and cytoplasm. It is vital in the regulation of neuronal protein synthesis, myelin production, and the metabolism of several neurotransmitters (Birken and Oldendorf 1989). NAA is also present in oligodendrocyte precursors, and thus may, theoretically, be elevated or reduced in processes involving oligodendrocytes and myelin, as well as those involving neurons and axons (Tzika et al. 1997; Urenjak et al. 1993). The NAA level is dependent on location (it is 10% lower in the normal cerebellum compared to cerebrum), maturity (increases as the brain develops and neurons mature), and neuronal health (decreased after injury or infiltration by neoplasm (Urenjak et al. 1995; Wang et al. 1996).

The Cho resonance is mainly composed of compounds in cell membranes, such as choline, phosphocholine, and glycerolphosphorylcholine (Waldrop et al. 1998). Choline protons within intact membranes (e.g., phosphatidylcholine), however, are immobile and do not contribute to MR signal (Dowling et al. 2001; Norfray et al. 1999; Waldrop et al. 1998). The Cho peak in the MR spectrum is composed of signal from these compounds during the processes of membrane synthesis and degradation (Dowling et al. 2001; Norfray et al. 1999; Waldrop et al. 1998); thus, elevated Cho is found in neoplasms, active infection, and regions containing inflammatory cells.

The Cr peak comes from methylamine peaks of creatine and phosphocreatine, compounds that provide a high-energy phosphate buffer for adenosine triphosphate synthesis (Norfray et al. 1999). In most disorders, it is not clear what processes produce changes in creatine concentrations. Cr can be depressed in high-grade or metabolically active neoplasm, due to the overwhelming requirements of the proliferating tumor cells (Tzika et al. 1996, 2001). It can also be depleted in regions of necrosis secondary to lack of metabolic needs and cell death (Taylor et al. 1996; Tzika et al. 1997, 2001; Yousem et al. 1992).

Lactate is an end product of anaerobic glycolysis that accumulates when the glycolytic rate exceeds lactate catabolism or overwhelms export by the blood stream (Norfray et al. 1999; Tomoi et al. 1997; Wang et al. 1995). It is a nonspecific marker seen in tumors, necrosis, ischemia, cysts, and treatment injury (Wang et al. 1995).

12.1.2 Technique

Currently at the University of California, San Francisco (UCSF) we obtain spectra from a large area of the brain (8×8×8 cm), and can resolve spectra from volumes of less than 1 cubic centimeter within that area in about 17 minutes (McKnight et al. 2001; Nelson et al. 1997, 1999). Using this technique, small foci of tumor can be identified in a large region of heterogeneous tissue. Moreover, post-processing allows the voxel to be placed in precisely the same region of interest as in prior studies, allowing increased confidence that the tumor has been sampled in precisely the same location (Nelson et al. 1994). On MR scanners without three-dimensional spectroscopic imaging (3D MRSI), 2D MRSI, commercially available from all major manufacturers, can be extremely useful. Coverage is permitted by 2D MRSI of a large area of tissue with small voxel size and an excellent signal to noise ratio (Dowling et al. 2001; Taylor et al. 1996). The only disadvantage is the necessity of acquiring separate spectra for each plane sampled.

12.1.3 Application

MRS is useful in the diagnosis and assessment of brain tumors because these tumors, as a rule, have elevated Cho levels and subnormal NAA levels compared to normal brain tissue. These features, however, are also found in other conditions in which membrane turnover is increased and the number of healthy mature neurons is decreased, such as immature brain, dysplastic brain, and inflammation. The concentration of NAA is normally 10% lower in the cerebellum than in cerebral white matter (Usenius et al. 1995; Wang et al. 1995). Cho concentrations in the cerebellum and pons are 70% higher than other areas (Usenius et al. 1995). Increased Cho in relation to NAA is even more dramatic in neonates (Tzika et al. 1996). Moreover, ratios of metabolites differ in different regions of the brain, even within different portions of the cerebral cortex (Wang et al. 1995). Thus, it is critical to correlate MRS with MRI and other tests in order to avoid false-positive diagnoses of tumor (Sutton et al. 1992). Indeed, one should never attempt to interpret MRS without MRI, as the MRS findings are entirely nonspecific by themselves.

Once the diagnosis of tumor is established, MRS can be of some use in grading astrocytic neoplasms. In general, the farther the metabolite peaks vary from normal, the more likely that the tumor is aggressive (Hunter and Wang 2001). In addition, the Lac peak magnitude tends to be more elevated in more aggressive neoplasms (Girard et al. 1998). It should be kept in mind, however, that juvenile pilocytic astrocytomas, among the most benign of brain tumors, have elevated choline and lactate, along with reduced NAA (Lazareff et al. 1999). In addition, similar grades of tumors of different histologic type may have very different spectra (e.g., a low-grade oligodendroglioma may have a spectrum very different from a low-grade astrocytoma). Thus, grading of neoplasms based on MRS has concentrated on determining peak magnitudes and ratios in tumors of the same histologic type (Cheng et al. 1998; Horska et al. 2001; Poptani et al. 1995; Shimizu et al. 1996; Tzika et al. 1996), and even in these cases it is not entirely reliable (Barker et al. 1993; Chang et al. 1998; Kimura et al. 2001; Lazareff et al. 1999; Shino et al. 1999; Tzika et al. 1996, 1997).

Rarely, tumors have unique spectra that can help narrow the differential diagnosis from that derived from routine MR imaging alone. For example, meningiomas often have an alanine peak not found in other neoplasms (Kinoshita and Yokota 1997; Kugel et al. 1992; Lehnhardt et al. 2001).

MRS can be helpful in selecting the best biopsy site in heterogeneous neoplasms (Dowling et al. 2001; Martin et al. 2001). However, for MRS to be useful in this regard, the voxel size must be small compared to the size of the neoplasm. Spectroscopic data obtained from a given volume of brain represents the average of the metabolic components of the volume. If the voxel is large or the tumor is small, the voxel might contain regions of both high and low grade or of neoplasm, normal brain, and necrosis (Tzika et al. 1996). The resultant spectrum reflects the percentage of each component and does not reflect the nature of the tumor. For example, the MRS of a highly aggressive neoplasm with a large component of necrosis or normal brain or low-grade tumor could mimic that of a low-grade neoplasm (Sijens et al. 1995; Venkatesh et al. 2001). Spectra can also be contaminated by adjacent CSF or by fat from the calvarium or scalp (Hunter and Wang 2001; Norfray et al. 1999; Sijens et al. 1995; Wang et al. 1996). Thus, it is imperative to use as small a voxel as possible. However, sampling many different voxels during a single exam necessitates excessively long scan times if each voxel is acquired separately. Thus, techniques have been developed to perform 3D MRSI, which allows a large volume of brain to be sampled during a single acquisition, with subsequent analysis of small areas within the volume during post-processing.

Although MRS can clearly distinguish abnormal from normal brain, it does not always correctly differentiate neoplasm from other processes (Kim et al. 1997; Sutton et al. 1992; Wilken et al. 2000), particularly those with a high concentration of inflammatory cells (Krouwer et al. 1998; Venkatesh et al. 2001). The literature contains many examples of inflammatory processes, such as demyelinating plaques, tuberculomas, xanthogranulomas, HIV encephalitis, and HSV encephalitis, that have MRS features nearly identical to neoplasia (Butzen et al. 2000; Krouwen et al. 1998; Shukla-Dave et al. 2001; Venkatesh et al.

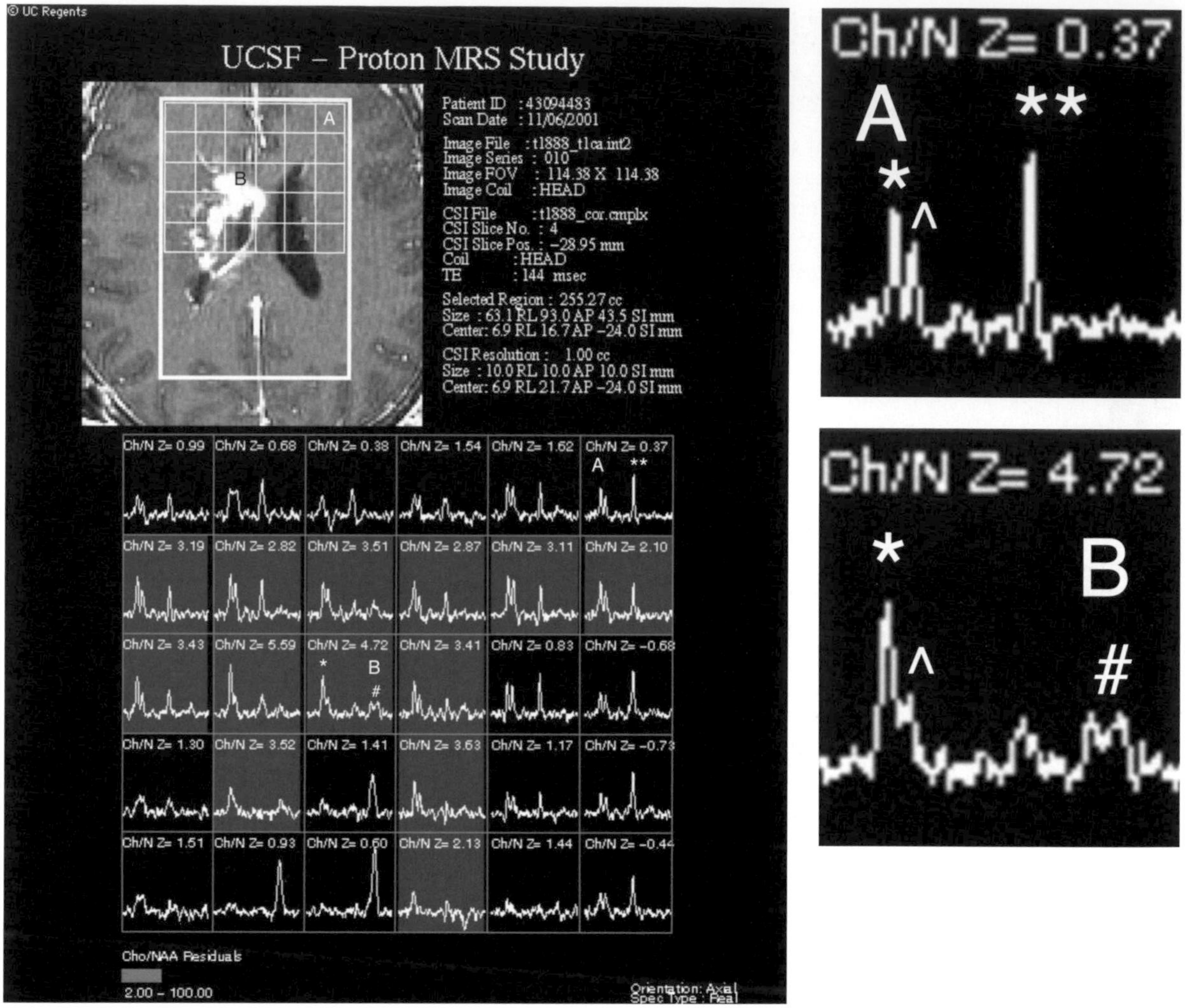

Figure 12.1a

High-grade glioma with both improved spectra and anatomic imaging after receiving radiation therapy. a Pre-treatment 3D CSI transposed on T$_1$-weighted gadolinium-enhanced axial image. Spectrum voxel labeled *A* is within normal left frontal white matter; choline (*), creatine (^) and NAA (**) peaks are normal for age and location. Spectrum voxel labeled *B* is within enhancing neoplasm; the spectrum shows elevated choline and lactate/lipid (#), with decreased NAA in the right splenium.

2001). These other processes should always be considered, particularly when the history or imaging characteristics are not classic for tumor or the patient has a history of a chronic illness.

However, MRS can be useful in differentiating abscess from tumor. Upregulated glycolysis and fermentation by bacteria produce elevated levels of lactate, acetate, and succinate, while proteolysis by enzymes produces valine, isoleucine, and leucine (Chang et al. 1998; Gupta et al. 2001; Kim et al. 1997). These compounds have protons that precess in the aliphatic region, upfield from NAA. Although ele-

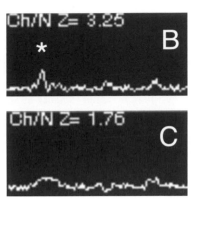

UCSF – Proton MRS Study

Patient ID   : 43094483
Scan Date   : 01/16/2002

Image File   : t1958_t1ca.int2
Image Series : 010
Image FOV   : 104.06 X 104.06
Image Coil   : HEAD

CSI File   : t1958_cor.cmplx
CSI Slice No. : 4
CSI Slice Pos. : –25.50 mm
Coil   : HEAD
TE   : 144 msec

Selected Region : 287.23 cc
Size : 83.4 RL 82.0 AP 42.0 SI mm
Center: 3.3 RL 16.1 AP –20.5 SI mm

CSI Resolution : 1.00 cc
Size : 10.0 RL 10.0 AP 10.0 SI mm
Center: 3.3 RL 16.1 AP –20.5 SI mm

Cho/NAA Residuals
2.00 – 100.00

Orientation: Axial
Spec Type : Real

Figure 12.1b

b Follow-up 3D CSI in the same location as image a. Choline peak (*) has decreased since the prior study, resulting in an improved Z-score, yet still has evidence of residual neoplasm; Spectrum voxel labeled *C* shows necrosis; all metabolites are decreased

---

vated lactate and succinate associated with radiation necrosis renders MRS nonspecific in the posttherapy patient (Kim et al. 1997; Yeung et al. 2001), the presence of these peaks is quite sensitive (92 to 100 %) and specific when MRS is performed at presentation (Grand et al. 1999; Gupta et al. 2001; Kim et al. 1997; Kimura et al. 2001; Shukla-Dave et al. 2001).

Distinguishing posttherapy injury from recurrent or residual neoplasm has been difficult for anatomic imaging techniques, as the enhancement and edema in both conditions can be nearly identical. This distinction is pivotal, since early recognition of recurrence can prolong survival or guide future treatment (Shtern 1992). MRS can be a useful technique in making this distinction, as injured brain produces a spectrum different from normal brain or tumor (Kamada et al. 1997). Early radiation injury produces elevated Cho from plasma and intracellular membrane disruption, but this usually clears quickly and a normal NAA peak remains (Szigety et al. 1993). A global decrease in peak amplitudes (NAA, Cho, and Cr peaks) is consistent with treatment injury without active neoplasm (Kimura et al. 2001; Ott et al. 1993; Taylor et al. 1996; Tzika et al. 1997; Yousem et al. 1992). Recurrence is suggested by new or persistent elevation of Cho and reduction of NAA (Fig. 12.1) (Lazareff et al. 1999; Sijens et al. 1995; Tzika et al. 1997).

There is no consensus as to how often patients should be evaluated. We believe that the most sensitive method to evaluate treatment efficacy and to screen for early recurrence or residual neoplasm is to perform serial exams, comparing them with a known baseline prior to treatment (Lazareff et al. 1999; Nelson et al. 1997, 1999; Norfray et al. 1999; Vigneron et al. 2001). It is important to remember that, although MRI/MRS is more sensitive than MRI alone, sensitivity is not 100%. Necrotic neoplasm with a paucity of viable tumor cells can have identical spectra to posttreatment necrosis (Taylor et al. 1996); differentiation can only be made when the Cho increases on subsequent exams. Serial follow-up studies are, therefore, essential to detect early growth of residual neoplasm.

MRS is a promising tool for assessing pediatric patients with brain tumors. In the appropriate setting, spectroscopy can improve the delineation of neoplastic brain involvement, increase the specificity of diagnosis, and help discriminate posttreatment injury from residual neoplasm. Research continues to define the role of MRS in grading neoplasms and possibly predicting treatment response (Girard et al. 1998; Lazareff et al. 1999; Lin et al. 1999; Negendank et al. 1996; Tzika et al. 2001; Waldrop et al. 1998).

12.2 MR Perfusion

12.2.1 Principles

Cerebral perfusion is defined as the delivery of nutrients and oxygen, via the blood, to brain tissue per unit volume. This is typically expressed in units of milliliters per 100 g of parenchyma per minute (Cha et al. 2002). With recent advances in fast imaging techniques and computer technology it is now possible to capture the dynamic changes in cerebral perfusion using MRI. MR perfusion imaging provides information on cerebral hemodynamic parameters that are reflective of tissue perfusion, including relative cerebral blood volume (rCBV), cerebral blood flow (CBF), and mean transit time (MTT).

Perfusion MR imaging (pMRI) has evolved from a research tool into a clinically useful technique due to wider availability of high performance MR gradients that allow faster imaging sequences (e.g., echo planar imaging) and improvement in computer image-processing algorithms. Quantitative analysis of perfusion parameters can now be derived from a clinically useful volume of brain using MR perfusion. In addition to the gathering of anatomical information as from conventional MR, this technique takes us one step closer to evaluating intracranial pathophysiology. A brief review of pMRI is presented for better understanding of the methodology and the basis for its clinical application.

12.2.2 Technique

There are several methods to derive perfusion parameters using MR imaging. Either endogenous (arterial water) or exogenous (gadolinium, deuterium oxide) contrast agents can be used in pMRI (Cha et al. 2002). Endogenous perfusion imaging (e.g., arterial spin labeling) provides absolute quantification of cerebral blood flow, but suffers from several pitfalls. These include long imaging time, extreme sensitivity to motion and low signal-to-noise ratio (SNR) (Cha et al. 2000a). This section will be limited to the discussion of pMRI using exogenous contrast (e.g., gadolinium-DTPA) due to its readily available clinical benefits and ease of use.

MR perfusion (e.g., dynamic susceptibility, weighted-contrast-enhanced perfusion MR imaging, DSC-pMRI) exploits the signal changes (T_2* signal loss) during bolus passage of a contrast agent through the cerebral vessels (Aronen et al. 1994; Ball and Holland 2001; Cha et al. 2000a; Ludemann et al. 2000; Siegal et al. 1997; Strong et al. 1993). Using tracer kinetic principles, the signal change is converted to an integral of tissue contrast agent concentration (Peters 1998; Rosen et al. 1990; Weisskoff et al. 1994). These values are then used to generate perfusion maps of various hemodynamic parameters.

To successfully image a large volume of brain during the finite time that contrast is within the cerebral vessels, faster imaging methods are necessary. Echo planar imaging (EPI) fulfills this requirement, with temporal resolution of 100 ms/slice. Several different pulse sequences can be used with EPI (e.g., spin echo, gradient echo). Spin echo images are thought to be more sensitive to signal changes from contrast agent within the capillaries (Weisskoff et al. 1994). Gradient echo images are more sensitive to medium to large vessels, and therefore greater signal drop is seen during the first-pass of a contrast agent. Although more prone to susceptibility artifact, gradient echo techniques are more sensitive to small changes in blood volume. Therefore, the gradient echo technique does not require higher doses of contrast agent as does spin echo to produce diagnostic images (Cha et al. 2002; Hunter and Wang 2001; Weisskoff et al. 1994).

12.2.3 Applications

DSC-pMRI, as adjunct imaging to conventional MR, has several potential applications. With the wide availability and application of faster imaging hardware and software, DSC-pMRI can be incorporated into the routine evaluation of intracranial lesions. Clinical roles for DSC-pMRI include grading neoplasms, directing stereotactic biopsies, and distinguishing therapy-related brain injury from residual/recurrent tumor (Cha et al. 2002; Knopp et al. 1999; Law et al. 2002; Maeda et al. 1993; Tzika et al. 2002).

Some advocate that DSC-pMRI may be helpful in adjusting chemotherapy dosing (Cha et al. 2000b).

Preliminary results on grading of gliomas with DSC-pMRI are promising. Although some authors using spin echo sequences have shown no statistical correlation between tumor grade and perfusion imaging, gradient echo-derived blood volumes have been more robust in distinguishing grades of glioma (Aronen et al. 1994; Ball and Holland 2001; Ludemann et al. 2000; Roberts et al. 2000; Rosen et al. 1991; Sugahara et al. 1998, 1999).

Separating high- from low-grade gliomas by histology relies on the presence of neovascularity and necrosis (Giannini and Scheithauer 1997; Plate and Mennel 1995). DSC-pMRI is a method that can noninvasively assess tumor vascularity and is complementary to histopathology in determining the grade and malignancy potential of a neoplasm (Fig. 12.2) (Gerlowski and Jain 1986).

Histology alone may not accurately predict tumor biology or patient prognosis. DSC-pMRI correlates with the degree of tumor angiogenesis and therefore may be able to predict aggressive biology (Aronen et al. 1994). Hence, the more aggressive the tumor, the larger the rCBV (Knopp et al. 1999; Sugahara et al. 1999). This technique offers a potentially powerful and noninvasive means of assessing tumor biology and serially monitoring changes in the tumor during therapy.

Most published reports in the literature for tumor grading using DSC-pMRI have been based on the adult population. Sensitivity for this technique may be reduced in children since certain benign tumors, such as pilocytic astrocytoma and choroid plexus papilloma, may have increased vascularity, i.e., high rCBV (Ball and Holland 2001; Giannini and Scheithauer 1997; Keene et al. 1999; Plate and Mennel 1995; Strong et al. 1993). Caution is also raised in interpretation of DSC-pMRI in heterogeneous tumors. Determining the rCBV can vary in these lesions depending on the location chosen to place the region of interest (ROI). An ROI placed in an area of necrosis or nonaggressive portion of the neoplasm could erroneously underestimate rCBV and result in under-grading of tumor. Alternatively, cortically based neoplasms that are contiguous with the brain surface vessels

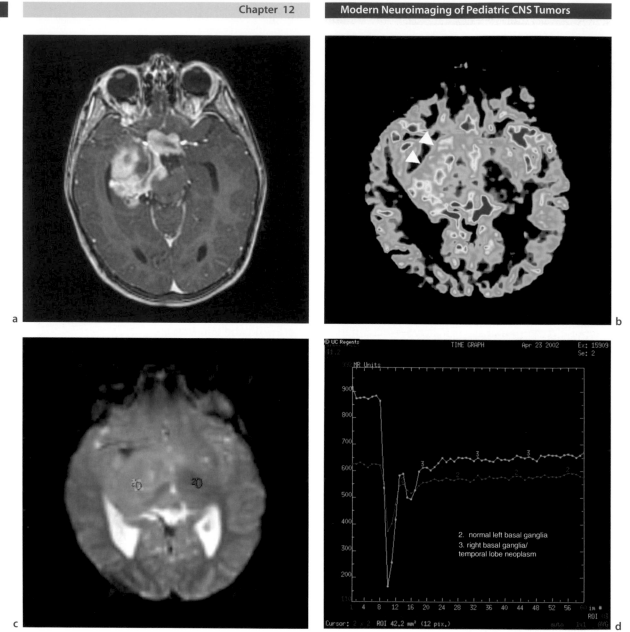

Figure 12.2 a–d

Right medial temporal lobe and chiasmatic glioma with pMRI characteristics of a vascular, intra-axial neoplasm. a Axial T$_1$-weighted gadolinium-enhanced image of the infiltrating, enhancing neoplasm. b Axial color map of the rCBV showing increased CBV within the neoplasm (*white arrowheads*) relative to normal vascularity on the contralateral side. c Axial T$_2$-weighted image shows the regions (*ovals*) that were sampled to calculate the time/signal curves (2 = normal left basal ganglia, 3 = neoplasm). d Time signal curve shows an intact BBB in region 2 (normal recovery of signal after the passage of the contrast bolus), but a partially disrupted BBB in region 3 (slower, incomplete recovery after the bolus due to contrast leaking through the BBB) may be falsely given a higher grade due to a high rCBV from an ROI placed over vessels (Sugahara et al. 2001). Larger studies are needed prior to DSC-pMRI's inclusion as a routine clinical practice for grading tumors in children.

A promising application for perfusion imaging is distinguishing treatment-induced brain injury from residual or recurrent neoplasm (Cha et al. 2000b, 2002; Roberts et al. 2000; Rosen et al. 1991; Siegal et al. 1997; Sugahara et al. 1999, 2000). With routine MRI, all of these can enhance and are indistinguishable until serial studies show growth, in the case of neoplasm. DSC-pMRI takes advantage of the pathophysiologic differences in vascularity to separate the entities. Posttreatment brain injury, in part, is believed to be the result of endothelial damage followed by vascular thrombosis and blood-brain barrier (BBB) breakdown. This ultimately leads to hypoperfusion of the affected tissue (Chan et al. 1999). The result of delayed radiation injury is vascular thrombosis and fibrinoid necrosis, which on DSC-pMRI manifests as a decrease in rCBV when compared to normal tissue (Cha et al. 2000b, 2002). On the other hand, tumor cells require a viable blood supply for growth and spread and, therefore, increased rCBV is seen in recurrent/residual neoplasm (Ball and Holland 2001; Cha et al. 2000b; Plate and Mennel 1995). Preliminary results show that decreased signal on DSC-pMRI correlates well with treatment-induced brain injury (Cha et al. 2000b, 2002; Siegal et al. 1997).

Exceptions still exist in making this important distinction between tumor and therapy-induced brain injury. Normal or even decreased rCBV in the area of residual tumor can occur if neoplastic tissue is mixed with hypovascular necrotic tissue. Treatment-induced injury can lead to aneurysmal dilation of vessels and formation of telangiectasias that can artificially elevate the rCBV, leading to false positives. Petechial hemorrhage or calcification in an area of residual tumor can produce susceptibility artifact that spuriously reduces the rCBV, resulting in a false negative (Sugahara et al. 2000). Further research is needed prior to standardized clinical use throughout multiple institutions.

DSC-pMRI continues to be investigated for use in guiding stereotactic biopsy of intracranial neoplasms. Traditionally, biopsies of brain neoplasm, guided by MR and CT, are directed to areas of conventional contrast enhancement. This approach, however, is prone to sampling error due to the intrinsic limitations of imaging enhancement to detect the most aggressive portion of a tumor (Cha et al. 2002; Joyce et al. 1978). In addition, limited tissue sample size can lead to erroneous grading and inadequate evaluation (Cappabianca et al. 1991; Chandrasoma et al. 1989).

Contrast enhancement on MR reflects the areas of breakdown within the BBB (Greenwood 1991). This is often in the rim adjacent to a necrotic portion of the neoplasm. Elevated rCBV is felt to represent the areas of vascular hyperplasia in the aggressive, viable neoplasm and may not always correspond to a contrast-enhancing portion (Cha et al. 2002). Using DSC-pMRI in addition to conventional anatomical images could result in reduced false negatives and errors in assessing tumor grade. Although still investigational, DSC-pMRI may be helpful in localizing the most aggressive portion of neoplasms and serve as a complementary tool to anatomic imaging (Aronen et al. 1994; Knopp et al. 1999; Rosen et al. 1991).

Future applications for DSC-pMRI under development include mapping dose distributions in neoplasms and following perfusion maps for therapy-outcomes research for new therapeutic agents (Cha et al. 2000b, 2002; Ludemann et al. 2000; Roberts et al. 2000).

In summary, DSC-pMRI is no longer primarily a research tool and promises to become an important diagnostic tool complementing conventional anatomical imaging. Clinical use for tumor grading, differentiating between residual neoplasm and treatment-associated injury, and assisting in therapy dosing and treatment follow-up are on the horizon. Guiding biopsies within heterogeneous tumors by perfusion imaging may reduce sampling errors and improve diagnostic accuracy.

12.2.4 Limitations

DSC-pMRI has several important constraints. Sensitivity to susceptibility artifact prevents its use in brain adjacent to the paranasal sinuses or the skull base (Ball and Holland 2001; Cha et al. 2002; Poussaint et al. 1995). The sequence is very sensitive to patient motion, and SNR is low in comparison to anatomic MR images (Aronen et al. 1994; Cha et al. 2002; Siegal et al. 1997). Only a limited volume of brain can be covered during the time it takes the contrast bolus to pass through the intracranial vasculature. Also, a compact delivery of the bolus may be difficult to attain in a patient who has limited intravenous access (Siegal et al. 1997). Furthermore, care must be taken to recognize false positives that are created by normal structures (e.g., choroid plexus and cortical veins) (Aronen et al. 1994; Sugahara et al. 1998).

Additional costs may be substantial, due to the stringent hardware and software requirements to acquire and process the MR data. An on-site physicist familiar with the MR technique is also beneficial, if not essential, to bring the system on line at a new facility and for continued support (Cha et al. 2002).

12.3 Nuclear Medicine

12.3.1 Principles

The role of radionuclide CNS imaging continues to evolve. The most commonly used techniques are single photon emission computed tomography (SPECT), which is readily available in most hospitals, and positron emission tomography (PET), which is more expensive and less readily available. Areas of current study include: differentiating lesions with similar imaging appearances (e.g., lymphoma from toxoplasmosis by thallium uptake), differentiating treatment injury from residual neoplasm, grading neoplasms, predicting response to therapy, and localizing eloquent cortices prior to surgery (Maria et al. 1998; Ricci et al. 1998).

The most widely practiced application is that of differentiating residual neoplasm from treatment injury. Without special techniques (such as MRSI; see previous section), this differentiation can be extremely difficult by conventional CT and MRI (Brunelle 2000; di Chiro et al. 1988; Valk and Dillon 1991). Both entities produce altered vasculature that can result in identical-appearing edema and enhancement. Even biopsy can lead to a false diagnosis. It is difficult to know if an area of enhancement represents an aggressive margin of neoplasm or just an area of active necrosis and BBB breakdown (Poussaint et al. 1995). If cognizant of the limitations, radionuclide imaging may be very helpful in select clinical scenarios.

Both SPECT and PET, utilizing several radionuclide imaging agents, have been studied in attempts to distinguish treatment injury from neoplasm. The most cited agents are Technetium-99m, thallium-201, fluorine-18, and carbon-11(Dadparvar et al. 2000; di Chiro et al. 1988; Go et al. 1994; Kim et al. 1992; Maria et al. 1994; Ogawa et al. 1991; Shinoura et al. 1997). Thallium-201 SPECT and ^{18}F-deoxyglucose (FDG) PET are currently the most promising methods (Loberboym et al. 1997; Maria et al. 1997); the remaining discussion is limited to these two.

12.3.2 Mechanism and Technique

The mechanism of thallium sequestration within tumor cells is unknown. The most accepted theories propose either passive uptake over a potential membrane gradient or high affinity for potassium-activated adenosine triphosphatase (Kaplan et al. 1987; Kim et al. 1992). Alteration of the BBB may also play a role (Kim et al. 1992). Whatever the mechanism, thallium seems to be incorporated into neoplastic glial cells considerably more than into non-neoplastic cells. A typical dose for a ^{201}Tl brain scan is 0.03 to 0.05 mCi/kg and images are obtained 5 to 10 minutes after administering the dose intravenously (O'Tuama 1998).

PET imaging for brain tumors is primarily with ^{18}FDG, a compound that has chemical properties similar to glucose and is therefore incorporated into astrocytes as an energy source. However, ^{18}FDG cannot be normally metabolized and, therefore, becomes entrapped within cells (Wang et al. 1996). Increased ^{18}FDG within tumor cells is attributed to the increased rate of glycolysis in rapidly growing neoplasms (de Witte et al. 2000; Shinoura et al. 1997). For pediatric brain scans, 0.14 mCi/kg of ^{18}FDG is given intravenously and images are usually obtained 30 minutes later (Kaplan et al. 1999; Kincaid et al. 1998).

12.3.3 Applications and Limitations

The usage of PET and SPECT to distinguish tumor from posttreatment injury has been studied extensively (Fig. 12.3). Both sensitivity and specificity of ^{18}FDG PET are in the range of 80 to 90% (di Chiro et al. 1988; Kim et al. 1992; Ricci et al. 1998; Valk and Dillon 1991). At least 80% of pediatric tumors have a high affinity for thallium. It may, therefore, be useful to distinguish neoplasm from posttreatment granulation tissue (Brunelle 2000; Maria et al. 1998). However, the grade of the neoplasm and histologic type do not always correlate with the amount of thallium uptake (Maria et al. 1994). Pilocytic astrocytoma has a very high metabolic rate and therefore often a high radiotracer uptake, even though it is a relatively benign neoplasm.

The data for PET is calculated from lesions that are at least 5 to 7 mm in dimension, the lower limits of resolution for this modality. This imposes a limitation on early detection of subtle neoplastic recurrence. Furthermore, the percentage of false negatives is rather high and, as a result, many authors do not consider this method acceptable for making therapeutic decisions (Barker et al. 1997; Kim et al. 1992; Ogawa et al. 1991; Valk et al. 1988). Other PET agents, such as ^{11}C choline and ^{11}C tyrosine, have had mixed success in detecting neoplastic recurrence and are still under investigation (Go et al. 1994; Shinoura et al. 1997).

Biopsy guidance by PET has been successful in the limited number of patients studied (Go et al. 1994; Massager et al. 2000). In theory, the most aggressive portion of a tumor has the highest glucose uptake and, thus, the highest ^{18}FDG uptake; PET can therefore assist in localizing the most aggressive portion of a heterogeneous neoplasm for proper staging. However, identification of the most aggressive portion of the tumor has not been reproducible at every institu-

tion. This may be due to difficulties in coregistering the PET images to anatomic imaging (e.g., MR imaging) and, perhaps, to the difficulty in identifying very small regions of high-grade tumor (Maria et al. 1994, 1998). Furthermore, it can be difficult to differentiate regions of cortex (which has higher ^{18}FDG uptake than normal white matter) from regions of tumor recurrence without additional MR imaging.

Accurately predicting tumor grade by imaging is imprecise and remains an elusive goal in practice. Some authors claim that radionuclide imaging is an equivalent, or occasionally better, predictor of survival in patients with a malignant glioma compared with a prediction based on histologic grade (Valk et al. 1988). Others believe that PET is at least adequate to distinguish high- from low-grade brain neoplasms (Black et al. 1994; Kincaid et al. 1998; Provenzale et al. 1999; Valk and Dillon 1991). However, most results indicate that nuclear imaging does not grade brain neoplasms with adequate accuracy to make it useful in clinical practice (Choi et al. 2000; de Witte et al. 2000; O'Tuama 1998). For example, high-grade neoplasms, often necrotic in part, will have low uptake in the necrotic regions so that when averaged with high-uptake regions may appear as low-grade neoplasms when calculating overall uptake. In addition, some low-grade pediatric neoplasms, such as pilocytic astrocytomas, have an increased uptake to make them appear as high-grade neoplasms.

Another potential application of radionuclides is as a means of segregating tumors amenable to anti-angiogenesis agents from those that would be resistant (O'Tuama 1998; Valk et al. 1988). Some authors suggest using PET to localize eloquent cortices preoperatively for patients unable to tolerate MR (Kaplan et al. 1999).

In general, radionuclide imaging is infrequently used for pediatric brain neoplasms at our institution, with conventional MRI, MRSI, perfusion imaging, and magnetic source imaging (MSI) being the imaging tools of choice. Each institution should determine the optimal tools for their patients depending upon their equipment and individual strengths.

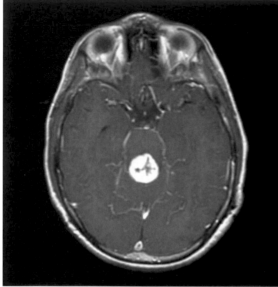

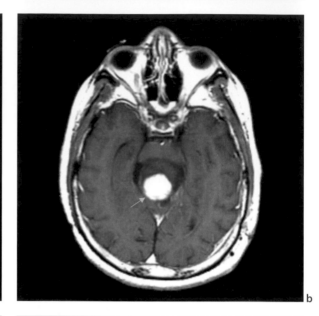

a

b

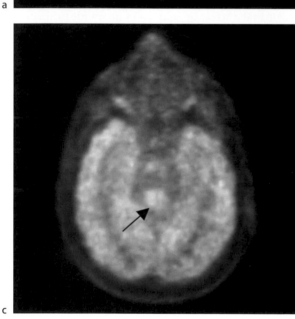

c

Figure 12.3 a–c

PET imaging complimenting anatomic MRI in a case of tumor recurrence. **a** Axial T_1-weighted gadolinium-enhanced image of a tectal glioma at presentation. **b** Axial T_1-weighted gadolinium-enhanced image of the same tectal glioma after radiation treatment. The enhancing mass may represent posttreatment granulation tissue or residual neoplasm. **c** Axial PET image showing increased activity (*black arrow*) within the tectal mass indicating residual active neoplasm

12.4 BOLD/MSI

12.4.1 Principles

Two techniques used for locating brain activity during specific tasks are blood oxygenation level dependent (BOLD) imaging and magnetic source imaging (MSI). Many clinical applications of these techniques are under investigation, including evaluating reorganization after injury and deterioration during progressive disease, evaluation of therapies, and cortical mapping prior to neurosurgery (Roberts et al. 2000; Vezina 1997). These techniques are well developed in adults, but are less useful in children, as they require a great deal of cooperation by the patient. Some authors have had success in children through the use of multiple training sessions. However, such training requires considerable time, personnel, and space, which are rarely available in most hospitals and outpatient centers. Task-related activations, which require that the patient perform specific tasks may be difficult or impossible in individuals with deficits such as reading disorders, mental retardation, hearing loss, and paralysis (Breier et al. 1999; Otsubo and Snead 2001; Simons et al. 1999). It is possible to perform some studies on sedated children, but it is not yet clear how much effect the sedation has on the results. Therefore, this section is composed based mainly on results in adults, in the hope that the difficulties in performing these studies in children will soon be overcome.

12.4.2 Mechanism of BOLD Imaging

In BOLD images, contrast is created by a local increase of oxygenated blood in activated tissue (Martin and Marcar 2001; Stippich et al. 1998). In theory, an activated group of neurons requires increased oxygenation. This increased need is fulfilled by local vasodilation, allowing more oxygenated blood to be transported to the activated cerebral cortex. The increase in blood flow more than compensates for the increased oxygen consumption, resulting in local increase in oxyhemoglobin and decrease in deoxyhemoglobin. As oxyhemoglobin is diamagnetic (does not alter the local magnetic field) and deoxyhemoglobin is paramagnetic (alters the local magnetic field and results in local signal loss); the reduced local concentration of deoxyhemoglobin results in less signal loss and increased local signal intensity (Beisteiner et al. 1995; Boxerman et al. 1995). This local signal alteration can be detected by susceptibility-weighted MR imaging sequences if multiple acquisitions are performed.

12.4.3 Mechanism of MSI

Neuronal activation results in electrical current, which can be measured with electroencephalography. The electrical current generates magnetic flux, the magnitude of which is in the order of a few picoteslas, a quantity that is eight orders of magnitude smaller than that produced from the earth's magnetic field and 12 orders smaller than that produced from MRI (Alberstone et al. 2000; Lev and Grant 2000). When performed in a room shielded from external magnetic fields, superconducting quantum interference devices (SQUIDs) (Ganslandt et al. 1999; Stippich et al. 1998) can be used to measure and localize these minute neuromagnetic signals using small receivers placed on the scalp (Alberstone et al. 2000; Papanicolaou et al. 2001). This technique is known as magnetoencephalography (MEG). MEG signal is generated from intracellular electron flux, not local vascular changes (as seen with functional MRI) (Roberts and Rowley 1997), and is distinguished from EEG, which detects extracellular currents and is therefore less precise than MEG (Alberstone et al. 2000). Superimposition of MEG data on co-localized MR images is referred to as magnetic source imaging (MSI) (Stippich et al. 1998).

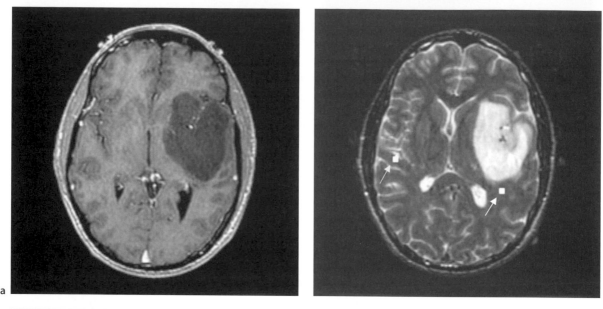

a   b

Figure 12.4 a,b

MSI for preoperative surgical planning in a patient who presented with grand mal seizure and aura, but without speech or motor deficits. **a** Axial T1-weighted gadolinium-enhanced image showing a non-enhancing left temporal lobe/basal ganglia low grade glioma. **b** Axial T_2-weighted image showing *white squares* that correspond to areas of auditory stimulation with a 1000 Hz frequency tone. The auditory cortex on the left side is displaced, but not invaded, by the neoplasm

12.4.4 Applications of BOLD and MSI

The most widely used clinical application of BOLD imaging and MSI is the localization of eloquent cortices for preoperative planning of brain surgery (Fig. 12.4) (Disbrow et al. 1999; Roberts and Rowley 1997). Both BOLD and MSI can accurately localize the primary motor cortex (Pujol et al. 1998; Roberts and Rowley 1997). Sensitivity varies from 82 to 100 % and often depends on whether the primary motor cortex is merely displaced or frankly invaded by the clinical process. Both techniques can also be used for localizing language centers prior to surgical resection of portions of the temporal lobe for epilepsy or tumor (Simos et al. 1999). BOLD may have the additional benefit over MEG in simultaneously localizing multiple areas involved in complex brain function (Roberts et al. 2000).

The accepted gold standard test to localize activated motor cortex is intraoperative cortical surface recording (Suzuki and Yasui 1992). For localizing hemispheric language centers, the Wada test (intracarotid amytal test) has been the standard examination for many years, but BOLD techniques have similar sensitivities and are less invasive.

BOLD imaging has two major advantages in comparison to intraoperative surface recording: (1) localization is obtained preoperatively, allowing prospective surgical planning; and (2) the study can be performed at the same time as the preoperative MRI instead of lengthening operating room time for an additional procedure. Both techniques suffer when anatomic landmarks are distorted by the tumor, as the surgeon may encounter inadequate surgical exposure of the primary motor cortex, and the navigation based on the MR may be changed by opening of the calvarium (Cedzich et al. 1996). Anesthetic agents may also influence the sensitivity of both the intraoperative and BOLD techniques (Cedzich et al. 1996), although older children and teens can generally undergo BOLD analysis without the need for sedation. In adults, overall sensitivity of intraoperatively localized eloquent cortices is roughly 91 to 94 % (estimated by postoperative deficits), which is similar to functional imaging (Ganslandt et al. 1999; Simos et al. 1999; Szymanski et al. 2001).

The Wada test requires an invasive catheter angiogram and sedation, both with inherent risks. Hemispheric dominance can be established in the majority of cases, but more specific cortical mapping is not possible (Simos et al. 1999). MSI and BOLD are both as sensitive and provide additional information that guides surgical approach and extent of resection (Alberstone et al. 2000; Dillon and Roberts 1999; Ganslandt et al. 1999; Pujol et al. 1998).

12.4.5 Limitations

Several pitfalls must be kept in mind when implementing these new techniques. Limitations of BOLD imaging include poor temporal resolution that can never be better than the time that is required to produce a hemodynamic response to activated neurons, roughly 2 to 5 seconds (Lev and Grant 2000; Martin and Marcar 2001; Roberts and Rowley 1997). The spatial resolution is dependent on the anatomic proximity of vessels to activated brain; high signal contribution by sulcal veins has a marked negative effect on resolution (Dillon and Roberts 1999; Holodny et al. 1999; Roberts and Rowley 1997). Infiltration by neoplasm and edema can further distort the anatomic relationship and possibly alter the autoregulation of local vessels (Dillon and Roberts 1999; Holodny et al. 1999; Pujol et al. 1998). Motion artifact, larger caliber vessels, and inflow effects can further distort localization (Beisteiner et al. 1995; Boxerman et al. 1995; Field et al. 2000; Holodny et al. 1999; Pujol et al. 1998). Despite these shortcomings, BOLD generally localizes activated groups of neurons within 1 to 2 cm of their anatomic location.

MSI is hindered by overwhelming susceptibility artifact from orthodontia and other ferromagnetic metals (Breier et al. 1999); BOLD imaging is also affected by such artifacts, but not as severely. The precision of labeling eloquent cortex by MEG is very good, but not perfect. The inaccuracies of transposing data from MEG to MRI reduces point localization by roughly 4 mm of dispersal (Szymanski et al. 2001). Overall error in localization is thought to be roughly a centimeter (Beisteiner et al. 1995), but this is superior to other accepted techniques, including BOLD. The largest drawback of MSI is the cost and lack of availability of the necessary equipment; whereas BOLD can be performed on a clinical magnet with software upgrade, MSI requires an expensive neuromagnetometer in addition to a clinical magnet.

In summary, functional imaging has some potential for use in pediatric brain tumor patients, but a number of problems need to be overcome before these techniques will be used routinely.

12.5 Diffusion Imaging

12.5.1 Principles

Diffusion-weighted imaging (DWI) is a technique that relies on the fact that the motion of water molecules causes decreased signal on specially acquired MR images (Mitchell 1999). A special type of diffusion-weighted imaging known as diffusion tensor imaging (DTI), which allows both the net direction and the magnitude of water motion in a voxel to be determined, has recently become clinically available. Both of these techniques have applications in the assessment of brain tumors.

12.5.2 Technique

The technique of DWI allows for the calculation of net water motion in a volume of tissue. Although it is not known how much of the imaged water is intra- versus extracellular, many authors have hypothesized that most of the signal in these images is derived from extracellular H_2O. Reduced diffusion reflects the net motion of all the free H_2O molecules within a given volume of tissue (Filippi et al. 2001; Inglis et al. 1999; Poupon et al. 1998).

The diffusion tensor is a mathematical probability function that calculates the precise net motion characteristics of the water protons in the voxel; in other words, it gives the probability that any molecule is moving in any direction at any velocity during the time of the imaging. If all of the water protons are equally free to move in all directions, the motion is said to be isotropic. If water protons move predominantly in one direction more than others (due to restricted movement in some directions or accentuated movement in others), the motion is said to be anisotropic. An example of a normal brain structure that has anisotropic features is an axon. Water motion is greater along the long axis than perpendicular to it, probably at least in part as a result of the surrounding hydrophobic myelin sheath. The characteristics of the motion can be displayed either as images or mathematically (Filippi et al. 2001; Gauvain et al. 2001; Melhem et al. 2000; Pierpaoli et al. 1996).

12.5.3 Applications

Few applications of diffusion imaging have been utilized for the analysis of pediatric brain tumors. One area in which it has been found to be helpful is in distinguishing between ring enhancing tumors and abscesses. In general, cystic tumors have increased water motion compared with surrounding brain, but abscesses have reduced water motion (Fig. 12.5) (Gauvain et al. 2001). DWI can also be helpful in distinguishing between cystic and solid tumors. For example, differentiation between an arachnoid cyst and an epidermoid tumor may be difficult by conventional MR sequences or CT. CSF freely moves in an arachnoid cyst and therefore is isointense to the subarachnoid space on DWI. An epidermoid tumor, on the other hand, is solid and therefore has diffusion characteristics similar to brain tissue. On diffusion-weighted images, which reflect both diffusion characteristics and T_2 characteristics, epidermoids are bright compared to both CSF and the surrounding brain, whereas on apparent diffusion coefficient (ADC) images, which reflect only diffusion, epider-

moids have a similar signal intensity to brain tissue (Gauvain et al. 2001).

A current area of research for the use of DWI in brain tumor patients is in evaluating postoperative injury (Tanner et al. 2000). Acutely injured tissue generally has reduced diffusion for several days after the injury. Areas of reduced diffusion around the surgical cavity in the first few days after tumor resection likely represents ischemic injury, possibly from damage to vessels in the region of the resection (Fig. 12.6). Such areas will generally show marked enhancement for more than six weeks after surgery and should not be mistaken for recurrent tumor.

DTI can potentially identify specific white matter tracts within the brain, a technique that has been called white matter tractography. Tractography may be able to localize the corticospinal tracts based on anatomic characteristics, which could help in preoperative planning. This technique could be especially helpful in the spinal cord, where normal anisotropic white matter tracts might be separable from disorganized neoplastic cells (Inglis et al. 1999). However, diffusion imaging in the spine is currently difficult, due to artifact created by the spinal column. Moreover, the small size of the spinal cord creates problems in resolution. One last potential application lies possibly in detecting loss of anisotropy in tumors; a few studies suggest that DTI may be able to distinguish between high- and low-grade neoplasms (Gauvain et al. 2001). In summary, diffusion imaging has relatively limited application in pediatric brain tumor imaging at this time, but may be helpful in the future.

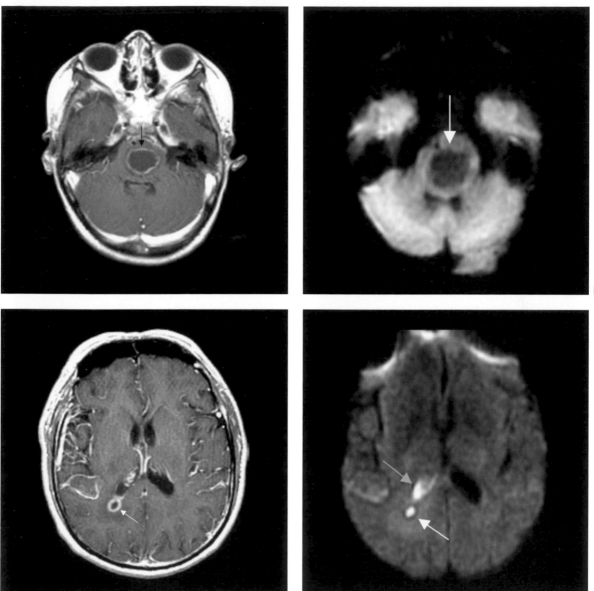

Figure 12.5 a–d

Diffusion-weighted images helping to distinguish abscess from necrotic glioma. **a** Axial T$_1$-weighted gadolinium-enhanced image showing a rim enhancing, centrally hypointense brainstem lesion (*black arrow*). **b** Axial diffusion-weighted image at the same level showing increased diffusion within the central portion of the lesion (*white arrow*) consistent with a necrotic glioma. **c** Different patient. Axial T$_1$-weighted gadolinium-enhanced image showing a deep right parietal ring-enhancing lesion (*white arrow*). **d** Axial diffusion-weighted image at the same level showing reduced diffusion within this lesion (*white arrow*) and adjacent ventricle (*gray arrow*) confirming that this was an abscess and not a neoplasm

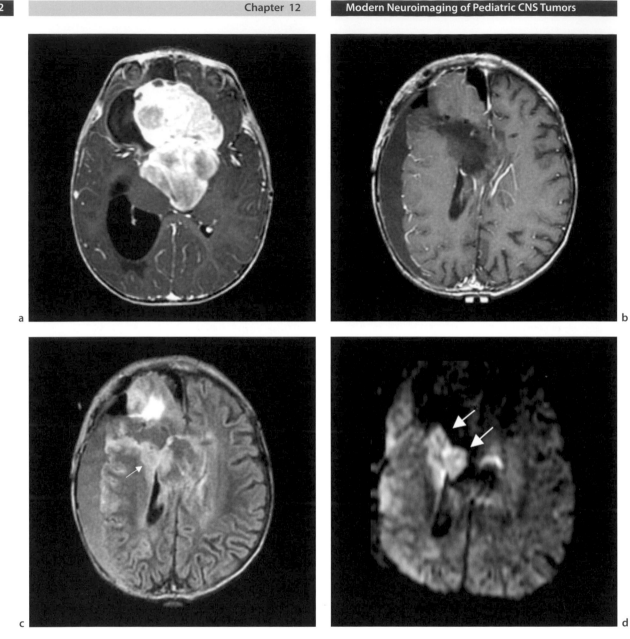

Figure 12.6 a–d

Large chiasmal/hypothalamic astrocytoma treated with partial surgical resection showing imaging evidence of postoperative ischemia. **a** Axial T_1-weighted gadolinium-enhanced image shows the enhancing tumor preoperatively. **b** Axial T_1-weighted gadolinium-enhanced image shows the postoperative resection cavity without evidence of residual enhancement. **c** Axial fluid attenuation inversion recovery (FLAIR) image of the resection cavity with thick posterolateral rim of high signal (*white arrow*) that may represent interstitial edema and/or injury. **d** Axial diffusion-weighted image at the same level shows high intensity (*arrows*), confirming that the area of increased signal on the FLAIR image was not edema, but postoperative ischemia

12.6 Magnetization Transfer

12.6.1 Principles

Magnetization transfer is a technique that allows imaging of molecules that interact with macromolecules in the brain (predominantly the components of myelin) separately from free, unbound water molecules. This technique gives us indirect information about the macromolecules that the water has interacted with. Although it is a useful technique in the assessment of patients with disorders of myelin, particularly multiple sclerosis, few applications to brain tumor imaging have been discovered.

12.6.2 Technique

Magnetization transfer images can be obtained by acquiring two sets of gradient echo scans with gradient spoilers. Data is best acquired using a repetition time of 300 ms, an echo time of 7 ms, a *theta* (flip angle) of 20°, a 3 mm partition thickness, a 12 cm field of view, and three-dimensional Fourier transform reconstruction techniques. A radio-frequency saturation band applied to the second set at 5 kHz off the resonance frequency of free water will saturate the pool of macromolecule-bound protons. Subtraction of the second data set from the first results in a magnetization transfer image. The amount of magnetization transfer in the different regions of the brain, which reflects the amount of water-binding macromolecules, can be calculated from region-of-interest measurements from those regions of brain [MTR = (Mo – Ms)/Mo, where MTR is the magnetization transfer ratio, M_o is the magnitude of signal without saturation by an off-frequency radio frequency pulse, and M_s is the magnitude of tissue signal with the saturation pulse on] (Graham and Henkelman 1997).

Alternatively, magnetization transfer images can be produced when the off-resonance RF pulse is applied during the imaging sequence. Application of this pulse negates the contribution of bound water protons to the overall MR image. As the binding of the macromolecules causes T1 shortening (by slowing the rotation and translation of the water molecules), the high signal of cerebral white matter is reduced on T1-weighted images.

12.6.3 Applications

The major application of MT imaging for brain tumors is to increase lesion conspicuity; by reducing the hyperintensity of white matter on T1-weighted images, enhancement becomes more conspicuous. The literature is mixed concerning the effect of MT imaging on lesion conspicuity after administration of low-dose gadolinium (Haba et al. 2001; Han et al. 1998; Knauth et al. 1996). It is generally accepted that lesion conspicuity after administration of a low gadolinium dose with MT is as good as high-dose imaging without MT in the evaluation of extra-axial neoplasms (Haba et al. 2001; Han et al. 1998). Only small series have been published to date. Higher sensitivity in defining the involvement of intra-axial neoplasms by MT, in comparison to routine MRI, has been proposed yet remains unproven (Grossman et al. 1994).

Other authors have explored the possibility that MT may distinguish cystic neoplasms from cystic infection. A potential role has been proposed in separating non-pyogenic abscesses (such as tuberculomas) from neoplasms (Gupta et al. 2001; Pui 2000). If proved in subsequent studies, this application would fill a void where MR spectroscopy is deficient. At present, bacterial abscesses are better evaluated by MR spectroscopy (Grand et al. 1999; Kim et al. 1997).

12.7 Improving Image Sensitivity with Surface Coils

Subtle or small neoplasms of the cortex (ganglioglioma, DNET), internal auditory canal (schwannoma in neurofibromatosis), and spinal cord (astrocytoma, ependymoma) can be missed on traditional MR sequences. There are primarily two methods to increase sensitivity to detect and characterize these neoplasms when they are small: higher resolution images obtained with a high-field-strength magnet (4+ Tesla) or by imaging with a routine-strength

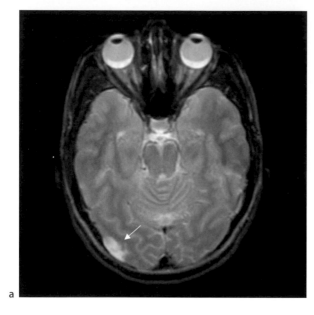

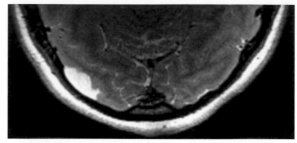

Figure 12.7 a,b

Surface coils utilized to prove that a presumed right oc-cipital arachnoid cyst was actually an intra-axial low-grade neoplasm (DNET). **a** Axial T_2-weighted image shows a hyperintense lesion (*white arrow*) on the sur-face of the right occipital lobe that is not clearly intra-axial. **b** T_2-weighted image obtained with surface coils shows the same lesion in better detail confirming that the lesion is an intra-axial mass

magnet and using special coils and software (Moyher et al. 1997). Use of phased-array surface coils and im-age-intensity correction algorithms can increase the signal-to-noise ratio for superficial lesions (Fig. 12.7). This technique may be helpful in the above cases (Grant et al. 1997, 1998).

12.8 Conclusion

Neuroradiologic evaluation of tumors has grown to include many more techniques than just anatomic imaging. Metabolic assessment, assessment of perfu-sion, and assessment of the function of surrounding brain can now be performed along with anatomic im-aging in a single visit to the MR suite. These tech-niques provide useful tools to assess the charac-teristics of pediatric brain tumors and their respons-es to therapy.

References

Alberstone CD, Skirboll SL, Benzel EC et al (2000) Mag-netic source imaging and brain surgery: presurgical and in-traoperative planning in 26 patients. J Neurosurg 92:1079–1090

Aronen HJ, Gazit IE, Louis DN et al (1994) Cerebral blood vol-ume maps of gliomas: comparison with tumor grade and histologic findings. Radiology 191:41–51

Ball WS Jr, Holland SK (2001) Perfusion imaging in the pediat-ric patient. MRI Clin North Am 9:207–216

Barker FG Jr, Chang SM, Valk PE et al (1997) 18-Fluorodeoxy-glucose uptake and survival of patients with suspected re-current malignant glioma. Cancer 79:115–26

Barker PB, Glickson JD, Bryan RN (1993) In vivo magnetic res-onance spectroscopy of human brain tumors. Top Magn Reson Imaging 5:32–45

Beisteiner R Gomiscek G, Erdler M et al (1995) Comparing lo-calization of conventional functional magnetic resonance imaging and magnetoencephalography. Eur J Neurosci 7:1121–1124

Birken DL, Oldendorf WH (1989) N-acetyl-L-aspartic acid: a literature review of a compound prominent in 1H-NMR spectroscopic studies of brain. Neurosci Biobehavioral Rev 13:23–31

Black KL, Emerick T, Hoh C et al (1994) Thallium-201 SPECT and positron emission tomography equal predictors of glioma grade and recurrence. Neurol Res 16:93–96

Boxerman JL, Bandettini PA, Kwong KK et al (1995) The intravascular contribution to fMRI signal change: Monte Carlo modeling and diffusion-weighted studies in vivo. Magn Reson Med 34:4–10

Breier JI, Simos PG, Zouridakis G et al (1999) Language dominance determined by magnetic source imaging: a comparison with the Wada procedure. Neurology 53:938–945

Brunelle F (2000) Noninvasive diagnosis of brain tumours in children. Childs Nerv Syst 16:731–734

Butzen J, Prost R, Chetty V et al (2000) Discrimination between neoplastic and nonneoplastic brain lesions by use of proton MR spectroscopy: the limits of accuracy with a logistic regression model. AJNR 21:1213–1219

Cappabianca P, Spaziante R, Caputi F et al (1991) Accuracy of the analysis of multiple small fragments of glial tumors obtained by stereotactic biopsy. Acta Cytol 35:505–511

Cedzich C, Taniguchi M, Schafer S et al (1996) Somatosensory evoked potential phase reversal and direct motor cortex stimulation during surgery in and around the central region. Neuroimage 4:201–209

Cha S, Lu S, Johnson G et al (2000a) Dynamic susceptibility contrast MR imaging: correlation of signal intensity changes with cerebral blood volume measurements. J Magn Reson Imaging 11:114–119

Cha S, Knopp EA, Johnson G et al (2000b) Dynamic contrast-enhanced T2-weighted MR imaging of recurrent malignant gliomas treated with thalidomide and carboplatin. AJNR 21:881–890

Cha S, Knopp EA, Johnson G et al (2002) Intracranial mass lesions: dynamic contrast-enhanced susceptibility-weighted echo-planar perfusion MR imaging. Radiology 223:11–29

Chan YL, Leung SF, King AD et al (1999Late radiation injury to the temporal lobes: morphologic evaluation at MR imaging. Radiology 213:800–807

Chandrasoma PT, Smith MM, Apuzzo ML (1989) Stereotactic biopsy in the diagnosis of brain masses: comparison of results of biopsy and resected surgical specimen. Neurosurgery 24:160–165

Chang KH, Song IC, Kim SH et al (1998) In vivo single-voxel proton MR spectroscopy in intracranial cystic masses. AJNR 19:401–405

Cheng LL, Chang IW, Louis DN et al (1998) Correlation of high-resolution magic angle spinning proton magnetic resonance spectroscopy with histopathology of intact human brain tumor specimens. Cancer Res 58:1825–1832

Choi JY, Kim SE, Shin HJ et al (2000) Brain tumor imaging with 99m Tc-tetrofosmin: comparison with 201Tl, 99mTc-MIBI, and 18F-fluorodeoxyglucose. J Neurooncol 46:63–70

Dadparvar S, Hussain R, Koffler SP et al (2000) The role of Tc-99m HMPAO functional brain imaging in detection of cerebral radionecrosis. Cancer 6:381–387

De Witte O, Lefranc F, Levivier M et al (2000) FDG-PET as a prognostic factor in high-grade astrocytoma. J Neurooncol 49:157–163

Dezortova M, Hajek M, Cap F et al (1999) Comparison of MR spectroscopy and MR imaging with contrast agent in children with cerebral astrocytomas. Childs Nerv Syst 15:408–412

Di Chiro G, Oldfield E, Wright DC et al (1988) Cerebral necrosis after radiotherapy and/or intraarterial chemotherapy for brain tumors: PET and neuropathologic studies. AJR 150:189–197

Dillon WP, Roberts T (1999) The limitations of functional MR imaging: a caveat. AJNR 20:536

Disbrow E, Roberts TP, Slutsky D et al (1999) The use of fMRI for determining the topographic organization of cortical fields in human and nonhuman primates. Brain Res 829:167–173

Dowling C, Bollen AW, Noworolski SM et al (2001) Preoperative proton MR spectroscopic imaging of brain tumors: correlation with histopathologic analysis of resection specimens. AJNR 22:604–612

Field AS, Yen YF, Burdette JH et al (2000) False cerebral activation on BOLD functional MR images: study of low-amplitude motion weakly correlated to stimulus. AJNR 21:1388–1396

Filippi M, Cercignani M, Inglese M et al (2001) Diffusion tensor magnetic resonance imaging in multiple sclerosis. Neurology 56:304–311

Ganslandt O, Fahlbusch R, Nimsky C et al (1999) Functional neuronavigation with magnetoencephalography: outcome in 50 patients with lesions around the motor cortex. J Neurosurg 91:73–79

Gauvain KM, McKinstry RC, Mukherjee P et al (2001) Evaluating pediatric brain tumor cellularity with diffusion-tensor imaging. AJR 177:449–454

Gerlowski LE, Jain RK (1986) Microvascular permeability of normal and neoplastic tissues. Microvascular Res 31:288–305

Giannini C, Scheithauer BW (1997) Classification and grading of low-grade astrocytic tumors in children. Brain Pathol 7:785–798

Girard N, Wang ZJ, Erbetta A et al (1998) Prognostic value of proton MR spectroscopy of cerebral hemisphere tumors in children. Neuroradiology 40:121–125

Go KG, Keuter EJ, Kamman RL et al (1994) Contribution of magnetic resonance spectroscopic imaging and L-[1–11C]tyrosine positron emission tomography to localization of cerebral gliomas for biopsy. Neurosurgery 34:994–1002

Graham SJ, Henkelman RM (1997) Understanding pulsed magnetization transfer. J Magn Reson Imaging 7:903–912

Grand S, Passaro G, Ziegler A et al (1999) Necrotic tumor versus brain abscess: importance of amino acids detected at 1H MR spectroscopy-initial results. Radiology 213:785–793

Grant PE, Barkovich AJ, Wald LL et al (1997) High-resolution surface-coil MR of cortical lesions in medically refractory epilepsy: a prospective study. AJNR 18:291–301

Grant PE, Vigneron DB, Barkovich AJ (1998) High-resolution imaging of the brain. Magn Reson Imaging Clin North Am 6:139–154

Greenwood J (1991) Mechanisms of blood-brain barrier breakdown. Neuroradiology 33:95–100

Grossman RI, Gomori JM, Ramer KN et al (1994) Magnetization transfer: theory and clinical applications in neuroradiology. Radiographics 14:279–290

Gupta RK, Vatsal DK, Husain N et al (2001) Differentiation of tuberculous from pyogenic brain abscesses with in vivo proton MR spectroscopy and magnetization transfer MR imaging. AJNR 22:1503–1509

Haba D, Pasco Papon A et al (2001) Use of half-dose gadolinium-enhanced MRI and magnetization transfer saturation in brain tumors. Eur Radiol 11:117–122

Han D, Chang KH, Han MH et al (1998) Half-dose gadolinium-enhanced MR imaging with magnetization transfer technique in brain tumors: comparison with conventional contrast-enhanced MR imaging. AJR 170:189–193

Holodny AI, Schulder M, Liu WC et al (1999) Decreased BOLD functional MR activation of the motor and sensory cortices adjacent to a glioblastoma multiforme: implications for image-guided neurosurgery. AJNR 20:609–612

Horska A, Ulug AM, Melhem ER et al (2001) Proton magnetic resonance spectroscopy of choroid plexus tumors in children. J Magn Reson Imaging 14:78–82

Hunter JV, Wang ZJ (2001) MR spectroscopy in pediatric neuroradiology. Magn Reson Imaging Clin North Am 9:165–189

Inglis BA, Neubauer D, Yang L et al (1999) Diffusion tensor MR imaging and comparative histology of glioma engrafted in the rat spinal cord. AJNR 20:713–716

Joyce P, Bentson J, Takahashi M et al (1978) The accuracy of predicting histologic grades of supratentorial astrocytomas on the basis of computerized tomography and cerebral angiography. Neuroradiology 16:346–348

Kamada K, Houkin K, Abe H et al (1997) Differentiation of cerebral radiation necrosis from tumor recurrence by proton magnetic resonance spectroscopy. Neurol Med Chir (Tokyo) 37:250–256

Kaplan AM, Bandy DJ, Manwaring KH et al (1999) Functional brain mapping using positron emission tomography scanning in preoperative neurosurgical planning for pediatric brain tumors. J Neurosurg 91:797–803

Kaplan WD, Takvorian T, Morris JH et al (1987) Thallium-201 brain tumor imaging: a comparative study with pathologic correlation. J Nucl Med 28:47–52

Keene DL, Hsu E, Ventureyra E (1999) Brain tumors in childhood and adolescence. Pediatr Neurol 20:198–203

Kim EE, Chung SK, Haynie TP et al (1992) Differentiation of residual or recurrent tumors from post-treatment changes with F-18 FDG PET. Radiographics 12:269–279

Kim SH, Chang KH, Song IC et al (1997) Brain abscess and brain tumor: discrimination with in vivo H-1 MR spectroscopy. Radiology 204:239–245

Kimura T, Sako K, Gotoh T et al (2001) In vivo single-voxel proton MR spectroscopy in brain lesions with ring-like enhancement. NMR Biomed 14:339–349

Kincaid PK, El-Saden SM, Park SH et al (1998) Cerebral gangliogliomas: preoperative grading using FDG-PET and 201 Tl-SPECT. AJNR 19:801–806

Kinoshita Y, Yokota A (1997) Absolute concentrations of metabolites in human brain tumors using in vitro proton magnetic resonance spectroscopy. NMR Biomed 10:2–12

Knauth M, Forsting M, Hartmann M et al (1996) MR enhancement of brain lesions: increased contrast dose compared with magnetization transfer. AJNR 17:1853–1859

Knopp EA, Cha S, Johnson G et al (1999) Glial neoplasms: dynamic contrast-enhanced T2*-weighted MR imaging. Radiology 211:791–798

Krouwer HG, Kim TA, Rand SD et al (1998) Single-voxel proton MR spectroscopy of nonneoplastic brain lesions suggestive of a neoplasm. AJNR 19:1695–1703

Kugel H, Heindel W, Ernestus RI et al (1992) Human brain tumors: spectral patterns detected with localized H-1 MR spectroscopy. Radiology 183:701–709

Law M, Cha S, Knopp EA et al (2002) High-grade gliomas and solitary metastases: differentiation by using perfusion and proton spectroscopic MR imaging. Radiology 222:715–721

Lazareff JA, Gupta RK, Alger J (1999) Variation of post-treatment H-MRSI choline signal intensity in pediatric gliomas. J Neurooncol 41:291–298

Lehnhardt FG, Rohn G, Ernestus RI et al (2001) 1H- and (31)P-MR spectroscopy of primary and recurrent human brain tumors in vitro: malignancy-characteristic profiles of water soluble and lipophilic spectral components. NMR Biomed 14:307–317

Lev MH, Grant PE (2000) MEG versus BOLD MR imaging: functional imaging, the next generation? AJNR 21:1369–1370

Lin A, Bluml S, Mamelak AN (1999) Efficacy of proton magnetic resonance spectroscopy in clinical decision making for patients with suspected malignant brain tumors. J Neurooncol 45:69–81

Lorberboym M, Mandell LR, Mosesson RE et al (1997) The role of thallium-201 uptake and retention in intracranial tumors after radiotherapy. J Nucl Med 38:223–226

Ludemann L, Hamm B, Zimmer C (2000) Pharmacokinetic analysis of glioma compartments with dynamic Gd-DTPA-enhanced magnetic resonance imaging. Magn Reson Imaging 18:1201–1204

Maeda M, Itoh S, Kimura H et al (1993) Tumor vascularity in the brain: evaluation with dynamic susceptibility-contrast MR imaging. Radiology 189:233–238

Maria BL, Drane WE, Quisling RG et al (1994) Value of thallium-201 SPECT imaging in childhood brain tumors. Pediatr Neurosurg 20:11–18

Maria BL, Drane WB, Quisling RJ et al (1997) Correlation between gadolinium diethylenetriamine-pentaacetic acid contrast enhancement and thallium-201 chloride uptake in pediatric brainstem glioma. J Child Neurol 12:341–348

Maria BL, Drane WE, Mastin ST et al (1998) Comparative value of thallium and glucose SPECT imaging in childhood brain tumors. Pediatr Neurol 19:351–357

Martin AJ, Liu H, Hall WA et al (2001) Preliminary assessment of turbo spectroscopic imaging for targeting in brain biopsy. AJNR 22:959–968

Martin E, Marcar VL (2001) Functional MR imaging in pediatrics. MRI Clin North Am 9:231–244

Massager N, David P, Goldman S et al (2000) Combined magnetic resonance imaging and positron emission tomography-guided stereotactic biopsy in brainstem mass lesions: diagnostic yield in a series of 30 patients. J Neurosurg 93:951–957

McKnight TR, Noworolski SM, Vigneron DB et al (2001) An automated technique for the quantitative assessment of 3D-MRSI data from patients with glioma. J Magn Reson Imaging 13:167–177

Melhem ER, Itoh R, Jones L et al (2000) Diffusion tensor MR imaging of the brain: effect of diffusion weighting on trace and anisotropy measurements. AJNR 21:1813–1820

Mitchell DG (1999) MRI principles. Saunders, Philadelphia, pp 199–203, 249–255

Moyher SE, Wald LL, Nelson SJ et al (1997) High resolution T2-weighted imaging of the human brain using surface coils and an analytical reception profile correction. J Magn Reson Imaging 7:512–517

Negendank WG, Sauter R, Brown TR et al (1996) Proton magnetic resonance spectroscopy in patients with glial tumors: a multicenter study. J Neurosurg 84:449–458

Nelson SJ, Nalbandian AB, Proctor E et al (1994) Registration of images from sequential MR studies of the brain. J Magn Reson Imaging 4:877–883

Nelson SJ, Huhn S, Vigneron DB et al (1997) Volume MRI and MRSI techniques for the quantitation of treatment response in brain tumors: presentation of a detailed case study. J Magn Reson Imaging 7:1146–1152

Nelson SJ, Vigneron DB, Star-Lack J et al (1997) High spatial resolution and speed in MRSI. NMR Biomed 10:411–422

Nelson SJ, Vigneron DB, Dillon WP (1999) Serial evaluation of patients with brain tumors using volume MRI and 3D 1H MRSI. NMR Biomed 12:123–138

Norfray JF, Tomita T, Byrd SE et al (1999) Clinical impact of MR spectroscopy when MR imaging is indeterminate for pediatric brain tumors. AJR 173:119–125

O'Tuama LA (1998) Childhood brain tumor: neuroimaging correlated with disease outcome. Pediatr Neurol 19:259–262

Ogawa T, Kanno I, Shishido F et al (1991) Clinical value of PET with 18F-fluorodeoxyglucose and L-methyl-11C-methionine for diagnosis of recurrent brain tumor and radiation injury. Acta Radiol 32:197–202

Otsubo H, Snead OC III (2001) Magnetoencephalography and magnetic source imaging in children. J Child Neurol 16:227–235

Ott D, Hennig J, Ernst T (1993) Human brain tumors: assessment with in vivo proton MR spectroscopy. Radiology 186:745–752

Papanicolaou AC, Simos PG, Breier JI et al (2001) Brain plasticity for sensory and linguistic functions: a functional imaging study using magnetoencephalography with children and young adults. J Child Neurol 16:241–252

Peters AM (1998) Fundamentals of tracer kinetics for radiologists. Br J Radiol 71:1116–1129

Pierpaoli C, Jezzard P, Basser PJ et al (1996) Diffusion tensor MR imaging of the human brain. Radiology 201:637–648

Plate KH, Mennel HD (1995) Vascular morphology and angiogenesis in glial tumors. Exp Toxicol Pathol 47:89–94

Poptani H, Gupta RK, Jain VK et al (1995) Characterization of intracranial mass lesions with in vivo proton MR spectroscopy. AJNR 16:1593–1603

Poupon C, Clark CA, Frouin V et al (2000) Regularization of diffusion-based direction maps for the tracking of brain white matter fascules. Neuroimage 12:184–195

Poussaint TY, Siffert J, Barnes PD et al (1995) Hemorrhagic vasculopathy after treatment of central nervous system neoplasia in childhood: diagnosis and follow-up. AJNR 16:693–699

Provenzale JM, Arata MA, Turkington TG, et al (1999) Gangliogliomas: characterization by registered positron emission tomography-MR images. AJR 172:1103–1107

Pui MH (2000) Magnetization transfer analysis of brain tumor, infection, and infarction. J Magn Reson Imaging 12:395–399

Pujol J, Conesa G, Deus J et al (1998) Clinical application of functional magnetic resonance imaging in presurgical identification of the central sulcus. J Neurosurg 88:863–869

Ricci PE, Karis JP, Heiserman JE et al (1998) Differentiating recurrent tumor from radiation necrosis: time for re-evaluation of positron emission tomography? AJNR 19:407–413

Roberts HC, Roberts TP, Brasch RC et al (2000) Quantitative measurement of microvascular permeability in human brain tumors achieved using dynamic contrast-enhanced MR imaging: correlation with histologic grade. AJNR 21:891–899

Roberts TP, Disbrow EA, Roberts HC et al (2000) Quantification and reproducibility of tracking cortical extent of activation by use of functional MR imaging and magnetoencephalography. AJNR 21:1377–1387

Roberts TP, Rowley HA (1997) Mapping of the sensorimotor cortex: functional MR and magnetic source imaging. AJNR 18:871–880

Rosen BR, Belliveau JW, Aronen HJ et al (1991) Susceptibility contrast imaging of cerebral blood volume: human experience. Magn Reson Med 22:293–299

Rosen BR, Belliveau JW, Vevea JM et al (1990) Perfusion imaging with NMR contrast agents. Magn Reson Med 14:249–265

Salibi N, Brown MA (1998) Clinical MR spectroscopy, first principles. Wiley-Liss, New York

Shimizu H, Kumabe T, Tominaga T et al (1996) Noninvasive evaluation of malignancy of brain tumors with proton MR spectroscopy. AJNR 17:737–747

Shino A, Nakasu S, Matsuda M et al (1999) Noninvasive evaluation of the malignant potential of intracranial meningiomas performed using proton magnetic resonance spectroscopy. J Neurosurg 91:928–934

Shinoura N, Nishijima M, Hara T et al (1997) Brain tumors: detection with C-11 choline PET. Radiology 202:497–503

Shtern F (1992) Clinical experimentation in magnetic resonance spectroscopy: a perspective from the national cancer institute. NMR Biomed 5:325–328

Shukla-Dave A, Gupta RK, Roy R et al (2001) Prospective evaluation of in vivo proton MR spectroscopy in differentiation of similar appearing intracranial cystic lesions. Magn Reson Imaging 19:103–110

Siegal T, Rubinstein R, Tzuk-Shina T et al (1997) Utility of relative cerebral blood volume mapping derived from perfusion magnetic resonance imaging in the routine follow up of brain tumors. J Neurosurg 86:22–27

Sijens PE, Vecht CJ, Levendag PC et al (1995) Hydrogen magnetic resonance spectroscopy follow-up after radiation therapy of human brain cancer. Invest Radiol 30:738–744

Simos PG, Papanicolaou AC, Breier JI et al (1999) Localization of language-specific cortex by using magnetic source imaging and electrical stimulation mapping. J Neurosurg 91: 787–796

Stippich C, Freitag P, Kassubek J et al (1998) Motor, somatosensory and auditory cortex localization by fMRI and MEG. Neuroreport 9:1953–1957

Strong JA, Hatten HP Jr, Brown MT et al (1993) Pilocytic astrocytoma: correlation between the initial imaging features and clinical aggressiveness. AJR 161:369–372

Sugahara T, Korogi Y, Kochi M et al (1998) Correlation of MR imaging-determined cerebral blood volume maps with histologic and angiographic determination of vascularity of gliomas. AJR 171:1479–1486

Sugahara T, Korogi Y, Shigematsu Y et al (1999) Value of dynamic susceptibility contrast magnetic resonance imaging in the evaluation of intracranial tumors. Top Magn Reson Imaging 10:114–124

Sugahara T, Korogi Y, Tomiguchi S et al (2000) Posttherapeutic intraaxial brain tumor: the value of perfusion-sensitive contrast-enhanced MR imaging for differentiating tumor recurrence from nonneoplastic contrast-enhancing tissue. AJNR 21:901–909

Sugahara T, Korogi Y, Kochi M et al (2001) Perfusion-sensitive MR imaging of gliomas: comparison between gradient-echo and spin-echo echo-planar imaging techniques. AJNR 22:1306–1315

Sutton LN, Wang Z, Gusnard D et al (1992) Proton magnetic resonance spectroscopy of pediatric brain tumors. Neurosurgery 31:195–202

Suzuki A, Yasui N (1992) Intraoperative localization of the central sulcus by cortical somatosensory evoked potentials in brain tumor. Case report. J Neurosurg 76:867–870

Szigety SK, Allen PS, Huyser-Wierenga D et al (1993) The effect of radiation on normal human CNS as detected by NMR spectroscopy. Int J Radiat Oncol Biol Phys 25:695–701

Szymanski MD, Perry DW, Gage NM et al (2001) Magnetic source imaging of late evoked field responses to vowels: toward an assessment of hemispheric dominance for language. J Neurosurg 94:445–453

Tanner SF, Ramenghi LA, Ridgway JP et al (2000) Quantitative comparison of intrabrain diffusion in adults and preterm and term neonates and infants. AJR 174:1643–1649

Taylor JS, Langston JW, Reddick WE et al (1996) Clinical value of proton magnetic resonance spectroscopy for differentiating recurrent or residual brain tumor form delayed cerebral necrosis. Int J Radiat Oncol Biol Phys 36:1251–1261

Tomoi M, Kimura H, Yoshida M et al (1997) Alterations of lactate(+lipid) concentration in brain tumors with in vivo hydrogen magnetic resonance spectroscopy during radiotherapy. Invest Radiol 32:288–296

Tzika AA, Vigneron DB, Dunn RS et al (1996) Intracranial tumors in children: small single-voxel proton MR spectroscopy using short- and long-echo sequences. Neuroradiology 38:254–263

Tzika AA, Vajapeyam S, Barnes PD (1997) Multivoxel proton MR spectroscopy and hemodynamic MR imaging of childhood brain tumors: preliminary observations. AJNR 18: 203–218

Tzika AA, Zurakowski D, Poussaint TY et al (2001) Proton magnetic spectroscopic imaging of the child's brain: the response of tumors to treatment. Neuroradiology 43:169–177

Tzika AA, Zarifi MK, Goumnerova L et al (2002) Neuroimaging in pediatric brain tumors: Gd-DTPA-enhanced, hemodynamic, and diffusion MR imaging compared with MR spectroscopic imaging. AJNR 23:322–333

Urenjak J, Williams SR, Gadian DG et al (1993) Proton nuclear magnetic resonance spectroscopy unambiguously identifies different neural cell types. J Neurosc 13:981–989

Usenius T, Usenius JP, Tenhunen M et al (1995) Radiation-induced changes in human brain metabolites as studied by 1H nuclear magnetic resonance spectroscopy in vivo. Int J Radiat Oncol Biol Phys 33:719–724

Valk PE, Dillon WP (1991) Radiation injury of the brain. AJNR 12:45–62

Valk PE, Budinger TF, Levin VA et al (1988) PET of malignant cerebral tumors after interstitial brachytherapy. Demonstration of metabolic activity and correlation with clinical outcome. J Neurosurg 69:830–838

Venkatesh SK, Gupta RK, Pal L et al (2001) Spectroscopic increase in choline signal is a nonspecific marker for differentiation of infective/inflammatory from neoplastic lesions of the brain. J Magn Reson Imaging 14:8–15

Vezina LG (1997) Diagnostic imaging in neuro-oncology. Pediatr Clin North Am 44:701–719

Vigneron D, Bollen A, McDermott M et al (2001) Three-dimensional magnetic resonance spectroscopic imaging of histologically confirmed brain tumors. Magn Reson Imaging 19:89–101

Waldrop SM, Davis PC, Padgett CA et al (1998) Treatment of brain tumors in children is associated with abnormal MR spectroscopic ratios in brain tissue remote from the tumor site. AJNR 19:963–970

Wang GJ, Volkow ND, Lau YH et al (1996) Glucose metabolic changes in nontumoral brain tissue of patients with brain tumor following radiotherapy: a preliminary study. JCAT 20:709–714

Wang Z, Sutton LN, Cnaan A et al (1995) Proton MR spectroscopy of pediatric cerebellar tumors. AJNR 16:1821–1833

Wang Z, Zimmerman RA, Sauter R (1996) Proton MR spectroscopy of the brain: clinically useful information obtained in assessing CNS diseases in children. AJR 167:191–199

Weisskoff RM, Zuo CS, Boxerman JL et al (1994) Microscopic susceptibility variation and transverse relaxation: theory and experiment. Magn Reson Med 31:601–610

Wilken B, Dechent P, Herms J et al (2000) Quantitative proton magnetic resonance spectroscopy of focal brain lesions. Pediatr Neurol 23:22–31

Yeung DK, Chan Y, Leung S et al (2001) Detection of an intense resonance at 2.4 ppm in 1H MR spectra of patients with severe late-delayed, radiation-induced brain injuries. Magn Reson Med 45:994–1000

Yousem DM, Lenkinski RE, Evans S et al (1992) Proton MR spectroscopy of experimental radiation-induced white matter injury. JCAT 16:543–548

Chapter 13

Current Surgical Management

N. Gupta · V. Perry · M. S. Berger

13.1 Introduction

For the majority of brain tumors in children, the extent of resection is the most important factor predicting long-term outcome. This conclusion has led many neurosurgeons to be as aggressive as possible during the initial surgical procedure in an effort to achieve gross total resection (GTR; Pollack 1999; Albright et al. 2000). It should be recognized that GTR is not the primary goal for tumors where sensitivity to adjuvant therapy is high (e.g., germinoma), or where there is clear extension into eloquent regions (e.g., brainstem and thalamic glioma). Fortunately, these latter groups represent a minority of pediatric brain tumors (Pollack 1994).

The majority of pediatric tumors are primary glial neoplasms arising within the cerebellar or cerebral hemispheres. Factors affecting extent of resection are: relation to functionally important structures, degree of infiltration, and presence or absence of tumor dissemination at time of presentation. Although the portions of infiltrative supratentorial tumors that extend into eloquent locations (primary motor, speech cortex, basal ganglia, or major white matter tracts such as the internal capsule) are likely to defy GTR, an argument can be made for extending resection sufficiently to allow a change to occur in the natural history of the disease (Keles et al. 2001). Previously, the definition of eloquent cortex relied mainly on variable anatomical maps, and resective procedures were limited by the inability to predict functional anatomy in specific patients. In the posterior fossa, GTR is limited either by involvement of the brainstem or the cranial nerves. Monitoring of virtually all cranial nerves is now possible, which greatly facilitates safe dissection of the tumor from normal structures. Infiltration into the brainstem by malignant tumors is not amenable to surgical resection.

Progress in various technologies has allowed maps to be created for individual patients that define the actual boundaries of eloquent cortex. These advances consist of neuronavigation coupled with high-resolution imaging modalities, non-invasive functional imaging, and adaptation of brain and spinal cord mapping techniques to the pediatric population.

13.2 Technical Adjuncts for Resection of Brain Tumors

13.2.1 Neuronavigation

Conventional magnetic resonance imaging (MRI) provides the necessary detail to assess the anatomical relationships of most intracranial tumors. Several manufacturers supply systems that use a preoperative MRI scan as the basis for an intraoperative three-dimensional guidance system. In their various configurations, these are all considered neuronavigation systems. A standard MRI may be complemented by techniques (see Chapter 12) such as MR spectroscopy, magnetic source imaging (MSI), high resolution sequences, and other modalities such as conventional angiography if necessary. These special sequences can also be incorporated into the standard MRI for intraoperative use.

Neuronavigation has impacted brain tumor surgery in three major ways. First, surgical routes can be simulated and planned preoperatively allowing maximum accuracy of craniotomy placements and cortical incisions. Mistakes in trajectory and depth during tumor resection are prevented. Second, the shortest and safest route through brain tissue that will avoid important neural and vascular structures can be determined well before the procedure. This reduces the risk of postoperative neurologic deficits, and improves assessment of risk preoperatively. Third, the use of neuronavigation improves the extent of tumor resection through providing "feedback" to augment the surgeon's perception of anatomical placement. Despite all of these advantages, the major limitation

of preoperative registered imaging data is obvious: intraoperative shifts of tissue cannot update a static set of data obtained prior to tumor resection.

The original intraoperative navigation systems used metal stereotactic frames rigidly attached to the calvarium. These are referred to as "frame-based" stereotactic devices. Target guidance relied upon anatomical coordinates as defined in anatomical atlases. Coordinates and targets could be refined modestly by imaging studies such as plain films and air ventriculograms. The inherent inaccuracy of this system is obvious in that patient-specific data is not used to guide the actual procedure. A critical advance occurred when CT or MRI scans were used in conjunction with frame-based systems (e.g., Leksell, BRW, CRW) to select targets and mathematically compute trajectories. These systems use guidance arcs that move directly over the surgical field and obstruct the surgeon if a large craniotomy is to be performed. These systems are, however, highly accurate and continue to be used widely in situations where target selection is critical such as Gamma Knife radiosurgery and functional procedures such as pallidotomy (both of which utilize refinements of the Leksell frame, Elekta AB, Stockholm, Sweden).

A major innovation occurred when advances in technology allowed sufficient computational power to allow manipulation and calculation of three dimensional image sets. This led to the creation of systems known as "frameless stereotaxy" that recreated a three dimensional volume space by using fiducials placed on the patient's head and registered to a preoperative imaging study. This allows "real time" intraoperative guidance and the ability to visualize the target in multiple planes (Fig. 13.1). A variety of tools, including surgical instruments, can also be registered and used as pointers that provide continuous updated information on a computer monitor as the tumor resection is performed. In children, the requirement for a preoperative MRI scan can limit the use of neuronavigation if general anesthesia is required for the imaging study. Nonetheless, many centers routinely use neuronavigation in all pediatric brain tumor cases.

The limitations of the technology for pediatric cases derive from the difficulty of obtaining preoperative MRI scans and maintaining constancy of fidu-

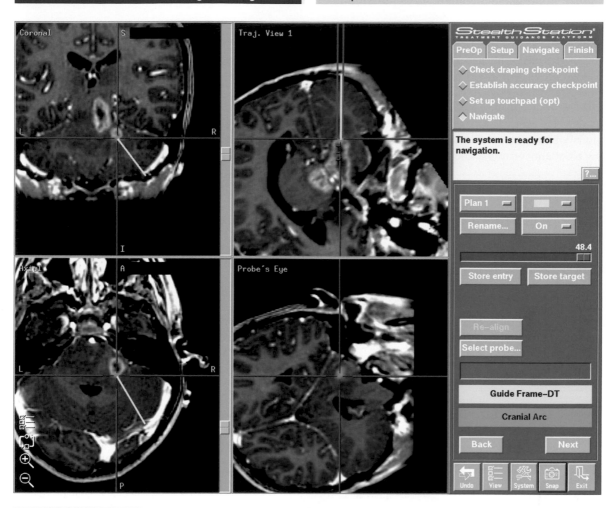

Figure 13.1

A screen capture image from a brainstem biopsy procedure. The biopsy trajectory is shown in three planes and the tip of the biopsy needle can be tracked in real time as it enters the brain ("Probes Eye" view, bottom right). StealthStation is a trademark of Medtronic Inc., Minneapolis, MN, USA

cial position. These obstacles have been largely surmounted by scheduling studies immediately prior to surgery, or in certain cases obtaining neuronavigation studies with the patient under general anesthesia and then moving the patient directly to the operating theatre for the procedure. More advanced technology has been put into practice at Brigham and Women's Hospital in Boston that allows imaging registration based upon surface anatomy (Gleason et al. 1994).

Intraoperative MRI (iMR), the next step in image-directed surgery, allows continual updating of preoperative image sets and adjustment of navigational parameters. Some reports indicate that the use of intraoperative imaging improves the extent of resection, although it is unclear whether such use results in improved outcomes (Fahlbusch et al. 2000; Schneider et al. 2001). This technique has been used to augment posterior fossa procedures (Lam et al. 2001). Currently, this technology remains labor and technology intensive and is not widely available. An intermediate step is the use of intraoperative ultrasound-assisted navigation as a means to update imaging data (Regelsberger et al. 2000). Integration with functional information (see below) will ultimately allow intraoperative "guideposts" for the surgeon, delineating regions amenable to resection and regions representing eloquent cortex or functional tracts.

13.2.2 Functional Imaging

Several imaging technologies have been adapted to create functional maps of the brain: functional MRI (fMRI), positron emission tomography (PET), and magnetoencephalography (MEG). Differences that occur in blood flow between active and inactive cortical areas are exploited by fMRI. These differences are magnified by instructing the patient to perform repetitive tasks – which may be as simple as repeatedly moving the fingers. Local increases in blood flow are then detected by specific MRI sequences. Patient cooperation is of course required. Diffusion tensor imaging (DTI) exploits the differences in the diffusion of water molecules depending upon the local environment of those molecules (e.g., water molecules within axons vs. those in the interstitial space). This information can then be extracted to create maps demonstrating the location and direction of white matter pathways. Some of these techniques are discussed in greater detail in Chapter 12.

Preoperative use of PET was originally presented by LeBlanc and Meyer (Leblanc and Meyer 1990; Leblanc et al. 1992). PET relies upon metabolic differences within active cortex to isolate functional areas. More recently, a variety of radiolabeled compounds such as $[^{18}F]$ fluorodeoxyglucose (FDG), $[^{11}C]$ L-methionine, and $[^{15}O]$ H_2O were used by Kaplan et al., to create functional maps prior to brain tumor resection in a pediatric population (Kaplan et al. 1999). Coregistering $[^{15}O]$ H_2O PET images with MRI allowed accurate determination of eloquent cortex prior to tumor resection.

Magnetoencephalography (MEG) relies on the ability to detect single dipole magnetic fields created by the pooled activity of groups of neurons to define potential areas of seizure activity (Chuang et al. 1995; Otsubo et al. 2001). Further refinement of these techniques, known as magnetic source imaging (MSI), al-

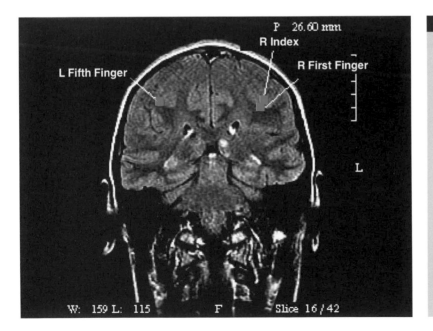

Figure 13.2

Magnetic source imaging (MSI) of a 15-year-old boy with an infiltrative anterior insular mass (not visible in this image). *Green squares* demonstrate sensory cortex representing left fifth finger, right index finger, and right first finger. These functional maps were integrated into the neuronavigation system prior to tumor resection

lows identification of functional areas of cortex and deep brain regions (Fig. 13.2). This information is especially valuable when correlated with tumor localization (Schiffbauer et al. 2001). Delineation of entire functional pathways using a combination of techniques may be possible in the near future.

13.2.3 Cortical Mapping for Supratentorial Tumors

The gold standard for functional mapping of the human brain remains direct electrical stimulation of the cortex and observation of its effect upon patient-directed actions during open craniotomy (Berger and Ojemann 1992). Although pioneered in the early part of the 20th century at the Montreal Neurological Institute, continual refinements are improving the sensitivity and accuracy of these techniques. For the most part, the vast majority of mapping cases are restricted to either motor or speech mapping. The major limitations of cortical mapping in children are the relative immaturity of the central nervous system in very young children, and the inability of children to cooperate in the execution of repetitive language tasks during speech-mapping procedures.

Motor mapping as described by Penfield remains the most robust electrical technique that can be practiced in the operating room (Penfield and Boldrey 1937). Patients remain under general anesthesia and direct systematic electrical stimulation of the precentral area permits the accurate mapping of primary motor cortex. Areas of cortex responsible for specific muscle groups (e.g., face, arm, hand, leg) can be reliably identified. A bipolar electrode with 5 mm spacing is used to deliver stimuli at 60 Hz with a duration of 1 ms (biphasic square wave pulse). In children less than five years of age, the cortex is generally less excitable by direct stimulation and motor cortex may not be clearly identified. An alternative method to detect the location of the central sulcus is by detecting a phase-reversal potential as one records over the motor and sensory cortex. Using subdural grids, mainly for the treatment of patients with epilepsy, Chitoku et al. were able to define the motor cortex in all children studied, using a variety of stimula-

tion thresholds (Chitoku et al. 2001). Younger children responded to stimuli in the vicinity of 8 to 12 mA while older children responded to stimuli in the range of 4 to 6 mA.

For language mapping, a basic surgical decision point is whether a child can tolerate an "awake craniotomy" (usually above 10 to 12 years of age). Language mapping is entirely dependent upon patient cooperation and, therefore, is the most difficult technique to accomplish in young children. During awake craniotomy, a handheld stimulator is used to directly inactivate the cortex while the patient names objects presented visually. Stimulation of Broca's area, which is usually adjacent to the primary motor cortex, usually leads to speech arrest although significant variability exists between individuals of different ages (Haglund et al. 1994; Ojemann et al. 2003).

In children unable to tolerate an awake craniotomy and for whom functional localization is crucial to the success of the procedure, placement of subdural grids will permit bedside cortical mapping. This requires two procedures for the patient, a substantial degree of patient cooperation, and close communication between child neurologists, psychologists, and nursing staff. Generally, this technique can be done in children above the age of four years, although it is most reliable in older children. The first procedure involves a craniotomy encompassing the area of resection and placement of an implantable subdural grid containing multiple electrical contacts. The contacts on the grid are then stimulated sequentially while the patient is led through specific language tasks such as naming, counting, and repeating. As with awake craniotomy, speech arrest during stimulation is the clue for identifying active cortex. Language paradigms have to be tailored to the age of the patient and level of comprehension. The procedure is time-consuming and laborious, often requiring sessions over two or three days. In the patient shown in Fig. 13.3, an infiltrative tumor was noted in the left fronto-parietal region. Although the patient was but five years old, he tolerated placement of subdural grids for several days and bedside mapping revealed the locations of the language and motor cortex allowing an extensive resection of the tumor.

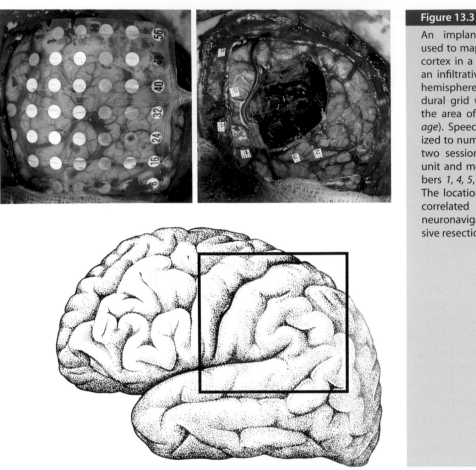

Figure 13.3

An implanted subdural grid used to map speech and motor cortex in a 5-year-old boy with an infiltrative tumor of the left hemisphere. A 64-contact subdural grid was implanted over the area of the tumor (*left image*). Speech cortex was localized to numbers *2* and *3* during two sessions in the telemetry unit and motor cortex to numbers *1, 4, 5,* and *6* (*right image*). The location of the tumor was correlated with intraoperative neuronavigation and an extensive resection was performed

13.2.4 Mapping of Seizure Foci

If seizures are particularly intractable or appear to be the dominant symptom associated with a brain tumor, the actual ictal focus may need to be identified. For epilepsy associated with a definite lesion, resection of the lesion will result in seizure control in the majority of cases (Mosewich et al. 2000). In some cases, the presence of a tumor is only detected after pathologic examination of the resected tissue. In one series, approximately 25 % of temporal lobe resections revealed a neoplasm, the majority of which were dysembryoblastic neuroepithelial tumors (DNET, see Chapter 8.2) (Hennessy et al. 2001).

Scalp electroencephalography is an essential first step in localization of seizure foci. This may be complemented by magnetoencephalography (MEG) or invasive monitoring with subdural grids and strip electrodes. Insertion of a subdural grid electrode array will provide ictal and interictal information. Strip electrodes are used for recordings from mesiobasal structures. In addition, recording along the hippocampus can be performed following the removal of lateral temporal cortex and entry into the temporal horn of the lateral ventricle. Strip electrodes may also be utilized for the orbitofrontal cortex or under the bone flap if the cortical exposure is not adequate. The recording may either be done for short time periods intraoperatively (5 to 20 min) prior to resection, or for prolonged periods postoperatively on the ward in specialized monitoring units. Intravenous infusion of methohexital (Brevital 0.5 to 1 mg/kg) may be used to chemically induce ictal discharges if epileptiform activity is sparse. Following tumor removal, post-resection electrocorticography is always performed in patients with identifiable pre-resection seizure foci. Infrequent spike activity is not pursued, especially when it involves functional cortex. Resected seizure foci are identified with respect to their geographic orientation to the tumor nidus and should be submitted separately for histopathological analysis.

13.3 Posterior Fossa Tumors

13.3.1 Surgical Principles

Posterior fossa tumors are among the most commonly encountered tumors in children and are located in the midline within the vermis, cerebellar hemisphere, and/or brainstem. Standard approaches to the posterior fossa are well developed and are described in various sources in the literature (Albright et al. 2001). Surgical planning is often modified by the pathology of the tumor. The three main pathological types that occur in this location are astrocytoma, medulloblastoma, and ependymoma. Medulloblastomas are characteristically midline tumors occupying the vermis and in some cases extending into the cerebellar hemisphere. Ependymomas of the posterior fossa can extend into the fourth ventricle and also may extend into the cerebellopontine angle closely associated with the cranial nerves. Both ependymoma and medulloblastoma can invade the brainstem.

For midline tumors, the standard approach is to position patients prone with the head flexed forward. A vertical incision allows access to most of the posterior fossa. If the tumor extends anterior to the cerebellum or brainstem, the tumor must be approached from a more lateral position; often with the head turned to allow a posterolateral trajectory. In the past, most surgeons would remove the overlying bone without replacement (craniectomy) although the current trend is to replace the bone flap at the conclusion of the procedure (craniotomy). There is some evidence that this reduces the risk of CSF leakage and pseudomeningocele formation (Gnanalingham et al. 2002). Dural opening is followed by definition of the boundary between the tumor and the normal cerebellum. The character of the interface between tumor and brain can vary across tumor types. In general, the interface is better defined with ependymomas as compared to medulloblastomas. Cerebellar astrocytomas have a clear margin between the tumor and the adjacent brain. The large size of most pediatric tumors and the need to avoid unnecessary brain retraction results in many tumors being resected piecemeal using either standard tools (cautery and suction) or ultrasonic aspirators that use a rapidly vibrating metal tip to disintegrate tissues. Removal of the central portion of the tumor then allows reflection of the deeper tumor tissue into the operative field and subsequent removal. For deep tumors, and those related to important structures, the use of frameless stereotaxy (neuronavigation) has revolutionized intra-operative guidance and structure localization (see Section 13.2.1).

Finally, additional safety can be obtained by monitoring various cranial nerves such as the facial nerve, oculomotor nerve, and hypoglossal nerves (Grabb et al. 1997; Sekiya et al. 2000). Tumors either infiltrating the floor of the fourth ventricle or along the anterior portion of the brainstem will involve cranial nerves. These nerves are sensitive to manipulation and can be difficult to identify when tumors surround them. Gradual dissection through tumor tissue requires careful identification of important structures.

13.3.2 Complications

Postoperative complications are discussed in greater detail in Chapter 2 (Section 2.9) in the context of cerebellar astrocytoma but can occur following any posterior fossa procedure. Some of these are briefly reviewed below.

13.3.2.1 Injury to Local Structures

Symptoms include long-tract signs of weakness and sensory loss, mutism, and cranial neuropathies (Cochrane et al. 1994). Ataxia and dysmetria are usually due to retraction injury or swelling of the cerebellum and improve after several weeks to months. Injury to the vermis can cause disabling truncal ataxia which may improve but can be permanent, particularly if large areas of the vermis have been involved. Impaired initiation of chewing, voiding, and eye opening may present after injury to areas of the cerebellum responsible for repetitive motor-movement memory. Approximately one-half of those with new deficits experience complete recovery of function (Pollack et al. 1995; Ersahin 1998).

13.3.2.2 Cerebellar Mutism

Injury to midline structures of the cerebellum can lead to mutism. Symptoms develop postoperatively and can worsen over a few days. Patients are unable to initiate speech without impairment of consciousness. Usually, there are no detectable cranial nerve deficits. The common pattern is for patients to have some preservation of speech function in the immediate postoperative period, with mutism developing within 24 to 94 hours (Pollack et al. 1995). The reported incidence is 8.5 % for all posterior fossa tumors and 12 % for vermian tumors (Catsman-Berrevoets et al. 1999). The incidence of mutism is higher in patients with malignant tumors (20 %) as compared to less invasive tumors (1 %; Ersahin et al. 1996; Doxey et al. 1999).

Recovery from complete mutism begins with profoundly dysarthric and abnormal speech, usually with isolated words and phrases, progressively improving to full sentences. The duration of recovery is variable, ranging from 2 weeks after onset of symptoms to several months. The average duration of mutism is 6 weeks (Aguiar et al. 1995; Pollack et al. 1995; Ersahin et al. 1996). Up to 20 % of patients may have permanent dysarthria following recovery from mutism.

13.3.2.3 Hydrocephalus

Hydrocephalus is the result of a mismatch between CSF production and absorption leading to an accumulation of CSF, with characteristic symptoms and ventricular enlargement. In the setting of a posterior fossa tumor, hydrocephalus is defined as "obstructive" because the ventricular CSF pathways are blocked by a mass lesion. Children can have hydrocephalus at presentation, or it can develop acutely in the postoperative period, usually in the setting of cerebellar swelling or a hematoma accumulating in the resection cavity. Acute symptomatic hydrocephalus, either pre- or postoperative, should be treated by immediate placement of an external ventricular drain. In most patients, complete removal of the mass lesion will result in resolution of the hydrocephalus. Most surgeons will attempt to "wean" a patient from the external drain following tumor resection. Following GTR, this is usually successful, although the need for placement of a permanent CSF shunt is increased in younger children (<3 years of age; Kumar et al. 1996).

Hydrocephalus can occur in a subacute manner following tumor resection even when GTR is achieved. These patients will usually have "communicating" hydrocephalus with enlargement of the entire ventricular system. This term is probably a misnomer since the presumed site of obstruction is the arachnoid villi where CSF is normally absorbed back into the venous system. The presumed etiology of this type of hydrocephalus is from localized inflammation secondary to subarachnoid blood or high CSF protein leading to loss of function of the arachnoid villi. Children should be observed carefully in the first few weeks following tumor resection for symptoms suggestive of hydrocephalus.

Asymptomatic ventricular enlargement resulting from a temporary alteration of CSF dynamics requires no immediate intervention, and the patient can be followed by clinical examination and serial CT scans. Placement of a shunt is indicated if symptoms develop, a persistent pseudomeningocele is present, and/or CSF leak occurs from the wound. The rate of CSF shunting following posterior fossa surgery ranges from 10 to 26 % of patients (Imielinski et al. 1998; Steinbok and Mutat 1999) to as high as 42 % (Gjerris et al. 1998). In the latter study, of 497 patients with a posterior fossa tumor, 68 (14%) were shunted prior to tumor resection, 94 (19%) after tumor resection, and 43 (9%) were treated by placement of shunt alone. Endoscopic third ventriculostomy, or fenestration of the floor of the third ventricle to bypass the posterior fossa obstruction, is another alternative to placement of a permanent shunt. One report suggests that this reduces the overall rate of shunt placement in patients with posterior fossa tumors (Sainte-Rose et al. 2001). The risk of extra-neural metastasis from shunting in children with cerebellar astrocytomas is virtually nonexistent (Berger et al. 1991).

13.3.3 Cognitive Consequences

Cerebellar lesions or injury result mainly in deficits of motor control and coordination. It is becoming clear, however, that in addition to these deficits, alterations in higher cognitive function and affect also occur. Neuropsychological changes at 2-year follow-up in a cohort of patients having had posterior fossa surgery included visual–spatial dysfunction in 37%, expressive language problems in 37%, verbal memory decline in 33%, and difficulty with affect control in 15 to 56% (Levisohn et al. 2000). These neuropsychological consequences appear to be temporary, but long-term studies are lacking. School performance and IQ are also affected by cerebellar surgery, but studies are confounded by the inability to separate the emotional and psychological effects of childhood illness and stress from the surgical procedure. The majority of patients (~60%) with benign or more indolent tumors such as cerebellar astrocytoma or histologically benign ependymoma will have normal IQ after surgery. This is in contrast to patients with medulloblastoma of whom only 10% will have IQ >90 after treatment (Hoppe-Hirsch et al. 1995).

13.4 The Role of Second Look Surgery

"Second-look" surgery refers to a planned second procedure to resect residual tumor prior to observation of radiographic progression. It may also be applied to situations where tissue is obtained for pathological diagnosis in patients previously treated by adjuvant therapy. The primary procedure may have been either a biopsy or an attempt at debulking. The general utility of performing second procedures remains unclear and few reports directly refer to its use for brain tumors. It may lead to improved rates of GTR for a subset of patients (Khan et al. 2001), but it has not been formally examined in a randomized clinical trial. Second-look surgery must be distinguished from procedures to remove "residual" disease, which can be defined as macroscopically visible tumor remaining after what was believed to be a GTR. In clear instances of residual disease remaining after the primary resection, the patient should be returned to the operating room for removal of the residual tumor.

Residual disease may be expected if GTR would lead to unacceptable morbidity. This is usually in the context of infiltration of eloquent areas and unresectable tissues (brainstem, cranial nerves, and vascular invasion). Interval adjuvant therapy may reduce the size of the tumor or vascularity, or may define the tumor/brain interface, ultimately facilitating the second surgical procedure (Foreman et al. 1997). A second procedure following chemotherapy has been advocated most forcefully in the treatment of intracranial germ cell tumors. Most of these tumors arise in the pineal region closely approximated to the deep cerebral veins and the brainstem. Subtotal resection is common and adjunctive therapy is frequently used. Excluding pure germinomas, which are sensitive to either radiation or chemotherapy, malignant nongerminomatous germ cell tumors (NGGCT) pose particularly difficult management problems. Most authors recommend tissue biopsy for marker-negative tumors with pathologic diagnosis guiding further treatment. Based upon favorable responses to chemotherapy, Weiner and Finlay (1999) advocate second-look surgery for any residual mass remaining after aggressive chemotherapy treatment. In another analysis of malignant germ cell tumors, neoadjuvant therapy followed by surgical resection for residual disease revealed that the majority had mature teratomas (Friedman et al. 2001). Outcomes following surgery were good in five of the six patients operated upon.

13.5 Conclusion

For most supra- and infratentorial brain tumors, gross total resection is associated with improved outcome. Cortical mapping, neuronavigation, and functional imaging can and should be utilized in children to increase the chances of a complete resection. Staged and second-look surgery may also facilitate the resection of unresectable tumors in conjunction with adjuvant therapy.

References

Aguiar PH, Plese JP, Ciquini O et al (1995) Transient mutism following a posterior fossa approach to cerebellar tumors in children: a critical review of the literature. Childs Nerv Syst 11:306–310

Albright AL, Pollack IF, Adelson PD (eds) (2001) Operative techniques in pediatric neurosurgery. Thieme, New York

Albright AL, Sposto R, Holmes E et al (2000) Correlation of neurosurgical subspecialization with outcomes in children with malignant brain tumors. Neurosurgery 47:879–885; discussion 885–887

Berger MS, Ojemann GA (1992) Intraoperative brain mapping techniques in neuro-oncology. Stereotact Funct Neurosurg 58:153–161

Berger MS, Baumeister B, Geyer JR et al (1991) The risks of metastases from shunting in children with primary central nervous system tumors. J Neurosurg 74:872–877

Catsman-Berrevoets CE, van Dongen HR, Mulder PG et al (1999) Tumour type and size are high risk factors for the syndrome of "cerebellar" mutism and subsequent dysarthria. J Neurol Neurosurg Psychiatry 67:755–757

Chitoku S, Otsubo H, Harada Y et al (2001) Extraoperative cortical stimulation of motor function in children. Pediatr Neurol 24:344–350

Chuang SH, Otsubo H, Hwang P et al (1995) Pediatric magnetic source imaging. Neuroimaging Clin North Am 5:289–303

Cochrane DD, Gustavsson B, Poskitt KP et al (1994) The surgical and natural morbidity of aggressive resection for posterior fossa tumors in childhood. Pediatr Neurosurg 20:19–29

Doxey D, Bruce D, Sklar, F et al (1999) Posterior fossa syndrome: identifiable risk factors and irreversible complications. Pediatr Neurosurg 31:131–136

Ersahin Y (1998) Transient cerebellar mutism. Childs Nerv Syst 14:687

Ersahin Y, Mutluer S, Cagli S et al (1996) Cerebellar mutism: report of seven cases and review of the literature. Neurosurgery 38:60–65

Fahlbusch R, Ganslandt O, Nimsky C (2000) Intraoperative imaging with open magnetic resonance imaging and neuronavigation. Childs Nerv Syst 16:829–831

Foreman NK, Love S, Gill SS et al (1997) Second-look surgery for incompletely resected fourth ventricle ependymomas: technical case report. Neurosurgery 40:856–860

Friedman JA, Lynch JJ, Buckner JC et al (2001) Management of malignant pineal germ cell tumors with residual mature teratoma. Neurosurgery 48:518–522

Gjerris F, Agerlin N, Borgesen SE et al (1998) Epidemiology and prognosis in children treated for intracranial tumours in Denmark 1960–1984. Childs Nerv Syst 14:302–311

Gleason PL, Kikinis R, Altobelli D et al (1994) Video registration virtual reality for nonlinkage stereotactic surgery. Stereotact Funct Neurosurg 63:139–143

Gnanalingham KK, Lafuente J, Thompaon D et al (2002) Surgical procedures for posterior fossa tumors in children: does craniotomy lead to fewer complications than craniectomy? J Neurosurg 97:821–826

Grabb PA, Albright AL, Sclabassi RJ et al (1997) Continuous intraoperative electromyographic monitoring of cranial nerves during resection of fourth ventricular tumors in children. J Neurosurg 86:1–4

Haglund MM, Berger MS, Shamseldin M et al (1994) Cortical localization of temporal lobe language sites in patients with gliomas. Neurosurgery 34:567–576

Hennessy MJ, Elwes RD, Honavar M et al (2001) Predictors of outcome and pathological considerations in the surgical treatment of intractable epilepsy associated with temporal lobe lesions. J Neurol Neurosurg Psychiatry 70:450–458

Hoppe-Hirsch E, Brunet L, Laroussinie F et al (1995) Intellectual outcome in children with malignant tumors of the posterior fossa: influence of the field of irradiation and quality of surgery. Childs Nerv Syst 11:340–345

Imielinski BL, Kloc W, Wasilewski W et al (1998) Posterior fossa tumors in children–indications for ventricular drainage and for V-P shunting. Childs Nerv Syst 14:227–229

Kaplan AM, Bandy DJ, Manwaring KH et al (1999) Functional brain mapping using positron emission tomography scanning in preoperative neurosurgical planning for pediatric brain tumors. J Neurosurg 91:797–803

Keles GE, Lamborn KR, Berger MS (2001) Low-grade hemispheric gliomas in adults: a critical review of extent of resection as a factor influencing outcome. J Neurosurg 95:735–745

Khan RB, Sanford RA, Kun LE et al (2001) Morbidity of second-look surgery in pediatric central nervous system tumors. Pediatr Neurosurg 35:225–229

Kumar V, Phipps K, Harkness W et al (1996) Ventriculo-peritoneal shunt requirement in children with posterior fossa tumours: an 11-year audit. Br J Neurosurg 10:467–470

Lam CH, Hall WA, Truwit CL et al (2001) Intra-operative MRI-guided approaches to the pediatric posterior fossa tumors. Pediatr Neurosurg 34:295–300

Leblanc R, Meyer E(1990) Functional PET scanning in the assessment of cerebral arteriovenous malformations. Case report. J Neurosurg 73:615–619

Leblanc R, Meyer E, Bub D et al (1992) Language localization with activation positron emission tomography scanning. Neurosurgery 31:369–373

Levisohn L, Cronin-Golomb A, Schmahmann JD (2000) Neuropsychological consequences of cerebellar tumour resection in children: cerebellar cognitive affective syndrome in a paediatric population. Brain 123:1041–1050

Mosewich RK, So EL, O'Brien TJ et al (2000) Factors predictive of the outcome of frontal lobe epilepsy surgery. Epilepsia 41:843–849

Ojemann SG, Berger MS, Lettich E et al (2003) Localization of language function in children: results of electrical stimulation mapping. J Neurosurg 98:465–470

Otsubo H, Ochi A, Elliott I et al (2001) MEG predicts epileptic zone in lesional extrahippocampal epilepsy: 12 pediatric surgery cases. Epilepsia 42:1523–1530

Penfield W, Boldrey E(1937) Somatic motor and sensory representation in the cerebral cortex of man as studied by electrical stimulation. Brain 60:389–443

Pollack IF (1994) Brain tumors in children. N Engl J Med 331:1500–1507

Pollack IF (1999) The role of surgery in pediatric gliomas. J Neurooncol 42:271–288

Pollack IF, Polinko P, Albright AL et al (1995) Mutism and pseudobulbar symptoms after resection of posterior fossa tumors in children: incidence and pathophysiology. Neurosurgery 37:885–893

Regelsberger J, Lohmann F, Helmke K et al (2000) Ultrasound-guided surgery of deep seated brain lesions. Eur J Ultrasound 12:115–121

Sainte-Rose C, Cinalli G, Roux FE et al (2001) Management of hydrocephalus in pediatric patients with posterior fossa tumors: the role of endoscopic third ventriculostomy. J Neurosurg 95:791–797

Schiffbauer H, Ferrari P, Rowley HA et al (2001) Functional activity within brain tumors: a magnetic source imaging study. Neurosurgery 49:1313–1320

Schneider JP, Schulz T, Schmidt F et al (2001) Gross-total surgery of supratentorial low-grade gliomas under intraoperative MR guidance. AJNR Am J Neuroradiol 22:89–98

Sekiya T, Hatayama T, Shimamura N et al (2000) Intraoperative electrophysiological monitoring of oculomotor nuclei and their intramedullary tracts during midbrain tumor surgery. Neurosurgery 47:1170–1166

Steinbok P, Mutat A (1999) Cerebellar astrocytoma. In: Albright AL, Pollack IF, Adelson PD (eds) Principles and practice of pediatric neurosurgery. Thieme, New York, p 1300

Weiner HL, Finlay JL (1999) Surgery in the management of primary intracranial germ cell tumors. Childs Nerv Syst 15:770–773

Chemotherapy

A. Banerjee · K. K. Matthay

Contents

14.1 Introduction

Chemotherapy treatment goals for pediatric brain tumors reflect the extreme heterogeneity of this group of malignancies. In the setting of average-risk medulloblastoma and germinoma, which have high cure rates with radiation treatment alone, chemotherapy is used to reduce radiation doses, yet maintain high cure rates. For infants with malignant brain tumors who are particularly vulnerable to radiation-related morbidity, chemotherapy has been used to delay or defer radiation treatment. Similarly, in the setting of unresectable, low-grade astrocytoma, chemotherapy can provide prolonged disease stabilization, perhaps allowing for delay or deferral of radiation.

While many clinical trials evaluating chemotherapy for the treatment of CNS tumors are exploratory, two randomized controlled trials have shown a survival benefit from the addition of chemotherapy to radiation therapy in comparison to radiation therapy alone in children with brain tumors. Sposto et al., reporting for the Children's Cancer Group, described a randomization of patients with newly diagnosed high-grade glioma between two treatment arms: postoperative radiation treatment alone versus treatment with postoperative radiation followed by chemotherapy (Sposto et al. 1989). Chemotherapy-treated patients had a 46% 5-year event-free survival (EFS), compared to radiation-only treated patients who had an 18% 5-year EFS More recently, a large scale, multi-institutional European trial reported improved 5-year EFS with the addition of chemotherapy to radiation therapy for average-risk medulloblastoma: 74% for radiation with chemotherapy vs. 59% for radiation alone (Taylor et al. 2003).

While most chemotherapeutic agents are initially tested in single-agent clinical trials to determine effectiveness against a particular tumor type, combination chemotherapy regimens are in widespread use. The goal of combination therapy is to maximize therapeutic effectiveness of chemotherapy by overcoming drug resistance, which exists in a high proportion of tumors. An optimally designed combination regimen combines agents with high response rates in single-agent trials, non-cross-resistant mechanisms of action in tumor cell subpopulations, and non-overlapping toxicity profiles.

This chapter will review important conventional chemotherapeutic agents in brain-tumor management, the use of combination chemotherapy for infants with brain tumors, high-dose myeloablative chemotherapy, and new classes of therapeutic agents. Disease-specific chemotherapy regimens are discussed separately in prior chapters.

14.2 General Principles of Chemotherapy

For most solid tumors such as CNS neoplasms, chemotherapy is considered most effective when used as an adjuvant to local-control measures, specifically surgery and radiation. Chemotherapy is most likely to contribute to long-term disease control when residual disease is minimal; this has been demonstrated in both medulloblastoma and high-grade glioma, where improved prognosis is clearly associated with gross total or near-total resection followed by radiation (Sposto et al. 1989; Packer et al. 1994). While adjuvant chemotherapy is important for preventing distant metastases in extracranial solid tumors (Ortega et al. 1975; Link et al. 1986; Eilber et al. 1987), the role of chemotherapy in preventing CNS dissemination or extraneural metastasis is unclear. Neo-adjuvant chemotherapy can also be used for patients who have disease that is unresectable or difficult to resect at diagnosis, with the hope of eliciting a tumor response that would allow improved, post-treatment resection (Rosen 1986; Trimble et al. 1993). While this strategy is used in the management of extracranial pediatric solid tumors, its utility in CNS tumors is uncertain. This rationale is being investigated in ongoing clini-

cal trials for infant embryonal tumors and ependymoma.

The blood-brain barrier (BBB) is an anatomic feature of the CNS consisting of specialized capillary endothelial cells that lack fenestrations and pinocytic vesicles, and express specialized transport proteins. The ability of a compound to cross the BBB is restricted by molecular weight, lipid solubility, and pH. Small, lipid-soluble molecules at physiologic pH readily cross the BBB (Rall and Zubrod 1962), but the properties of most chemotherapeutic compounds prevent movement across the BBB. Despite this fact, the objective response of some CNS tumors to chemotherapy alone suggests that systemically administered agents are still able to reach brain tumor cells. Based on this observation, as well as the ability of CNS tumors to enhance with gadolinium on MRI (in which gadolinium must cross the BBB) suggests that the BBB is physiologically disrupted in the tumor environment, and that tumor concentrations of systemically administered drugs are likely to be higher than those in normal brain (Stewart 1994). Nevertheless, concerns about the role of the BBB in resistance to chemotherapy has resulted in the development of various treatment strategies to overcome it, which are summarized below.

14.3 Specific Chemotherapeutic Agents

14.3.1 Platinums

Cisplatin and carboplatin are non-cell-cycle-specific alkylating agents. The cytotoxic (free or unbound) fraction of drug acts to form a platinum-DNA adduct which produces inter- and intra-strand cross-links by alkylating the N7 position of guanine (Zwelling and Kohn 1979). When used as a single agent, cisplatin has been shown to produce disease responses in medulloblastoma, germinoma, ependymoma, and astrocytoma (Sexauer et al. 1985; Walker and Allen 1988; Bertolone et al. 1989). Used adjuvantly with lomustine (CCNU) and vincristine, cisplatin has been shown to improve disease-free survival in medulloblastoma (Packer et al. 1991, 1994). The toxicity of cisplatin is substantial, including hearing loss, nephrotoxicity, myelosuppression, nausea and vomiting, and peripheral neuropathy (Jorg and Hans-Peter 2003).

Carboplatin, an analogue of cisplatin, has similar efficacy but a somewhat different toxicity profile. While less ototoxic and nephrotoxic than cisplatin, carboplatin is more myelosuppressive. Carboplatin also has less associated peripheral neuropathy and is less emetogenic than cisplatin (Duffful and Robinson 1997). Single-agent treatment results in moderate tumor responses in recurrent childhood brain tumors (Walker and Allen 1988; Gaynon et al. 1990). In combination with vincristine, carboplatin has been shown to be an active agent in pediatric low-grade astrocytoma (Packer et al. 1997; Mahoney et al. 2000), and plays a role in the combination chemotherapy of infant brain tumors as well. A new strategy using carboplatin in conjunction with a blood-brain barrier disrupting agent is discussed later in this chapter.

14.3.2 Nitrosoureas

CCNU (lomustine) and BCNU (carmustine), the most commonly utilized nitrosoureas, are non-cell-cycle-specific alkylators. Both are pro-drugs that spontaneously decompose into two active metabolites: an isocyanate group and a chloroethyldiazohydroxide. The chloroethyldiazohydroxide alkylates DNA, resulting in cross-linking followed by cellular instability. Nitrosoureas are small, lipophilic molecules that penetrate the blood-brain barrier easily, and are among the few systemically administered agents found in moderate to high concentrations in the brain (reviewed in Middleton 2003). Nitrosourea-based combination therapy has appeared in some trials to have a modest impact on survival in pediatric patients with high-grade astrocytoma (Sposto et al. 1989; Finlay et al. 1995; Levin et al. 2000). A single-agent phase II trial of high-dose BCNU for pediatric high-grade glioma showed only modest tumor response with substantial toxicity (Bouffet et al. 1997). CCNU, in combination with vincristine, is clearly beneficial in the adjuvant, post-radiation treatment of medulloblastoma, and in one study was the rationale for reduction of the neuraxis radiation dose from 36 Gy to 23.4 Gy, with preservation of good dis-

ease-free survival in average-risk medulloblastoma (Packer et al. 1994). Nitrosourea-based therapy has also been shown to produce disease responses and prolong stable disease in pediatric low-grade astrocytoma when used in combination with procarbazine, 6-thioguanine, and vincristine (Prados et al. 1997). The major toxicities of nitrosoureas include nausea, myelosuppression and, less commonly, pulmonary fibrosis and nephrotoxicity. The myelosuppression is typically delayed, seen approximately three to five weeks following administration of the dose, and is frequently cumulative (Balis et al. 2002).

14.3.3 Cyclophosphamide and Ifosfamide

These parenterally administered pro-drug members of the nitrogen mustard family of drugs are thought to have the same mechanism of activity as most classic alkylators, i.e., by forming covalent bonds with nucleophilic groups, resulting in cross-linking between DNA strands or intrastrand linking, thus impairing DNA replication (Pratt et al. 1994). These agents have produced responses and stable disease in both primary and recurrent pediatric brain tumors, including medulloblastoma/PNET, high-grade astrocytoma, and germ cell tumors. These agents also compose an important part of combination chemotherapy for infants with malignant brain tumors (Friedman et al. 1986; Longee et al. 1990; Packer et al. 1999; Zeltzer et al. 1999). Toxicities are substantial, including nausea, myelosuppression, hemorrhagic cystitis, and in the case of ifosfamide, nephrotoxicity (Balis et al. 2002). Impaired fertility has been reported in patients treated with these agents (Byrne et al. 1987). Secondary leukemia has recently been described in a cohort of infants with malignant brain tumors treated with high cumulative doses of cyclophosphamide and etoposide (Duffner et al. 1998; Smith et al. 1999).

14.3.4 Temozolomide

Temozolomide is a rapidly absorbed, oral pro-drug that undergoes spontaneous hydrolysis to form its active metabolite, 3-methyl-(triazen-1-yl)-imidazole-4-carboxamide (MTIC). Its mechanism of action is via the methylation of DNA, largely at the O6 position of guanine (Newlands et al. 1997). While adult patients with glioblastoma multiforme have been shown to have some survival advantage when treated at diagnosis with radiation and temozolomide (Stupp et al. 2002), the role of this agent in pediatric brain tumors has not yet been established. Responses to temozolomide have been reported in pediatric patients with recurrent high-grade astrocytoma, and in a small series of patients with ependymoma, PNET, and germ cell tumor (Pollack et al. 1999). This early promise of temozolomide is undergoing further investigation in ongoing trials to evaluate safety and toxicity of temozolomide in combination with other agents, including radiation, CCNU, and thalidomide. Temozolomide is well tolerated although its reported toxicities include nausea, constipation, and myelosuppression (Nicholson et al. 1998; Friedman et al. 2000).

14.3.5 Etoposide

Etoposide is a semisynthetic derivative of a plant extract, podophyllotoxin, which binds to tubulin. Etoposide interacts with DNA topoisomerase II, causing single- and double-stranded breaks and a cell-cycle arrest in G_2 and mitosis (Hande 1998). Despite its highly lipophilic properties, it does not cross the blood-brain barrier easily due to its large size (Newton et al. 1999). Etoposide can be administered orally or parenterally. It is active against many pediatric brain tumors, including medulloblastoma/PNET, ependymoma, and germ cell tumor (Allen et al. 1985; Bouffet and Foreman 1999; Kobrinsky et al. 1999; Chamberlain 2001). It has been used in combination with cisplatin, carboplatin, ifosfamide, and cyclophosphamide with acceptable toxicity in the treatment of childhood brain tumors (Busca et al. 1997; Gururangan et al. 1998; White et al. 1998; Duffner et

al. 1999; Kortmann et al. 2000). Daily oral etoposide has produced modest responses and prolonged stable disease in patients with recurrent PNET and high-grade astrocytoma (Ashley et al. 1996; Fulton et al. 1996; Chamberlain and Kormanik 1997; Needle et al. 1997).

Toxicities of etoposide include nausea and myelosuppression, as well as diarrhea and mucositis when administered in high doses (Mathew et al. 1994; Taylor et al. 2003). High cumulative doses have been associated with an increased risk of secondary leukemia in infants with malignant brain tumors as well as other childhood cancers (Smith et al. 1999; Duffner et al. 1998).

14.3.6 Vincristine

Vincristine is a plant alkaloid that binds tubulin and induces metaphase arrest in a cell-cycle-specific fashion (Jordan 2002). It has limited CNS penetration, and has never been rigorously evaluated as a single agent in pediatric brain tumors (Kellie et al. 2002). Nevertheless, it has shown activity in multiagent regimens, and is widely used in combination treatment regimens for medulloblastoma/PNET, low-grade astrocytoma, and infant brain tumors (Packer et al. 1994, 1997; Duffner et al. 1999). Its toxicities include constipation, peripheral neuropathy, and the syndrome of inappropriate antidiuretic hormone (SIADH) (Balis et al. 2002).

14.4 Combination Chemotherapy for Infant Brain Tumors

Combination chemotherapy is in widespread use for almost all types of childhood CNS tumors. Specific regimens targeted at individual tumor types are discussed in the prior individual disease-specific chapters (Chapters 1 to 11). Infants and very young children, however, are especially susceptible to complications of CNS irradiation, including neuro-cognitive decline, neuro-endocrine deficits, and hearing loss (Miettinen et al. 1997; Siffert and Allen 2000; Mulhern et al. 2001; Packer 2002; Spoudeas et al. 2003). In order to delay or defer radiation treatment, chemotherapy has been investigated for infants and very young patients with primary malignant brain tumors as the primary adjuvant therapy following surgery. Because malignant brain tumors in infants are rare, most infant studies include a broad range of diagnoses, often including both embryonal (e.g., medulloblastoma/PNET) and astrocytic tumors, as well as ependymoma. The largest clinical trial for infants, "Baby POG 1," done by the Pediatric Oncology Group (POG 8633) reported on 198 patients less than 36 months of age. The patients in this study were treated with one (patients 25 to 36 months of age) or two (patients 0 to 24 months of age) years of pre-radiation chemotherapy, followed by radiation therapy. Chemotherapy consisted of multiple cycles of a four-drug regimen (cisplatin, etoposide, vincristine, and cyclophosphamide) prior to radiation (Duffner et al. 1993, 1999). The overall 5-year survival for all patients was 32%; survival for those who had gross total resection (GTR) was 62% compared with 31% for patients with subtotal resection. These figures were similar when patients with medulloblastoma and ependymoma were examined independently (Duffner et al. 1993, 1999).

In another trial that demonstrated the feasibility of pre-radiation chemotherapy in infants, Mason et al. (1998) attempted to achieve further gains by increasing the dose intensity of chemotherapy. They utilized induction chemotherapy similar to that of the Baby POG 1 study, and then added high-dose treatment with stem cell rescue, with radiation therapy reserved for patients with progressive or residual disease following chemotherapy. Sixty-two patients under the age of six were enrolled; the 3-year progression free survival was 27%. Degree of resection was again found to be an important prognostic feature; 3-year overall survival for children with GTR was 59%, in comparison to 30% for children who had only subtotal resection or biopsy. The proportion of patients undergoing GTR between the studies of POG 8633 and Mason et al. was similar, 34% and 35 %, respectively. The high-dose chemotherapy-based regimen had substantial toxicity with a mortality rate of 6% attributed to toxicity, although it is important to recognize that the Baby POG 1 patients were sig-

nificantly younger (<36 months) than those reported by Mason, et al (<72 months).

The Australian and New Zealand Children's Cancer Study Group (CCG) reported on a chemotherapy-alone protocol for patients less than 36 months old utilizing combination chemotherapy with vincristine, etoposide, and cyclophosphamide for 64 weeks without radiation therapy. Forty patients were enrolled; progression-free survival (PFS) was reported at 11% (White et al. 1998). Geyer et al. reported on the CCG 921 experience in infants with PNET and malignant ependymoma who were enrolled in a randomized trial of two chemotherapy regimens ("8 drugs in one" vs. prednisone, vincristine, and lomustine), with radiation treatment at investigator discretion. Ninety-six patients were treated (only 13 were irradiated); after 3 years of follow up PFS was 23% (Geyer et al. 1994). It is important to note that long-term disease control with surgery and chemotherapy alone has been reported in a small number of children, typically with medulloblastoma. In a series reported by Ater et al. (1997), infants less than three were treated with mechlorethamine, vincristine, procarbazine, and prednisone. Eight of 12 patients with medulloblastoma survived more than 10 years without radiation therapy. Nevertheless, the majority of patients treated with chemotherapy alone in larger-scale cooperative group studies develop recurrent disease.

In summary, while these preliminary results have shown the dose-intensive approach to be feasible, albeit with increased toxicity over the standard schedule, the survival benefit is unknown. There is no clear standard chemotherapy approach for infants with malignant brain tumors. One strategy currently under investigation includes combination chemo-radiotherapy protocols. Incorporation of intrathecal mafosfamide and conformal radiation is currently under investigation by the Pediatric Brain Tumor Consortium. An alternative strategy under investigation is high-dose therapy with hematopoietic stem cell rescue.

14.5 High Dose Chemotherapy with Hematopoietic Stem Cell Rescue

14.5.1 Rationale

Many CNS tumors fail to respond to standard-dose chemotherapy, or fail to demonstrate a sustained response. Potential reasons for this failure include inherent or acquired drug resistance and poor CNS penetration of drug. High-dose, myeloablative chemotherapy with autologous stem cell rescue is an investigational strategy designed to overcome some of these barriers by maximizing dose intensity and achieving high systemic drug concentrations, hopefully improving CNS penetration. The initial transplant chemotherapy regimens were nitrosourea based, but dose-limiting neurotoxicity prevented adequate dose escalation (Burger et al. 1981; Hochberg et al. 1981; Bashir et al. 1988). More contemporary regimens under investigation typically use alkylating agents, often in combinations with etoposide (Mahoney et al. 1996; Busca et al. 1997; Gururangan et al. 1998; Papadopoulos et al. 1998). Other current conditioning regimens are based on either thiotepa, a highly lipophilic alkylator with excellent CNS penetration, or melphalan (reviewed in Dunkel and Finlay 2002).

The two patient groups targeted for high-dose therapy are those with recurrent disease following standard therapy (either chemotherapy or radiation), and infants with malignant brain tumors. High-dose therapy is of particular interest for infants as they typically have a poor prognosis and are especially susceptible to delayed post-radiation toxicity. Multiple investigators have established the feasibility of this approach, and the initial results have been modestly encouraging.

14.5.2 Recurrent Medulloblastoma

High-dose therapy for recurrent medulloblastoma has shown the most promising results to date, with sustained complete responses in a few patients, often for many months (Mahoney et al. 1996; Graham et al. 1997). Dunkel and colleagues report 3-year progression-free survival of 34% in a series of patients with recurrent medulloblastoma treated with high-dose therapy. Patients with the best outcome were those with no evidence of disease at the time of transplant (Dunkel et al. 1998a). Graham et al. reporting on a heterogeneous group of patients with recurrent malignant tumors treated with high-dose chemotherapy regimens described 18 patients with recurrent medulloblastoma, 4 of whom were surviving 27 to 49 months at the time of reporting. All four patients had local recurrences while patients with metastatic disease in this cohort had uniformly poor outcomes (Graham et al. 1997; Grovas et al. 1999).

14.5.3 Gliomas

Results for glioma have been less encouraging, however, with fewer long-term disease responses reported. Two clinical trials utilizing high-dose therapy following radiation for patients with diffuse pontine glioma showed no impact on survival in comparison to historical controls (Dunkel et al. 1998b; Bouffet et al. 2000). An early study treated 11 patients with newly diagnosed and recurrent high-grade astrocytoma with thiotepa and cyclophosphamide following surgery (limited to biopsy in 6 patients), followed by radiation for those patients who had stable disease or better. Although one complete response and two partial responses were observed, median progression-free survival remained disappointingly short at 9 months (Heideman et al. 1993). The Children's Cancer Group reported on 18 patients with recurrent malignant astrocytoma treated with thiotepa and etoposide, 5 of whom had PFS ranging from 39 to 59 months (Finlay et al. 1996). A follow-up phase II pilot conducted by the Children's Cancer group added carmustine to thiotepa and etoposide, followed by radiation therapy for newly diagnosed glioblastoma multiforme. Although 2-year PFS was promising at 46%, accrual was closed early because of unacceptable pulmonary and neurological toxicities (Grovas et al. 1999). There have been no clinical trials prospectively comparing standard chemotherapy to high-dose therapy for childhood brain tumors.

14.5.4 Other Tumor Types

High-dose chemotherapy has been shown to be feasible for the treatment of pineoblastoma. Gururangan et al. (1998) reported on 12 patients with newly diagnosed pineoblastoma (age 0.3 to 43.7 years), who were treated with surgery, radiation (all but two patient received radiation), and high dose chemotherapy. Four-year progression-free survival was 69%. A group of Japanese investigators reported a small series of 6 patients with intracranial non-germinomatous germ cell tumors treated with myeloablative chemotherapy alone, all of whom are surviving without tumor recurrence with follow-up of 1 to 7 years (Tada et al. 1999).

Toxicity of stem-cell transplant is considerable, with mortality rates from 3% to 16% (Mahoney et al. 1996; Dunkel et al. 1998b; Gururangan et al. 1998; Papadopoulos et al. 1998). Current strategies under investigation include the use of multiple, tandem high-dose treatments, with multiple stem-cell infusions, the incorporation of temozolomide into myeloablative regimens, and the use of high-dose therapy in infants and very young children with newly diagnosed disease. While high-dose therapy has promise as a treatment approach in a select group of patients, it remains investigational, and its role outside of clinical trials is unclear.

14.6 New Strategies

14.6.1 Radiation Sensitizers

Numerous investigational chemotherapy treatment strategies are designed to maximize the known benefit of radiation therapy in CNS tumors. Multiple potentiating effects of platinum agents on radiation have been described. Hypoxic cells (typically radiation resistant) are more sensitive to radiation following exposure to platinum agents in vitro (Skov and MacPhail 1991). Platinum agents may also have a role in preventing the development of radiation-resistant clones by inhibiting "potentially lethal damage recovery," a mechanism by which tumor cells are able to repair lethal or sub-lethal DNA damage following radi-

ation exposure (Wilkins et al. 1993). Clinical trials evaluating toxicity and response to combination chemo-radiotherapy with carboplatinum are currently underway for newly diagnosed high-risk PNET and for brainstem glioma through the Children's Oncology Group (COG) .

Gadolinium-texaphyrin is a metalloporphyrin-like compound, currently being tested as a radiation sensitizer in brainstem glioma by the COG. Gadolinium-texaphyrin is preferentially taken up by tumor cells, and has been shown to produce radiosensitization in vitro by prolonging the half-life of cytotoxic radicals formed following exposure to ionizing radiation (Young et al. 1996). An ongoing COG trial administers Gadolinium-texaphyrin simultaneously with radiation.

As discussed in Chapter 15, tyrosine kinase receptor inhibitors, specifically of the epidermal growth factor receptor, and farnesyl transferase inhibitors designed to inhibit signal transduction in the Ras pathway also have promising pre-clinical data to suggest radiosensitizing properties. Phase I clinical trials are underway through the Pediatric Brain Tumor Consortium to further investigate the safety and tolerability of these agents in combination with radiation.

14.6.2 Targeting Drug Resistance

14.6.2.1 P-glycoprotein Pump

Many brain tumors are resistant to conventional chemotherapeutic agents. Investigators have identified mechanisms of drug resistance amenable to pharmacologic treatment that would render tumor cells more sensitive to chemotherapy. The P-glycoprotein pump (PGP) is the protein product of the multi-drug resistance gene (MDR-1), which is amplified in many resistant and refractory tumors, including glioblastoma, medulloblastoma, and ependymoma (Chou et al. 1995, 1996; von Bossanyi et al. 1997; Decleves et al. 2002). The PGP serves as an efflux pump, allowing the cell to transport specific toxins, including chemotherapeutic agents (Sikic et al. 1997). In mice, capillary endotchlial cells composing the blood-brain barrier have high concentrations of PGP (Schinkel et al. 1994). Cyclosporine A is a potent inhibitor of PGP and effectively sensitizes high-PGP-expressing cells in vitro (Sikic et al. 1997). Clinical trials using cyclosporine A in combination with chemotherapy, largely in the setting of adult myeloid leukemia, have shown high toxicity with unclear therapeutic benefit (Chauncey 2001). The only trial in pediatric CNS tumors was a phase I clinical trial of cyclosporine A in combination with intravenous etoposide for patients with intrinsic pontine glioma, following radiation therapy. The results of this trial have not yet been published.

14.6.2.2 Alkylguanine-DNA-alkyltransferase

Alkylguanine-DNA-alkyltransferase (AGT) is a DNA repair enzyme that plays an important role in tumor resistance to alkylnitrosoureas and temozolomide. AGT reverses DNA methylation and chloroethylation (induced by chemotherapy) at the O^6 position of guanine, thus rescuing the cell from lethal injury. Many brain tumors have high levels of AGT, and these high levels are associated with poor survival in clinical trials in adults with malignant glioma (Wiestler et al. 1984; Pegg 1990; Pegg and Byers 1992; Hongeng et al. 1997). Experiments in brain tumor cell lines as well as tumor xenografts have shown that depletion of AGT with O^6-benzylguanine (acting as an alternate substrate for AGT) increases tumor cell sensitivity to chemotherapy (Jaeckle et al. 1998). A phase I clinical trial in malignant glioma of O^6-benzylguanine (O^6BG) administered preoperatively as a single agent showed reduced levels of AGT in the resected tumor, suggesting that combination treatment with O^6BG and nitrosourea or temozolomide would increase tumor-cell sensitivity (Friedman et al. 1998). A phase I clinical trial of temozolomide in combination with O^6BG is currently underway for recurrent or refractory pediatric brain tumors.

14.6.3 Molecular Targets and Signal Transduction Inhibition

The enormous expansion in knowledge of the detailed molecular basis of neoplastic transformation has led to the development of a new class of agents designed to inhibit specific intracellular biochemical pathways. The majority of these agents function through the inhibition of receptor tyrosine kinases, a class of cellular proteins that bind a specific ligand through their extracellular domains. Activation of the intracellular tyrosine kinase catalytic domain of the receptor after ligand binding subsequently triggers a cascade of biochemical signals. This ligand-dependent tyrosine kinase activation mediates a host of cellular properties, including proliferation, survival, and differentiation. In normal cellular homeostasis, these functions are tightly regulated. In oncogenesis, unregulated ligand-independent kinase phosphorylation and subsequent receptor activation is a common event and is likely a key mechanism in maintaining the malignant phenotype. Receptor tyrosine kinases known to be important in CNS tumors include the epidermal growth factor receptor (EGFR), the platelet derived growth factor receptor (PDGFR), and vascular endothelial growth factor receptor (VEGFR). Small-molecule and monoclonal-antibody inhibitors of these receptors are discussed in greater detail in Chapter 15.

14.6.4 Angiogenesis Inhibitors

The role of angiogenesis in supporting tumor cell proliferation and survival has been extensively investigated since the hypothesis of "angiogenesis dependency" of tumors was first proposed by Judah Folkman (Folkman 1971; Balis et al. 2002). The angiogenesis hypothesis proposes that tumor-induced proliferation of blood vessels is necessary to support ongoing proliferation and survival. Tumor-cell-induced angiogenesis appears to have multiple mechanisms. Tumor cells produce pro-angiogenic cytokines, including acidic and basic fibroblast growth factor (aFGF, bFGF), angiogenin, vascular endothelial growth factor (VEGF), platelet derived growth factor (PDGF), and interleukin 8 (IL-8). Additionally, tumor cells produce matrix metalloproteinases (MMP), which can induce breakdown in extracellular matrix, again allowing for release of pro-angiogenic peptides. Finally, tumor cells recruit inflammatory cells that subsequently produce pro-angiogenic cytokines (Bicknell and Harris 1996; Pluda 1997; Paku 1998).

A number of therapeutic agents have been shown to inhibit neovascularization in vitro and in vivo. Thalidomide, initially developed as a sedative and subsequently found to be a potent teratogen in humans, has anti-angiogenic properties (D'Amato 1994). It has been shown to inhibit bFGF-induced corneal vascularization in animals (Kenyon et al. 1997). In a single-agent clinical trial of recurrent gliomas, objective response rates (partial response and stable disease) of up to 45% were reported (Fine et al. 2000).

The role of cyclooxygenase inhibitors as an anti-angiogenic treatment strategy is also under investigation. Cyclooxygenase 2 (COX-2) induces vascular proliferation following trauma or stimulation with growth factor, and is highly expressed in some human tumors, including high-grade glioma (Joki et al. 2000). Treatment of glioma cell cultures with a specific COX-2 inhibitor was found to produce diminished proliferation and invasion and increased apoptosis (Joki et al. 2000). Celecoxib is a specific inhibitor of COX-2, with a highly favorable toxicity profile. While celecoxib is not currently under investigation in large-scale pediatric clinical trials, its ease of use and low toxicity make it an interesting agent to pursue in combination with other agents.

Specific anti-angiogenesis agents are under development. The largest class of agents are small-molecule tyrosine kinase inhibitors, which block VEGF-mediated signaling (Glade-Bender et al. 2003). Additionally, matrix metalloproteinases inhibitors and integrin antagonists are under investigation (reviewed in Drevs et al. 2002). Finally, the use of conventional cytotoxic agents given in low-dose, metronomic regimens is being piloted. These regimens are based on the principle that while endothelial cell proliferation appears to be sensitive to chronic but low-dose exposure, it has ample recovery time during the recovery phase of dose-intensive therapy schedules. Growing evidence from pilot clinical trials support this hypothesis (Einhorn 1991; Ashley et al. 1996; Kushner and Cheung 1999; Klement et al. 2000). Therapies directed against angiogenesis for pediatric brain tumors are currently entering clinical trials.

14.6.5 Overcoming the Blood Brain Barrier

The blood-brain barrier (BBB) is composed of tight endothelial cell junctions that exclude most large molecules and is freely permeable only to small molecules that are highly lipophilic. This barrier limits the ability of many systemically administered chemotherapeutic agents to penetrate the CNS. Radiographic evidence based on heterogeneous uptake of gadolinium on magnetic resonance imaging suggests, however, that the BBB is only partially intact in many CNS tumors. Further support of tumor degradation of the BBB lies in the responsiveness of tumors to large, water-soluble molecules such as the platinum agents. Nevertheless, resistance of CNS tumors to therapy may partially lie in the infiltrative, nonenhancing portions of tumor that presumably have an intact BBB, and thus are able to escape cytotoxicity of systemically administered agents. This is supported by the propensity of many tumors to recur locally at the infiltrating edge of the tumor. A number of strategies are under investigation with the intent to disrupt or bypass the BBB.

14.6.5.1 BBB Disruption

Mannitol was one of the first agents used to attempt disruption of the blood brain barrier. Increased osmotic pressure transiently opens the BBB, allowing entry of molecules otherwise unable to penetrate the CNS (Neuwelt et al. 1983). Increased disease response has been reported following BBB disruption, largely in adult patients with non-AIDS CNS lymphoma (Neuwelt et al. 1981). The Children's Cancer Group reported on the only pediatric experience with this strategy, using mannitol in combination with etoposide for recurrent or refractory CNS tumors. They were unable to document a clear benefit (Kobrinski et al. 1999).

RMP-7 (Cereport) is a bradykinin analogue, which, on binding to specific B_2 bradykinin receptors on the surface of endothelial cells, transiently increases permeability of the BBB. While increased concentration of carboplatin when administered with this agent has been documented in animals (Dean et al. 1999), a randomized, placebo-controlled, phase II trial in adults with malignant glioma showed no survival benefit from the addition of Cereport to carboplatin alone (Prados et al. 2003). A phase II pediatric trial conducted by the Children's Oncology Group for patients with recurrent or refractory brain tumors is ongoing.

14.6.5.2 Intra-arterial Delivery

Intra-arterial delivery of chemotherapy, often delivered in conjunction with mannitol, may provide improved delivery of drug and minimal systemic toxicity, possibly allowing for the use of lower doses delivered directly to the tumor. A number of studies have investigated the use of intra-arterial carmustine, cisplatin, and carboplatin. While modest responses have been reported, neurologic toxicities are substantial, including irreversible encephalopathy and vision loss (Bashir et al. 1988; Mahaley et al. 1989; Newton et al. 1989).

14.6.5.3 Intratumoral Drug Delivery

A variety of novel techniques to deliver drug directly to the tumor or resection cavity are under investigation. The use of carmustine-impregnated "wafers" (Gliadel) has been reported on in adults with malignant glioma. This strategy allows for the passive diffusion of high concentrations of BCNU from wafers surgically implanted in the resection cavity to surrounding tumor cells, with minimal systemic exposure. Modest improvements in survival have been shown with this intervention (Brem et al. 1995; Valtonen et al. 1997), and a phase I trial of Gliadel in com-

bination with O^6BG has recently begun accruing patients in the Pediatric Brain Tumor Consortium.

Passive diffusion, however, is limited by minimal ability of the drug to penetrate beyond the margin of the tumor resection cavity. Convection-enhanced delivery (CED) is a novel delivery strategy that overcomes this barrier, and allows for delivery of larger molecules intra- or peri-tumorally. CED requires the surgical placement of catheters intra- or peri-tumorally, through which a therapeutic agent is infused under positive pressure (Bobo et al. 1994), which allows for a substantially larger area of brain to be treated. This approach has been largely used to deliver biologic cytotoxins targeted to high-grade glioma cells. The first such agent to be reported was a conjugate of transferrin (highly expressed in GBM) with truncated diphtheria toxin. The infusions were relatively tolerated, and the treatment produced 9 objective responses in 15 evaluable patients (Laske et al. 1997). Another promising agent for CED is IL13-PE38QQR, a conjugate molecule of IL13 and inactivated pseudomonas exotoxin, capitalizing on the high expression of IL13 receptor in malignant glioma with minimal expression in normal brain (Debinski et al. 1999). Direct intratumoral infusion in glioblastoma xenografts produces complete regression of tumor. Convection-enhanced delivery of this agent is currently in phase I clinical trials for both pediatric and adult patients with high-grade glioma.

14.6.6 Differentiation of Neoplastic Cells

Agents that induce differentiation of tumor cells, thereby suppressing neoplastic proliferation, may have a role in the management of brain tumors. Experiments in cell culture using both retinoic acid and phenylacetate show both differentiation and inhibition of proliferation of astrocytoma-derived and medulloblastoma-derived cell lines (Mukherjee and Das 1990; Rodts and Black 1994). Treatment of adult patients with malignant glioma with single-agent 13-cis-retinoic acid showed a modest partial response plus a stable disease rate of 46%, with tolerable toxicity (Yung et al. 1996). A recent phase II study investigated the combination of temozolomide with 13-cis-retinoic acid for recurrent malignant glioma in adults. A slight improvement in 6-month progression-free survival was observed over historical controls, suggesting that the combination is active in recurrent malignant glioma (Jaeckle et al. 2003). In a randomized trial adding retinoic acid to combination therapy for high-risk neuroblastoma, patients treated with retinoic acid had a better outcome (Matthay et al. 1999). Based on these findings, its favorable toxicity and ease of administration, retinoic acid is a feasible agent to be used in future combination-regimen clinical trials for medulloblastoma and high-grade glioma. Phenylacetate and its analogue phenylbutyrate have also entered clinical trials. Chang et al. (1999) published results of a phase II trial showing 75% failure rate after 2 months in adult patients with recurrent malignant glioma, and a median survival of 8 months, suggesting no improvement from treatment over historical controls. Toxicities were mild, but the future impact of this agent is uncertain.

14.6.7 Gene Therapy

The goal of gene therapy is to transfer genetic material into a tumor cell to achieve a targeted therapeutic effect with minimal toxicity to surrounding normal cells. The genetic material is typically transferred using a modified viral vector. A number of genetic events can be introduced to achieve this goal. "Suicide gene therapy" involves the introduction of a gene that encodes for a protein that will make the tumor cell more vulnerable to toxicity from a specific drug. The herpes simplex virus thymidine kinase (HSV-tk) ganciclovir (GCV) model has been used in clinical trials (Culver et al. 1992). The *HSV-tk* gene encodes an enzyme whose substrate range is greater than that of its host. Its function is to phosphorylate purine pentosides and a wide variety of nucleoside analogues. Initial gene therapy directed against brain tumors used retrovirally delivered *HSV-tk*. Cells transfected with the *HSV-tk* gene become susceptible to treatment by GCV. Phosphorylation of GCV by HSV-tk produces a nucleotide-like precursor that blocks replication, thereby causing death of those cells expressing HSV-tk. Cells not transfected by *HSV-tk* are

unaffected by GCV. This strategy has been used for both adult and pediatric recurrent gliomas, with minimal success (Viola and Martuza 1996). Poor efficiency of transfection of virus into tumor cells appears to be one of the major barriers. Packer et al. demonstrated the feasibility of this approach in a Phase I clinical trial using this strategy for children with recurrent, supratentorial tumors. Twelve children with recurrent malignant glioma, ependymoma, or PNET were treated with local injections into a resection cavity. While four episodes of transient neurologic deterioration were described, no irreversible toxicity was noted (Packer et al. 2000).

A number of other gene therapy strategies are in development. One exploits the function of tumor-suppressor genes in brain tumors. A number of tumor-suppressor genes (TSGs) have been characterized in human malignancies, and many are important in gliomagenesis as well as in CNS embryonal tumors (von Deimling et al. 1995; Cogen and McDonald 1996). Tumor-suppressor genes encode proteins that inhibit cell growth; absent or nonfunctional proteins result in loss of inhibition and unchecked tumor growth. Among the important TSGs in CNS tumors are *p53* and *PTEN*. Both genes have been found to be mutated or deleted in a large number of adult high-grade glioma specimens (Koga et al. 1994; Li et al. 1997, 1998; Rasheed et al. 1997). Replacement of *p53* function by transfecting tumor cell lines that have mutated or deleted *p53* reverses the malignant phenotype in cell culture and animal experiments, suggesting that TSG replacement is a feasible gene-therapy strategy (Hsiao et al. 1997; Kokunai et al. 1997). Results of a recently published Phase I trial utilizing an adenoviral vector to introduce the p53 TSG into tumor cavities of patients with recurrent glioma support this strategy, although the strategy was found to be limited by an inadequate volume of transduced cells (Lang et al. 2003). Similar experiments have been done with tumor cells containing mutations in *PTEN*, another important gene in adult glioma, again showing reversal of the malignant phenotype (Cheney et al. 1998; Tamura et al. 1998). One of many challenges impeding the progress of TSG-replacement gene therapy is the heterogeneous nature of many gliomas, in which only a subset of tumor cells carry the TSG mutation while other tumor cells may have different genetic changes supporting their malignant behavior.

Antisense gene therapy is designed to block the expression of pro-oncogenic proteins. A molecule with a gene encoding a nucleotide sequence complementary to the target tumor gene is introduced into the tumor cell with a viral vector; the transcript of the transfected gene binds to the target gene mRNA and impedes protein translation (Yung 1994; Alama et al. 1997). Preclinical studies of this strategy in an animal models of non CNS tumors have targeted the K-*ras* oncogene with mixed success (Aoki et al. 1997; Wickstrom 2001). Problems with this technique include poor stability of antisense oligonucleotides.

Gene therapy remains an exciting prospect for future development. The ability to target and disrupt not only genes that modulate tumor proliferation and survival, but also tumor angiogenesis and invasion all require further investigation. Vector design also requires substantial further development to overcome such challenges as poor transfection efficiency and risk of pathogenic infection. Importantly, the improved characterization of the genetics of childhood brain tumors will be critical as specific gene-therapy targets move closer to clinical trials.

14.6.8 Immunotherapy

The goal of immunologically directed anti-tumor therapy is to eradicate tumor cells either by stimulating host immunologic anti-tumor reactions, or by blocking tumor related local immunosuppression. Immunotherapy can be broadly divided into four categories: cytokine-based therapy, serotherapy, adoptive transfer (of activated lymphocytes), and active immunotherapy (i.e., tumor vaccines; Parney et al. 2000). Cytokine-based therapy is the systemic administration of immunomodulatory cytokines. A number of cytokines have shown anti-tumor activity in preclinical studies, including IL-2, IL-4, IFN-α, and TNF-α (Merchant et al. 1990; Lapena et al. 1991; Iwasaki et al. 1993; Kondo et al. 1994). Systemic administration of IL-2 at high doses did show anti-tumor effect in clinical trials, but was associated with substan-

tial toxicity, including cerebral edema (Rosenberg et al. 1987; Merchant et al. 1990). Clinical trials of other immunostimulatory cytokines have been disappointing, with minimal or no anti-tumor effect seen (reviewed in Parney et al. 2000).

Serotherapy utilizes anti-tumor antibodies, systemically or locally administered. Tenascin and gp240 are glioma antigens for which monoclonal antibodies have been developed and tested in clinical trials. Phase I/II clinical trials of I[131]-radiolabeled antibodies directed against tenascin and gp240 have shown promising early results with objective response rates up to 50% and modest prolongation of survival in adult patients (Riva et al. 1997; Bigner et al. 1998). EGFRvIII-directed monoclonal antibody therapy shows promise in pre-clinical studies (Mishima et al. 2001; Ohman et al. 2002; Mamot et al. 2003).

Adoptive transfer therapy, in which ex-vivo-activated lymphocytes are administered intratumorally, has been disappointing in clinical trials (Barba et al. 1989; Lillehei et al. 1991; Sankhla et al. 1995). Autologous tumor vaccines, one of the earliest forms of immunotherapy, have had equivocal benefit in clinical trials, but no clear benefit has been demonstrated (Bloom et al. 1973; Mahaley et al. 1983). Gene-therapy techniques have recently been incorporated into tumor vaccine development. Here, immunostimulatory genes are transferred to target cells to enhance anti-tumor immune function. Animal studies have shown successful vaccination with GM-CSF (a pro-inflammatory cytokine) transduced melanoma cells, resulting in resistance to repeat tumor challenge (Sampson et al. 1996; Yu et al. 1997). An anti-sense strategy to block glioma-derived local immunosuppressant cytokines has also been used successfully with anti-tumor effect in animal models. Many other immunotherapeutic strategies are under investigation, including local or intratumoral infusion of pro-inflammatory cytokines, and dendritic cell therapy, which involves the genetic manipulation of these antigen-presenting cells to stimulate host cytotoxic T cells (reviewed in Parney et al. 2000). Although relatively few immunotherapies have entered pediatric clinical trials, ongoing research in this field carries future promise.

14.7 Conclusion

While prognosis for malignant brain tumors of childhood has improved somewhat in the past decades, 5-year survival for all tumors except low-grade astrocytoma remains suboptimal at 60%. The incorporation of chemotherapy into pediatric brain tumor management has allowed for advances in survival and reduction of morbidity, and is now the standard of care for many childhood brain tumors. Critical to the further improvement of prognosis and long-term outcome is the continued effort of multi-institutional, cooperative group clinical trials. The largest clinical trials group conducting pediatric brain-tumor trials is the National Cancer Institute (NCI)-sponsored Children's Oncology Group (COG). The COG includes the majority of pediatric cancer treatment centers in the United States, and incorporates programs in Canada, Europe, and Australia. Research activities include clinical trials for the majority of newly diagnosed and recurrent brain tumors, as well as studies of new agents. To further expedite the development of new agents for pediatric patients with high-risk brain tumors, the NCI established the Pediatric Brain Tumor Consortium (PBTC), with the goal of bringing novel agents and translational research to the pediatric brain tumor community. Information on the COG and the PBTC can be found on the internet at *www.childrensoncologygroup.org* and *www.pbtc.org*.

References

Alama AB, Cagnoli F, Schettini G (1997) Antisense oligonucleotides as therapeutic agents. Pharmacol Res 36:171–178

Allen JC, Gosl G, Walker R (1985) Chemotherapy trials in recurrent primary intracranial germ cell tumors. J Neurooncol 3:147–152

Aoki K, Yoshida T, Matsumoto N et al (1997) Suppression of Ki-ras p21 levels leading to growth inhibition of pancreatic cancer cell lines with Ki-ras mutation but not those without Ki-ras mutation. Mol Carcinog 20:251–258

Ashley DM, Meier L, Kerby T et al (1996) Response of recurrent medulloblastoma to low-dose oral etoposide. J Clin Oncol 14:1922–1927

Ater JL, Van Eys J, Woo SY et al (1997) MOPP chemotherapy without irradiation as a primary postsurgical therapy for brain tumors in infants and young children. J Neurooncology 32:243–252

Balis FM, Holcenberg JS, Blaney S (2000) General principles of chemotherapy. In: Pizzo PA (ed, Polack DG) Principles and practice of pediatric oncology. Lippincott, Williams and Wilkins, Philadelphia, pp 237–308

Barba D, Saris SC, Holder C et al (1989) Intratumoral LAK cell and interleukin-2 therapy of human gliomas. J Neurosurg 70:175–182

Bashir R, Hochberg FH, Linggood RM et al (1988) Preirradiation internal carotid artery BCNU in treatment of glioblastoma multiforme. J Neurosurg 68:917

Bertolone SJ, Baum ES, Krivit W, Hammond GD (1989) A phase II study of cisplatin therapy in recurrent childhood brain tumors. A report from the Children's Cancer Study Group. J Neurooncol 7:5–11

Bicknell R, Harris AL (1996) Mechanisms and therapeutic implications of angiogenesis. Curr Opin Oncol 8:60–65

Bigner DD, Brown MT, Friedman AH et al (1998) Iodine-131-labeled anti-tenascin monoclonal antibody 81C6 treatment of patients with recurrent malignant glioma. J Clin Oncol 16:2202–2212

Bloom HJ, Peckham MJ, Richardson AE et al (1973) Glioblastoma multiforme: a controlled trial to assess the value of specific active immunotherapy in patients treated by radical surgery and radiotherapy. Br J Cancer 27:253–267

Bobo RH, Laske DW, Akbasak A et al (1994) Convection-enhanced delivery of macromolecules in the brain. Proc Natl Acad Sci USA 91:2076–2080

Bouffet E, Foreman N (1999) Chemotherapy for intracranial ependymomas. Childs Nerv Syst 15:563–570

Bouffet E, Khelfaoui F, Philip I et al (1997) High dose carmustine for high grade gliomas in childhood. Cancer Chemother Pharmacol 39:376–379

Bouffet E, Raquin M, Doz F et al (2000) Radiotherapy followed by high dose busulfan and thiotepa: a prospective assessment of high dose chemotherapy in children with diffuse pontine gliomas. Cancer 88:685–692

Brem H, Piantadosi S, Burger PC (1995) Placebo-controlled trial of safety and efficacy of intraoperative controlled delivery by biodegradable polymers of chemotherapy for recurrent gliomas. The Polymer-brain Tumor treatment group. Lancet 345:1008–1012

Burger P, Komenar I, Schold S (1981) Encephalomyelopathy following high-dose BCNU therapy. Cancer 48:1318

Busca A, Miniero R, Besenzon L et al (1997) Etoposide-containing regimens with autologous bone marrow transplantation in children with malignant brain tumors. Childs Nerv Syst 13:572–577

Byrne J, Mulvihill JJ, Myers MH et al (1987) Effects of treatment on fertility in long-term survivors of childhood or adolescent cancer. N Engl J Med 317:1315–1321

Chamberlain M (2001) Recurrent intracranial ependymoma in children: salvage therapy with oral etoposide. Pediatr Neurol 24:117–121

Chamberlain MC, Kormanik PA (1997) Chronic oral VP-16 for recurrent medulloblastoma. Pediatr Neurol 17:230–234

Chang SM, Kuhn JG, Robins HI et al (1999) Phase II study of phenylacetate in patients with recurrent malignant glioma: a North American Brain Tumor Consortium report. J Clin Oncol 17:984–990

Chauncey T (2001) Drug resistance mechanisms in acute leukemia. Curr Opin Oncol 13:21–26

Cheney IW, Johnson DE, Vaillancourt MT et al (1998) Suppression of tumorigenicity of glioblastoma cells by adenovirus-mediated MMC1/PTEN gene transfer. Cancer Res 58:2331–2334

Chou PM, Barquin N, Gonzalez-Crussi F et al (1996) Ependymomas in children express the multidrug resistance gene: immunohistochemical and molecular biologic study. Pediatr Pathol Lab Med 16:551–561

Chou PM, Reyes-Mugica M, Barquin N et al (1995) Multidrug resistance gene expression in childhood medulloblastoma: correlation with clinical outcome and DNA ploidy in 29 patients. Pediatr Neurosurg 23:291–292

Cogen PH, McDonald JD (1996) Tumor suppressor genes and medulloblastoma. J Neurooncol 29:103–112

Culver KW, Ram Z, Wallbridge S et al (1992) In vivo gene transfer with retroviral vector-producer cells for treatment of experimental brain tumors. Science 256:1550–1552

D'Amato R (1994) Thalidomide is an inhibitor of angiogenesis. Proc Natl Acad Sci USA 91:4082–4085

Dean RL, Emerich DF, Hasler BP et al (1999) Cereport (RMP-7) increases carboplatin levels in brain tumors after pretreatment with dexamethasone. Neurooncology 1:268–274

Debinski W, Gibo DM, Hulet SW et al (1999) Receptor for interleukin 13 is a marker and therapeutic target for human high grade gliomas. Clin Cancer Res 5:985–990

Decleves X, Fajac A, Lehmann-Che J et al (2002) Molecular and functional MDR1-Pgp and MRPs expression in human glioblastoma multiforme cell lines. Int J Cancer 98:173–180

Drevs J, Laus C, Medinger M et al (2002) Antiangiogenesis: current clinical data and future perspectives. Onkologie 25:520–527

Duffner PK, Horowitz ME, Krischer JP et al (1993) Postoperative chemotherapy and delayed irradiation in children less than three years of age with malignant brain tumors. N Engl J Med 328:1725–1731

Duffner PK, Horowitz ME, Krischer JP et al (1999) The treatment of malignant brain tumor in infants and very young children: an update of the Pediatric Oncology Group experience. Neurooncology 1:152–161

Duffner PK, Krischer JP, Horowitz ME et al (1998) Second malignancies in young children with primary brain tumors following treatment with prolonged postoperative chemotherapy and delayed irradiation: a Pediatric Oncology Group Study. Ann Neurol 44:313–316

Dufful SB, Robinson BA (1997) Clinical pharmacokinetics and dose optimisation of carboplatin. Clin Pharmacokinet 33:161–183

Dunkel IJ, Finlay JL (2002) High-dose chemotherapy with autologous stem cell rescue for brain tumors. Crit Rev Oncol Hematol 41:197–204

Dunkel IJ, Boyett JM, Yates A, et al (1998a) High-dose carbolatin, thiotepa, and etoposide with autologous stem-cell rescue for patients with recurrent medulloblastoma. Children's Cancer Group. J Clin Oncol 16:222–228

Dunkel IJ, Boyett JM, Yates A et al (1998b) High dose chemotherapy with autologous bone marrow rescue for children with diffuse pontine brain stem tumors. Children's Cancer Group. J Neurooncol 37:67–73

Eilber F, Giuliano A, Eckardt J et al (1987) Adjuvant chemotherapy for osteosarcoma: a randomized prospective trial. J Clin Oncol 5:21–26

Einhorn L (1991) Daily oral etoposide in the treatment of cancer. Semin Oncol 18 [Suppl 2]:42–47

Fine HA, Figg WD, Jaeckle K et al (2000) Phase II trial of the antiangiogenic agent thalidomide in patients with recurrent high-grade gliomas. J Clin Oncol 18:708–715

Finlay JL, Boyett JM, Yates AJ et al (1995) Randomized phase III trial in childhood high-grade astrocytoma comparing vincristine, lomustine and prednisone with the eight-drugs-in-one-day regimen. J Clin Oncol 13:112–123

Finlay JL, Goldman S, Wong MC et al (1996) Pilot study of high-dose thiotepa and etoposide with autologous bone marrow rescue in children and young adults with recurrent CNS tumors. The Children's Cancer Group. J Clin Oncol 14:2495–2503

Folkman J (1971) Tumor angiogenesis: therapeutic implications. N Engl J Med 285:1182–1186

Friedman HS, Mahaley MS, Schold SC et al (1986) Efficacy of vincristine and cyclophosphamide in the therapy of recurrent medulloblastoma. Neurosurgery 18:335–340

Friedman HS, Kokkinakis DM, Pluda J et al (1998) Phase I trial of O^6-benzylguanine for patients undergoing surgery for malignant glioma. J Clin Oncol 16:3570–3575

Friedman HS, Kerby T, Calvert H (2000) Temozolomide and treatment of malignant glioma. Clin Cancer Res 6:2585–2597

Fulton D, Urtasun R, Forsyth P (1996) Phase II study of pro-longed oral therapy with etoposide (VP16) for patients with recurrent malignant glioma. J Neurooncol 27:149–155

Gaynon PS, Ettinger LJ, Baum, ES et al (1990) Carboplatin in childhood brain tumors. A Children's Cancer Study Group Phase II trial. Cancer 66:2465–2469

Geyer JR, Zeltzer PM, Boyett JM et al (1994) Survival of infants with primitive neuroectodermal tumors or malignant ependymomas of the CNS treated with eight drugs in 1 day: a report from the Children's Cancer Group. J Clin Oncol 12:1607–1615

Glade-Bender J, Kandel JJ, Yamashiro DJ (2003) VEGF blocking therapy in the treatment of cancer. Exp Opin Biol Ther 3:236–276

Graham ML, Herndon JE 2nd, Casey JR et al (1997) High-dose chemotherapy with autologous stem-cell rescue in patients with recurrent and high-risk pediatric brain tumors. J Clin Oncol 15:1814–1823

Grovas AC, Boyett JM, Lindsley K et al (1999) Regimen-related toxicity of myeloablative chemotherapy with BCNU, thiotepa, and etoposide followed by autologous stem cell rescue for children with newly diagnosed glioblastoma multiforme: report from the Children's Cancer Group. Med Pediatr Oncol 33:83–87

Gururangan S, Dunkel IF, Goldman S et al (1998) Myeloablative chemotherapy with autologous bone marrow rescue in young children with recurrent malignant brain tumors. J Clin Oncol 16:2486–2493

Hande K (1998) Etoposide: four decades of development of a topoisomerase II inhibitor. Eur J Cancer 34:1514–1521

Heideman RL, Douglass EC, Krance RA et al (1993) High-dose chemotherapy and autologous bone marrow rescue followed by interstitial and external-beam radiotherapy in newly diagnosed pediatric malignant gliomas. J Clin Oncol 11:1458–1465

Hochberg FH, Parker LM, Takvorian T (1981) High-dose BCNU with autologous bone marrow rescue for recurrent glioblastoma multiforme. J Neurosurg 54:455–460

Hongeng S, Brent TP, Sanford RA et al (1997) O^6-Methylguanine-DNA methyltransferase protein levels in pediatric brain tumors. Clin Cancer Res 3:2459–2463

Hsiao M, Tse V, Carmel J et al (1997) Intracavitary liposome-mediated p53 gene transfer into glioblastoma with endogenous wild-type p53 in vivo results in tumor suppression and long term survival. Biochem Biophys Res Commun 233:359–364

Iwasaki K, Rogers LR, Estes ML et al (1993) Modulation of proliferation and antigen expression of a cloned human glioblastoma by interleukin-4 alone and in combination with tumor necrosis factor-a and/or interferon-g. Neurosurgery 33:489–494

Jaeckle KA, Eyre HJ, Townsend JJ et al (1998) Correlation of tumor O^6-methylguanine-DNA methyltransferase levels with survival of malignant astrocytoma patients treated with bischoloroethylnitrosourea: a Southwest Oncology Group study. J Clin Oncol 16:3310–3315

Jaeckle KA, Hess KR, Yung WK et al (2003) Phase II evaluation of temozolomide and 13-cis-retinoic acid for the treatment of recurrent and progressive malignant glioma: a North American Brain Tumor Consortium study. J Clin Oncol 21:2305–2311

Joki T, Heese O, Nikas DC et al (2000) Expression of cyclooxygenase 2 (COX-2) in human glioma and in vitro inhibition by a specific COX-2 inhibitor, HS-398. Cancer Res 60:4926

Jordan M (2002) Mechanism of action of antitumor drugs that interact with microtubules and tubulin. Curr Med Chem Anti Cancer Agents 2:1–17

Jorg TH, Hans-Peter L (2003) Expert opinion on pharmacotherapy. Toxicity Platinum Compounds 4:889–901

Kellie SJ, Barbaric D, Koopmans P et al (2002) Cerebrospinal fluid concentrations of vincristine after bolus intravenous dosing: a surrogate marker of brain penetration. Cancer 94:1815–1820

Kenyon BM, Browne F, D'Amato RJ (1997) Effects of thalidomide and related metabolites in a mouse corneal model of neovascularization. Exp Eye Res 64:971–978

Klement G, Baruchel S, Rak J et al (2000) Continuous low dose therapy with vinblastine and VEGF receptor 2 antibody induces sustained tumor regression without overt toxicity. J Clin Invest 105:15–24

Kobrinsky N, Packer RJ, Boyett JM et al (1999) Etoposide with or without mannitol for the treatment of recurrent of primarily unresponsive brain tumors: a Children's Cancer Group Study. J Neurooncol 45:47–54

Koga H, Zhang S, Kumanishi T et al (1994) Analysis of p53 mutations in low-and high-grade astrocytomas by polymerase chain reaction assisted single strand conformation polymorphism and immunohistochemistry. Acta Neuropathol (Berl) 83:225–232

Kokunai T, Kawamura A, Tamaki N (1997) Induction of differentiation by wild-type p53 gene in a human glioma cell line. J Neurooncol 32:125–133

Kondo S, Yin D, Takeuchi J et al (1994) Tumor necrosis factor-a induces an increase in susceptibility of human glioblastoma U87MG cells to natural killer cell-mediated lysis. Br J Cancer 69:627–632

Kortmann RD, Kuhl J, Timmermann B et al (2000) Postoperative neoadjuvant chemotherapy before radiotherapy as compared to immediate radiotherapy followed by maintenance chemotherapy in the treatment of medulloblastoma in childhood: results of the German prospective randomized trial HIT'91. Int J Radiat Oncol Biol 46:269–279

Kushner BK, Cheung NK (1999) Oral etoposide for refractory and relapsed neuroblastoma. J Clin Oncol 17:3221–3225

Lang FF, Bruner JM, Fuller GN et al (2003) Phase I trial of adenovirus-mediated p53 gene therapy for recurrent glioma: biological and clinical results. J Clin Oncol 21:2508–2518

Lapena P, Isasi C, Vaquero J et al (1991) Modulation by interferon-a of the decreased natural killer activity in patients with glioblastoma. Acta Neurochir (Wein) 109:109–113

Laske DW, Youle RJ, Oldfield EH (1997) Tumor regression with regional distribution of the targeted toxin TF-CRM 107 in patients with malignant brain tumors. Nature Med 12:1362–1368

Levin VA, Lamborn K, Wara W et al (2000) Phase II study of 6-thioguanine, procarbazine, dibromodulcitol, lomustine, and vincristine chemotherapy with radiotherapy for treating malignant glioma in children. Neurooncology 2:22–28

Li J, Yen C, Liaw D et al (1997) PTEN, a putative protein tyrosine phosphatase gene mutated in human brain, breast, and prostate cancer. Science 275:1943–1947

Li Y, Millikan RC, Carozza S et al (1998) p53 mutations in malignant gliomas. Cancer Epidemiol Biomarkers Prev 7:303–308

Lillehei KO, Mitchell DH, Johnson SD et al (1991) Long-term follow-up of patients with recurrent malignant gliomas treated with adjuvant adoptive immunotherapy. Neurosurgery 28:16–23

Link MP, Goorin AM, Miser AW et al (1986) The effect of adjuvant chemotherapy on relapse-free survival in patients with osteosarcoma of the extremity. N Engl J Med 314:1600–1606

Longee DC, Friedman HS, Albright RE Jr et al (1990) Treatment of patients with recurrent gliomas with cyclophosphamide and vincristine. J Neurooncol 72:583–588

Mahaley MS, Bigner DD, Dudka LF et al (1983) Immunobiology of primary intracranial tumors, part 7. Active immunization of patients with anaplastic human glioma cells: a pilot study. J Neurosurg 59:201–207

Mahaley MS Jr, Hipp SW, Dropcho EJ et al (1989) Intracarotid cisplatin chemotherapy for recurrent gliomas. J Neurosurg 70:371

Mahoney DH Jr, Strother D, Camitta B et al (1996) High-dose melphalan and cyclophosphamide with autologous bone marrow rescue for recurrent/progressive malignant brain tumors in children: a pilot Pediatric Oncology Group study. J Clin Oncol 14:382–388

Mahoney DH Jr, Cohen ME, Friedman HS et al (2000) Carboplatin is effective therapy for young children with progressive optic pathway tumors: a Pediatric Oncology Group phase II study. Neurooncology 2:213–230

Mamot C, Drummond DC, Greiser U et al (2003) Epidermal Growth Factor Receptor (EGFR)-targeted immunoliposomes mediate specific and efficient drug delivery to EGFR- and EGFRvIII-overexpressing tumor cells. Cancer Res 63:3154–3161

Mason WP, Goldman S, Yates AJ et al (1998) Survival following intensive chemotherapy with bone marrow reconstitution for children with recurrent intracranial ependymoma – a report of the Children's Cancer Group. J Neurooncol 37:135–143

Matthay KK, Villablanca JG, Seeger RC et al (1999) Treatment of high-risk neuroblastoma with intensive chemotherapy, radiotherapy, autologous bone marrow transplantation, and 13-cis-retinoic acid. N Engl J Med 341:1165–1173

Mathew P, Ribeiro RC, Sonnichsen D et al (1994) Phase I study of oral etoposide in children with refractory solid tumors. J Clin Oncol 12:1452–1457

Merchant RE, Ellison ED, Young HF (1990) Immunotherapy for malignant glioma using human recombinant interleukin-2 and activated autologous lymphocytes. J Neurooncol 8:173–188

Middleton M (2003) Improvement of chemotherapy efficacy by inactivation of a DNA-repair pathway. Lancet Oncol 4:37–44

Miettinen S, Laurikainen E, Johansson R et al (1997) Radiotherapy enhanced ototoxicity of cisplatin in children. Acta Otolaryngol [Suppl] 529:90–94

Mishima K, Johns TG, Luwor RB et al (2001) Growth suppression of intracranial xenografted glioblastomas overexpressing mutant epidermal growth factor receptors by systemic administration of monoclonal antibody (mAb) 806, a novel monoclonal antibody directed to the receptor. Cancer Res 61:5349–5354

Mukherjee P, Das SK (1990) Antiproliferative action of retinoic acid in cultured human brain tumour cells G1-As-14(S). Cancer Lett 52:83–80

Mulhern RK, Palmer SL, Reddick WE et al (2001) Risks of young age for selected neurocognitive deficits in medulloblastoma are associated with white matter loss. J Clin Oncol 19:472–479

Needle MN, Molloy PT, Geyer JR et al (1997) Phase II study of daily oral etoposide in children with recurrent brain tumors and other solid tumors. Med Pediatr Oncol 29:28–32

Neuwelt EA, Diehl JT, Vu LH et al (1981) Monitoring of methotrexate delivery in patients with malignant brain tumors after osmotic blood-brain barrier disruption. Ann Intern Med 94:449–454

Neuwelt EA, Specht HD, Howieson J et al (1983) Osmotic blood-brain barrier modification: clinical documentation by enhanced CT scanning and/or radionuclide brain scanning. Am J Roentgenol 4:907–913

Newlands ES, Stevens MF, Wedge SR et al (1997) Temozolomide: a review of its discovery, chemical properties, pre-clinical development and clinical trials. Cancer Treat Rev 23:35–61

Newton HB, Page MA, Junck L et al (1989) Intra-arterial cisplatin for the treatment of malignant gliomas. J Neurooncol 7:39

Newton HB, Turowski RC, Stroup TJ et al (1999) Clinical presentation, diagnosis, and pharmacotherapy of patients with primary brain tumors. Ann Pharmacother 33:816–832

Nicholson HS, Krailo M, Ames MM et al (1998) Phase I study of temozolomide in children and adolescents with recurrent solid tumors: a report from the Children's Cancer Group. J Clin Oncol 16:3037–3043

Ohman L, Gedda L, Hesselager G et al (2002) A new antibody recognizing the vIII mutation of human epidermal growth factor receptor. Tumour Biol 23:61–69

Ortega JA, Rivard GE, Isaacs H et al (1975) The influence of chemotherapy on the prognosis of rhabdomyosarcoma. Med Pediatr Oncol 1:227–234

Packer RJ (2002) Radiation-induced neurocognitive decline: the risks and benefits of reducing the amount of whole-brain irradiation. Curr Neurol Neurosci Rep 2:131–133

Packer RJ, Sutton LN, Goldwein JW et al (1991) Improved survival with the use of adjuvant chemotherapy in the treatment of medulloblastoma. J Neurosurg 74:433–440

Packer RJ, Sutton LN, Elterman R et al (1994) Outcome for children with medulloblastoma treated with radiation and cisplatin, CCNU, and vincristine chemotherapy. J Neurosurg 81:690–698

Packer RJ, Ater J, Allen J et al (1997) Carboplatin and vincristine chemotherapy for children with newly diagnosed progressive low-grade gliomas. J Neurosurg 86:747–754

Packer RJ, Goldwein J, Nicholson HS et al (1999) Treatment of children with medulloblastomas with reduced-dose craniospinal radiation therapy and adjuvant chemotherapy: a Children's Cancer Group study. J Clin Oncol 17:2127–2136

Packer RJ, Raffel C, Villablanca JG et al (2000) Treatment of progressive or recurrent pediatric malignant supratentorial brain tumors with herpes simplex virus thymidine kinase gene vector-producer cells followed by intravenous ganciclovir administration. J Neurosurg 92:249–254

Paku S (1998) Current concepts of tumor-induced angiogenesis. Pathol Oncol Res 4:62–75

Papadopoulos KP, Garvin JH, Fetell M et al (1998) High-dose thiotepa and etoposide-based regimens with autologous hematopoietic support for high-risk or recurrent CNS tumor in children and adults. Bone Marrow Transplant 7:661–667

Parney I, Hao C, Petruk K (2000) Glioma immunology and immunotherapy. Neurosurgery 46:778–791

Pegg A (1990) Regulation and importance in response to alkylating carcinogenic and therapeutic agents. Cancer Res 50:6119–6129

Pegg AE, Byers T (1992) Repair of DNA containing O^6-alkylguanine. FASEB J 6:2302–2310

Pluda JM (1997) Tumor-associated angiogenesis: mechanisms, clinical implications, therapeutic strategies. Semin Oncol 24:203–218

Pollack IF, Boyett JM, Finlay J (1999) Chemotherapy for high-grade gliomas of childhood. Childs Nerv Syst 15:529–544

Prados MD, Edwards MS, Rabbit J (1997) Treatment of pediatric low grade gliomas with a nitrosourea-based multiagent chemotherapy regimen. J Neurooncol 32:235–241

Prados MD, Schold SC Jr, Fine HA et al (2003) A randomized, double-blind placebo-controlled, phase 2 study of RMP-7 in combination with carboplatin administered intravenously for the treatment of recurrent malignant glioma. Neurooncology 5:96–103

Pratt WB, Ruddon RW, Ensminger WD et al (1994) The anticancer drugs. Oxford University Press, New York

Rall D, Zubrod C (1962) Mechanisms of drug absorption and excretion: passage of drugs in and out of the central nervous system. Annu Rev Pharmacol 2:109–128

Rasheed BK, Stenzel TT, McLendon RE et al (1997) PTEN gene mutations are seen in high-grade but not in low-grade gliomas. Cancer Res 57:4187–4190

Riva P, Franceschi G, Arista A et al (1997) Local application of radiolabeled monoclonal antibodies in the treatment of high grade malignant gliomas: a six-year clinical experience. Cancer 80:2733–2742

Rodts GE, Black KL (1994) Trans retinoic acid inhibits in vivo tumor growth of C6 glioma in rats: effect negatively influenced by nerve growth factor. Neurol Res 16:184–186

Rosen G (1986) Neoadjuvant chemotherapy for osteogenic sarcoma: a model for the treatment of other highly malignant neoplasms. Rec Res Cancer Res 103:148–157

Rosenberg SA, Lotze MD, Muul ML et al (1987) A progress report on the treatment of 157 patients with advanced cancer using lymphokine-activated killer cells and interleukin-2 or high dose interleukin-2 alone. N Engl J Med 316:889–897

Sampson JH, Archer GE, Ashley DM et al (1996) Subcutaneous vaccination with irradiated, cytokine-producing tumor cells located in the "immunologically privileged" central nervous system. Proc Natl Acad Sci USA 93:10399–10404

Sankhla SK, Nadkarni JS, Bhagwati SN (1995) Adoptive immunotherapy using lymphokine-activated (LAK) cells and interleukin-w for recurrent malignant primary brain tumors. J Neurooncol 27:133–140

Schinkel AH, Smit JJ, van Tellingen O et al (1994) Disruption of the Mouse mdr 1a P-glycoprotein gene leads to a deficiency in the blood brain barrier and to increased sensitivity to drugs. Cell 77:491–502

Sexauer CL, Khan A, Burger PC et al (1985) Cisplatin in recurrent pediatric brain tumors. A POG Phase II study. A Pediatric Oncology Group Study. Cancer 56:1497–1501

Siffert J, Allen JC (2000) Late effects of therapy of thalamic and hypothalamic tumors in childhood: vascular, neurobehavioral and neoplastic. Pediatr Neurosurg 33:105–111

Sikic BI, Fisher GA, Lum BL et al (1997) Modulation and prevention of multidrug resistance by inhibitors of P-glycoprotein. Cancer Chemotherapy Pharmacology 40 [Suppl]:13–19

Skov K, MacPhail S (1991) Interaction of platinum drugs with clinically relevant x-ray doses in mammalian cells: a comparison of cisplatin, carboplatin, iproplatin, and tetraplatin. Int J Radiat Oncol Biol 20:221–225

Smith MA, Rubinstein L, Anderson JR et al (1999) Secondary leukemia or myelodysplastic syndrome after treatment with epipodophyllotoxins. J Clin Oncol 17:569–577

Sposto R, Ertel IJ, Jenkin RD et al (1989) The effectiveness of chemotherapy for treatment of high grade astrocytoma in children; results of a randomized trial. A report from the Children's Cancer Study Group. J Neurooncol 7:165–177

Spoudeas HA, Charmandari E, Brook CG (2003) Hypothalamo-pituitary-adrenal axis integrity after cranial irradiation for childhood posterior fossa tumours. Med Pediatr Oncol 40:224–229

Stewart D (1994) A critique of the role of the blood-brain barrier in the chemotherapy of human brain tumors. J Neurooncol 20:121–139

Stupp R, Dietrich PY, Ostermann Kraljevic S et al (2002) Promising survival for patients with newly diagnosed glioblastoma multiforme treated with concomitant radiation plus temozolomide followed by adjuvant temozolomide. J Clin Oncol 20:1375–1382

Tada T, Takizawa T, Nakazato F et al (1999) Treatment of intracranial nongerminomatous germ-cell tumor by high-dose chemotherapy and autologous stem-cell rescue. J Neurooncol 44:71–76

Tamura M, Gu J, Matsumoto K, Aota S, Parsons R, Yamada KM (1998) Inhibition of cell migration, spreading and focal adhesions by tumor suppressor gene PTEN. Science 280:1614–1617

Taylor RE, Bailey CC, Robinson K et al (2003) Results of a randomized study of preradiation chemotherapy versus radiotherapy alone for nonmetastatic medulloblasotma: the International Society of Paediatric Oncology/United Kingdom Children's Cancer Study Group PNET-3 study. J Clin Oncol 21:1581–1591

Trimble EL, Ungerleider RS, Abrams JA et al (1993) Neoadjuvant therapy in cancer treatment. Cancer 72:3515–3524

Valtonen S, Timonen U, Toivanen P et al (1997) Interstitial chemotherapy with carmustine-loaded polymers for high-grade gliomas: a randomized double-blind study. Neurosurgery 41:44–48

Viola JJ, Martuza RL (1996) Gene therapies for glioblastomas. Bailleres Clin Neurol 5:413–424

Von Bossanyi P, Diete S, Dietzmann K et al (1997) Immunohistochemical expression of P-glycoprotein and glutathione S-transferases in cerebral gliomas and response to chemotherapy. Acta Neuropathol (Berl) 94:605–611

Von Deimling A, Louis DN, Wiestler OD (1995) Molecular pathways in the formation of gliomas. Glia 15:328–338

Walker RW, Allen JC (1988) Cisplatin in the treatment of recurrent childhood primary brain tumors. J Clin Oncol 6:62–66

White L, Kellie S, Gray E et al (1998) Postoperative chemotherapy in children less that 4 years of age with malignant brain tumors: promising initial response to a VETOPEC-based regimen. A Study of the Australian and New Zealand Children's Cancer Study Group. J Pediatr Hematol Oncol 20:125–130

Wickstrom E (2001) Oligonucleotide treatment of ras induced tumors in nude mice. Mol Biotechnol 18:35–55

Wiestler O, Kleihues P, Pegg AE (1984) O^6-Alkylguanine-DNA alkyltransferase activity in human brain and brain tumors. Carcinogenesis 5:121–124

Wilkins DE, Heller DP, Raaphorst GP (1993) Inhibition of potentially lethal damage recovery by cisplatin in a brain tumor cell line. Anticancer Res 13:2137–2142

Young SW, Quing F, Harriman A et al (1996) Gadolinium (III) texaphyrin: a tumor selective radiation sensitizer that is detectable by MRI. Proc Natl Acad Sci USA 93:6610–6615

Yu JS, Burwick JA, Dranoff G et al (1997) Gene therapy for metastatic brain tumor by vaccination with granulocyte-macrophage colony-stimulating factor-transduced tumor cells. Hum Gene Ther 8:1065–1072

Yung W (1994) New approaches in brain tumor therapy using gene transfer and antisense oligonucleotides. Curr Opin Oncol 6:171–178

Yung WK, Kyritsis AP, Gleason MJ et al (1996) Treatment of recurrent malignant gliomas with high-dose 13-cis-retinoic acid. Clin Cancer Res 2:1931–1935

Zeltzer PM, Boyett JM, Finlay JL et al (1999) Metastasis stage, adjuvant treatment, and residual tumor are prognostic factors for medulloblastoma in children: conclusions from the Children's Cancer Group 921 randomized phase III study. J Clin Oncol 17:832–845

Zwelling LA, Kohn KW (1979) Mechanism of action of cis-dichlorodiammineplatinum(II). Cancer Treatment Rep 63:1439–1444

Advances in Radiation Therapy

D. Haas-Kogan · B. M. Frisch

Contents

15.1 Introduction

Despite the known effects of ionizing radiation on the nervous system, most children with brain tumors will receive radiation therapy at some point during treatment. As advances in neurosurgery, chemotherapy, and radiotherapy enter clinical practice, multimodality therapy has become the norm. For any given tumor, the incorporation of radiation therapy into such treatment must consider the timing of radiation, the most appropriate radiation modality, short- and long-term toxicities both for radiation alone and for radiation in conjunction with chemotherapy, and, finally, the integration of novel antineoplastic agents with radiation.

15.2 Radiobiology

The biologic effects of ionizing radiation primarily result from the formation of double-strand breaks in cellular DNA (Hall 2000). Although most radiation-induced single-strand DNA breaks are efficiently repaired, double-strand breaks cause irreparable damage, resulting in mitotic cell death. Photon radiation (x-ray or gamma ray) can cause damage by direct interaction with the DNA molecule, or indirectly by the formation of free radicals that then interact chemically with DNA leading to double-strand breaks. Charged particles such as helium, carbon, or neon predominantly cause damage by direct interactions. High-energy neutrons, although not charged, also interact with the nucleus of an atom, resulting in the creation of densely ionizing recoil protons, alpha particles, and nuclear fragments. Linear energy transfer

(LET) measures the average energy deposited in tissue per unit distance traveled by a particle or photon. While conventional radiation is sparsely ionizing (low LET), fast neutrons and heavy particles are more densely ionizing (high LET) (Hall 2000).

Tissue oxygenation influences the response of tumors and normal tissues to ionizing radiation (Brown and Giaccia 1994; Brown 1999). Poorly oxygenated tissues are two to three times more resistant to radiation compared to normally oxygenated tissue. Oxygen is thought to mediate indirect damage, combining with free radicals to make DNA damage irreversible. The effect of tissue oxygenation is measured by the oxygen enhancement ratio (OER). This is the ratio of doses under hypoxic versus aerated conditions required to produce a given level of cell kill. As LET increases, the magnitude of the OER decreases (Hall 2000).

Radiation causes complex cascades of molecular events, affecting cell cycle check points, apoptosis, DNA damage response, and DNA repair. These effects offer many potential approaches to enhance radiation damage of tumor cells and to protect normal tissues. These techniques will be discussed further in this chapter.

15.3 Three-Dimensional Conformal Radiation Therapy

While radiation therapy plays a key role in the treatment of pediatric brain tumors, delivery of adequate therapy must always be balanced against potential treatment-related toxicity. As radiation therapy has evolved, treatment modalities have emerged that allow for more precise planning and delivery (Suit 2002). Advances in imaging technologies, including magnetic resonance imaging (MRI) and computed tomography (CT), have allowed better identification of both tumor and surrounding critical structures.

The development of three-dimensional conformal radiation therapy (3DCRT), and more recently, intensity modulated radiation therapy (IMRT), have allowed clinicians to decrease the doses delivered to critical structures while maintaining or increasing the dose to tumor (Weil 2001). While the concept of conformal therapy is not new, dramatic improvements in the power and availability of computers have allowed more complex treatment planning systems. The advent of other technical advances such as multi-leaf collimation (MLC), digitally reconstructed radiographs (DRRs), and electronic portal imaging has contributed to the integration of conformal radiation delivery. The planning process for 3DCRT is significantly more complex than for conventional radiation therapy and requires multiple well-coordinated steps.

15.3.1 Immobilization and Imaging

The initial step of the planning process is to place the patient in a reproducible position that optimizes treatment of the entire tumor volume while sparing surrounding critical structures. This position may be different for each individual patient, and is dependent upon the specific location, shape and size of the tumor, and areas at increased risk for suspected microscopic disease. A variety of customizable immobilization devices are available, including thermoplastic facemasks, alpha cradles, and vacuum bags. It is important to note that as a planned course of radiation therapy becomes increasingly conformal, the importance of reliable and reproducible immobilization becomes critical. Once the patient has been optimally and reproducibly positioned, localization marks are placed on the skin. With the patient in the treatment position, CT images are then obtained of the area of interest. These data are then transferred to the planning system, at which point the clinician can define target volumes as well as critical structures. While some well-defined structures can be contoured automatically, most structures must be defined manually. A pre-treatment CT scan is generally used for treatment planning, although other modalities such as MRI images can be co-registered with the CT data.

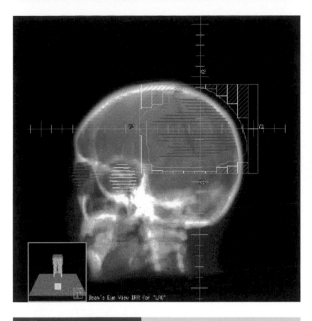

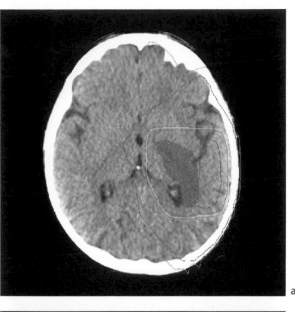

a

Figure 15.1

Beam's-eye view of a left anterior oblique field in a patient with a supratentorial primitive neuroectodermal tumor (PNET). (Courtesy of Clayton Akazawa, CMD, Department of Radiation Oncology, UCSF)

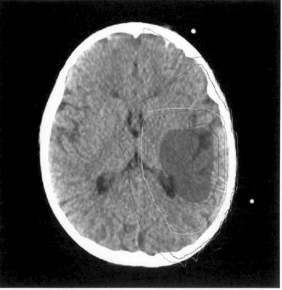

b

15.3.2 Target Definition and Planning

The CT images are analyzed jointly by radiation oncologists, diagnostic radiologists, and occasionally by other treating physicians such as medical oncologists and surgeons. The treatment volume is dictated by the natural history of the tumor. Gross tumor volume (GTV) is defined by physical exam and imaging studies and encompasses the macroscopic extent of the tumor. Clinical target volume (CTV) contains both the GTV and areas at risk for microscopic spread of disease. The planning target volume (PTV) is defined as the CTV surrounded by adequate margin to account for variation in patient position, organ motion, and other movement (Hall 2000; Purdy 1999).

Figure 15.2 a,b

Isodose curves of a 3-dimensional conformal plan on serial axial slices in a patient with a supratentorial primitive neuroectodermal tumor (PNET). The *red line* depicts the 99% isodose line, *light blue* represents 95%, *yellow* depicts 93%, *green* depicts 90%, *blue* depicts 60%, and *gold* depicts 50%. (Courtesy of Clayton Akazawa, CMD, Department of Radiation Oncology, UCSF) ▶

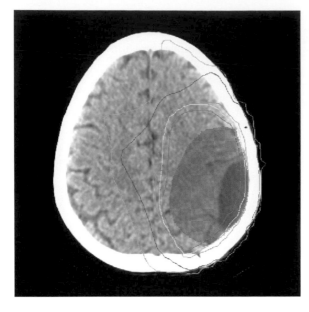

Figure 15.2 c

Isodose curves of a 3-dimensional conformal plan on serial axial slices in a patient with a supratentorial primitive neuroectodermal tumor (PNET). The *red line* depicts the 99% isodose line, *light blue* represents 95%, *yellow* depicts 93%, *green* depicts 90%, *blue* depicts 60%, and *gold* depicts 50%. (Courtesy of Clayton Akazawa, CMD, Department of Radiation Oncology, UCSF)

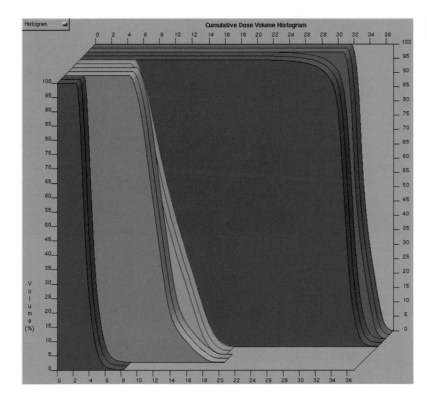

Figure 15.3

A dose–volume histogram for an intensity-modulated radiation therapy (IMRT) plan in a patient with a medulloblastoma. Clinical target volume (CTV) is depicted in *orange*, planning target volume (PTV) in *pink*, left ear in *turquoise*, right ear in *gold*, and optic chiasm in *dark blue*. (Courtesy of Pam Akazawa, CMD, Department of Radiation Oncology, UCSF)

Once target volumes and critical structures are defined, beam geometry and weighting are defined and dose distribution is calculated (Purdy 1999). Selection of beam angles can be done by referencing axial images or by use of beams-eye view (BEV; Fig. 15.1). BEV allows the visualization of the relationship of tumor volumes to those of critical normal tissues as if looking from the origin of the beam. This allows beam angles and beam shaping to be selected more intelligently. Once an initial plan has been developed, the resulting dose distributions are calculated and evaluated by the clinician. The plan can then be altered to improve on initial results, if necessary. The beam directions as well as their relative weights and shapes are modified to finally optimize the 3DCRT plan.

Plans are evaluated by viewing isodose curves on serial images of a CT scan (Fig. 15.2a–c), as well as by the generation of dose-volume histograms (DVHs; Fig. 15.3). DVHs can be generated for a tumor volume or other organs of interest, allowing the clinician to evaluate the dose delivered to the total volume. DVHs typically graph percent volume of a given tissue on the Y-axis and dose on the X-axis. This allows a clinician to visualize what percentage of a defined structure is receiving a given dose. This data allows plans to be modified as needed to either increase dose to tumor or decrease dose to a nearby critical structure.

15.3.3 Treatment Verification and Delivery

Once a satisfactory plan has been generated, DRRs corresponding to the planned radiation fields are generated. These DRRs typically display field shapes and tumor volumes as well as standard radiographic information, such as anatomy. These serve as templates for design of cut blocks. Alternately, block shape information can be transferred directly to the computer system that controls the MLC. Using a complex three-dimensional plan, an MLC allows for rapid change of field shape under computer control, dramatically shortening the time needed to treat a patient. Of note, studies have shown that dose distributions produced with MLC are equivalent to those with cut blocks.

A verification simulation can be performed to check the validity and accuracy of the fields. First-day portal films are also generated to confirm accuracy of patient positioning and beam angles. This can be done with conventional portal films or with the use of an electronic portal imaging device (EPID). Because there is no development time (as there is with conventional portal images), the use of an EPID can significantly shorten the time needed to take portal images of complex multi-field plans.

15.4 New Technical Approaches

15.4.1 Intensity Modulated Radiation Therapy

While 3DCRT allows for selection of beam shapes and angles to conform to a selected tumor volume, intensity modulated radiation therapy (IMRT) allows modulation of intensity within each given beam (Purdy 1999; Webb 2000). The initial form this approach took was the use of "beam within beam" planning with standard 3DCRT systems to treat static-shaped fields. The use of MLC makes this fairly easy to achieve. This process is typically referred to as "forward-planned" IMRT (Verhey 1999). More recently, a process called inverse planning has been developed. As with forward-planning, critical structures and tumor volumes are identified. The desired dose distribution is then defined, including desired tumor dose and maximum allowable dose to critical structures. The planning algorithm then computes a plan that attempts to achieve results compatible with the desired distribution. Optimization of inverse-planned plans requires adjustment of the dose parameters (Verhey 1999).

A number of techniques developed to deliver IMRT treatments have become commercially available in recent years. Most of these use MLCs to treat several static field shapes from each beam angle. Each MLC shape is referred to as a segment. Greater numbers of segments lead to longer treatment times. Other techniques include computer-controlled dynamic MLC, the use of custom compensators, and rotational therapy combined with dynamic MLC.

Using these techniques can result in dramatic dose gradients, allowing high doses to tumor, with rapid dose fall-off (Verhey 1999). An example of an IMRT

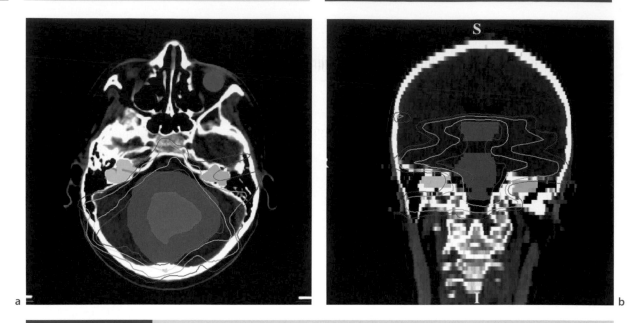

Figure 15.4 a,b

Axial (a) and coronal (b) images showing isodose curves for an intensity-modulated radiation therapy (IMRT) plan in a patient with medulloblastoma. The *blue line* depicts the 83% isodose line, *yellow* depicts 70%, *green* depicts 50%, and *red* depicts 40%. (Courtesy of Ping Xia, PhD, Department of Radiation Oncology, UCSF)

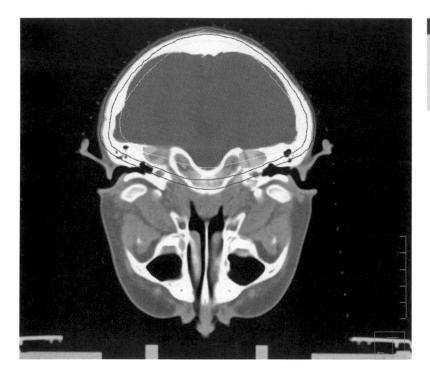

Figure 15.5 a

Comparison of axial sections planned with either 3DCRT (a) or IMRT (b), demonstrating the sparing of normal structures, most notably the inner ears

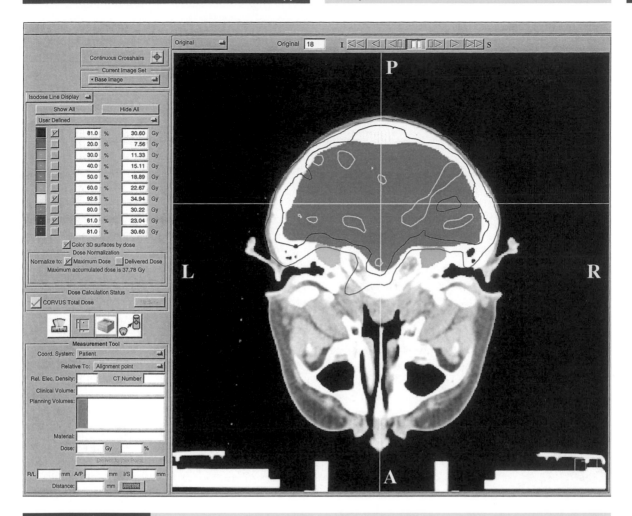

Figure 15.5b

Comparison of axial sections planned with either 3DCRT (a) or IMRT (b), demonstrating the sparing of inner structures achieved with IMRT without compromising the dose delivered to the target volume

plan is shown in Fig. 15.4. The rapid fall-off of dose must be considered when immobilization systems are being devised prior to treatment. Another issue that must be noted when IMRT is used is integral dose. With IMRT, the total number of monitor units delivered to the patient is higher than with conventional treatments. Due to an increase in dose inhomogeneity, more total dose is delivered. The long-term significance of this increased integral dose has

not yet been determined. Dose inhomogeneity also results in hot spots within the treated volume. Although these hot spots typically fall within the tumor volume, the significance of having regions of extremely high dose is unclear.

In the use of any of these conformal therapies, it is important to consider anatomy. Particularly in the use of inverse planning, if an area is not contoured as tumor, it will likely receive sub-optimal dose. Areas of subclinical disease must also be taken into account. Only through careful consideration of anatomy and dose can IMRT be safely applied. Figure 15.5 compares axial sections planned with either 3DCRT or IMRT, demonstrating the sparing of inner structures achieved with IMRT without compromise of the dose delivered to the target volume.

15.4.2 Proton Beam Therapy

Although proton radiation is not significantly more biologically effective than conventional radiation, it has physical characteristics that allow precise control of dose fall-off, especially beyond the target volume (Yang 1999). Specifically, a properly focused proton beam demonstrates rapid fall-off of delivered dose immediately beyond the target (a feature known as the "Bragg peak"). This allows for potential sparing of critical structures. It is conventionally accepted that proton beam therapy is superior to standard radiotherapy for skull base chondrosarcomas and chordomas, but its effectiveness compared to radiosurgery or conformal radiotherapy has not been tested rigorously.

15.4.3 Intraoperative Radiotherapy (IORT)

Intraoperative radiotherapy typically involves the delivery of a single large fraction of radiation therapy at the time of open surgery (Willett 2001). Radiation is most commonly given to the resection cavity using electrons. Depth of dose is controlled by choice of electron energy. Fall-off is rapid beyond the effective range of the selected electron energy.

15.4.4 Temporary or Permanent Brachytherapy

Interstitial brachytherapy allows for the delivery of high doses of radiation to a tumor region. Brachytherapy entails the placement of radiation sources either directly in tissues, or into catheters placed within tissues. As dose falls off with the square of the distance away from the radiation sources, and is further attenuated by tissue, normal structures can be spared (Hall 2000).

Temporary brachytherapy typically entails the implantation of catheters in the tumor or tumor bed. Following placement of catheters, radiation sources are loaded into the catheters to deliver the desired dose. Historically, a variety of radioactive sources, including radium and cesium have been used. In current practice an ^{192}Ir source is frequently used, utilizing a robotic remote afterloading system to minimize dose to medical personnel.

Permanent brachytherapy implants can also be performed. Radioactive sources are inserted into tumor tissue or placed in regions surrounding a resection cavity. Sources containing ^{125}I and ^{103}Pd are frequently used in clinical practice. Both of these approaches can allow delivery of a very high dose of radiation, while limiting dose to normal tissue.

A recent retrospective study reported a large series of pediatric brain tumors treated with ^{125}I brachytherapy (Sneed et al. 1996). Twenty-eight children were treated with temporary, high-activity ^{125}I brachytherapy for recurrent or persistent supratentorial, unifocal, well-circumscribed tumors less than 6 cm in diameter that had previously received external beam radiation therapy. Exclusion criteria included tumors with diffuse margins, corpus callosum involvement, or subependymal spread. The most useful information to come from this study is the documentation of acute and late toxicities. Outcome data, however, are less reliable given the variety of brain tumors included in the analysis. No grade 3 or grade 4 acute or late toxicities occurred. However, 22 patients (79% of 28 total patients) required at least one reoperation following brachytherapy and 17 of these 22 patients had evidence of necrosis in the resected specimen.

15.4.5 Radiosurgery

Conceptually, radiosurgery consists of multiple beams of radiation, all converging at the designated target volume. A Gamma Knife® with 201 collimated beams of cobalt-60 radiation or a specially adapted linear accelerator delivers a single high-dose fraction of focused radiation to a small intracranial target. Frequently, sensitive normal structures lie in near proximity to the target volume. Rapid fall-off of radiation dose outside the target spares adjacent normal tissues and maintains a safe, acceptable level of irradiation. The value of radiosurgery has been demonstrated by many retrospective studies, which included a variety of benign and malignant brain tumors (Kondziolka et al. 2000). Benign tumors tend to shrink slowly over years after radiosurgery, while brain metastases generally shrink more rapidly. With the exception of metastases less than 1 cm in diameter, tumors, whether benign or malignant, generally do not disappear completely following radiosurgery treatment.

15.4.6 Neutron Beam Therapy

Neutrons deposit their dose more densely than conventional photon radiation and the increased relative biological effect results in greater cell death. In addition, hypoxic cells exhibit less resistance to neutron radiation than to conventional photon radiation. Although clinical trials of neutrons in the treatment of malignant gliomas have resulted in higher control rates than treatment with photons, no improvement in survival has been demonstrated, likely due to increased necrosis associated with neutron therapy (Laramore et al. 1988; Battermann 1980; Catteral et al. 1980; Griffin et al. 1983). In a randomized study examining the optimal dose of neutrons for a limited-volume neutron boost combined with photon whole-brain radiotherapy, no beneficial combination was documented (Laramore et al. 1988).

15.4.7 Boron Neutron Capture Therapy (BNCT)

Boron neutron capture therapy was first proposed in 1936 but has yet to make a significant mark on the clinical treatment of human malignancies. A stable isotope of boron, ^{10}B, is administered to patients in a pharmacologic preparation and accumulates in tumor cells. Normal and tumor tissue are then irradiated by broad-beam low-energy thermal or epithermal neutron irradiation. The ^{10}B nuclei have a high probability of thermal neutron capture that results in nuclear fission. High LET particles are created with a range of only one cell diameter, killing only the cells in the immediate vicinity of the boron compound. The clinical utility of BNCT rests on achieving higher concentrations of a ^{10}B-containing compound within tumor cells than within blood, scalp, and normal brain tissues (Diaz 2000). The major compound used in clinical trials to date, p-boronophenylalanine (BPA), produces ^{10}B concentrations 3.5-fold higher in tumor and 1.5-fold higher in scalp than in blood (Chadha et al. 1998). The promise of BNCT in clinical practice rests on the implementation of newer compounds that accumulate more selectively in tumor cells.

15.5 Toxicity of Radiation Therapy

A wide range of potential toxicities complicates the implementation of radiation therapy in the treatment of tumors of the craniospinal axis. These toxicities can be severe and debilitating, particularly in pediatric patients (Syndikus et al. 1994; Kalapurakal and Thomas 1997; Donahue 1992). Care should be taken to minimize these effects. Treatment of intracranial tumors can result in damage to the eye, ear, brain, and hypothalamic-pituitary axis, as well as affecting normal growth. Treatment of the spine can result in growth deficits and damage to the spinal cord. Specific potential acute side-effects of radiation to the central nervous system include epilation, skin reactions, otitis, hematopoietic depression, and somnolence. Specific late toxicities of such radiation include radionecrosis, myelopathy, leukoencephalopathy, vascular injury, neuropsychologic sequelae, endocrine dysfunction, bone and tooth abnormalities, ocular complications, ototoxicity, and induction of second primary tumors (Syndikus et al. 1994; Kalapurakal and Thomas 1997; Donahue 1992). Table 15.1 delineates the radiation doses associated with late toxicities that may result from radiation therapy to the central nervous system.

Table 15.1. Late toxicities of CNS irradiation

Structure	Late effect	Threshold dose
Spinal cord	Chronic progressive myelitis	45 Gy
Brain	Radiation necrosis	60 Gy
	Intellectual deficits	12–18 Gy
Eye		
Lens	Cataract formation	8 Gy
Retina	Radiation retinopathy	45 Gy
Retina	Optic neuritis	50 Gy
Inner ear	Sensorineural hearing loss	40–50 Gy

15.5.1 Spinal Cord

Severe damage to the spinal cord can result following radiation therapy, with functional transection of the cord at the affected level being the most severe result, taking the form of chronic progressive myelitis. This complication is rare, due to the care taken by radiation oncologists to avoid it. Wara et al. reported a 1% incidence of spinal cord damage at 42 Gy, and a 5% incidence at 45 Gy. A number of reports have indicated that tolerance of the cervical spinal cord to radiation toxicity is somewhat higher than 45 Gy in adults (Wara et al. 1975). However, it is unclear what the cervical spinal cord tolerance is in pediatric patients. Radiation to the spinal cord can also result in Lhermitte's syndrome, which is characterized by tingling, numbness, and a sensation of electric shock. Symptoms are often present only with neck flexion. Lhermitte's syndrome is typically self-limiting, presenting within the first one to three months following radiation, and having an average duration of three to four months.

Craniospinal radiation can result in decreased truncal, or sitting, height. This is due to decreased growth of the vertebral bodies following radiation therapy, and becomes clinically evident at doses greater than 20 Gy.

15.5.2 Brain

Acute reactions during radiation therapy, thought to result from disruption of the blood-brain barrier, are uncommon. However, there are reports of edema following single conventional fractions (Kramer and Lee 1974). Clinically apparent acute changes are more common with hypofractionated doses, such as used in radiosurgery (Loeffler et al. 1990). Steroids can be administered to address edema.

Subacute reactions are more common, and are thought to be due to transient demyelination (Boldrey and Sheline 1966). These effects typically occur within the first few months following radiation and usually resolve within six to nine months. This syndrome is seen in a large number of patients receiving prophylactic cranio-spinal radiation along with intrathecal chemotherapy for acute lymphoblastic lymphoma (ALL) (Littman et al. 1984). Severe subacute effects such as rapidly progressive ataxia are more rare, and are generally associated with fractions larger than 2.0 Gy and total doses larger than 50 Gy (Lampert and Alegria 1964).

The late effects of radiation are primarily due to radiation necrosis. Symptoms are related to the neuroanatomical location of necrosis (sensory, motor, speech/receptive deficits, seizures) and may, in addition, be due to increased intracranial pressure. Focal necrosis is uncommon with doses below 60 Gy given with conventional fractionation (Halperin and Burger 1985).

With large-volume radiation therapy, diffuse white matter changes can be seen. Clinically, these can result in lassitude, personality change, or neurocognitive deficits. Multiple studies have examined the effect of whole-brain radiation therapy on intellect in patients treated for leukemia. Radiation-associated depression in IQ has been noted by a number of authors (Rowland et al. 1984; Copeland et al. 1985). Halberg et al. (1992) compared three groups of patients. The first group received 18 Gy (1.8 Gy per fraction) cranial irradiation, while the second received 24 Gy cranial irradiation. The third group consisted of other oncology patients who did not receive cranial irradiation. Lower IQ scores were noted in the group receiving 24 Gy (Halberg et al. 1992). High-dose methotrexate and female sex appear to increase risk of intellectual deficits (Waber et al. 1992). The effects of cranial irradiation are also more severe in younger children. Intellectual deficits resulting from radiation most commonly result in difficulty acquiring new knowledge, decreased processing speed, and memory deficits (most frequently short-term; Mulhern et al. 1992).

Children irradiated for primary brain tumors have also shown intellectual deficits. Effects of radiation are more difficult to evaluate in this setting, as most of these patients have also had surgical resection. However, similar to patients with ALL, younger age appears to result in a higher rate of neurocognitive deficits. Larger fields and higher doses also appear to cause a higher rate of toxicity.

15.5.3 Eye

The lens of the eye is exquisitely sensitive to radiation. Radiation-induced cataracts are caused by damage to the germinal zone at the equator of the lens. Initially, this results in a central opacity that progresses to an opaque cortex. The threshold for radiation damage is 8 Gy in a single fraction, or 10 Gy to 15 Gy in fractionated doses. More rapid cataract formation is associated with higher doses of radiation. Radiation-induced retinopathy appears to have a threshold of 46 Gy at conventional fractionation (1.8 to 2.0 Gy per fraction), but is rare below doses of 50 to 60 Gy. Retinopathy is typically seen beginning from 6 months to 3 years following radiation. It is characterized by macular edema, non-perfusion, and neovascularization. The optic nerves and chiasm are also at risk for damage from radiation. Damage to the optic nerve is characterized by a pale optic disc, abnormal papillary response, and visual deficits. Damage to the optic nerve or chiasm is potentially blinding. The threshold for this damage is 50 Gy. Every effort should be made to keep these structures below their tolerated doses (Emami et al. 1991).

15.5.4 Ear

Radiation-induced sensorineural hearing loss is dose-dependant and is more severe in younger patients. Hearing loss can result from doses greater than 40 to 50 Gy, usually developing within 6 to 12 months of treatment (Grau et al. 1991; Grau and Overgaard 1996). High frequency hearing loss is seen in 25 to 50% of patients who received greater than 50 to 60 Gy to inner ear structures (Anteunis et al. 1994). Hearing loss is typically attributed to radiation changes induced in the cochlea and vasculature. Ototoxicity related to cisplatinum chemotherapy is well-documented (Schell et al. 1989). Cranial irradiation prior to or concurrent with cisplatinum chemotherapy enhances ototoxicity (Schell et al. 1989; Walker et al. 1989). Chronic otitis can also develop following radiation therapy, due to obstruction of the Eustachian canal.

15.5.5 Endocrine

Whole cranial irradiation or focal radiation that includes the hypothalamic-pituitary axis can result in neuroendocrine abnormalities. The neuroendocrine complications that can result from radiation therapy are summarized in Table 15.2. Growth hormone (GH) production appears to be the most prone to disruption by radiation therapy. GH deficiency worsens over time and may follow radiation doses as low as 12 Gy (Merchant et al. 2002). This appears to be a result of decreased GH-releasing hormone (GHRH) in the hypothalamus, as GH deficiency is seen in patients undergoing hypothalamic radiation with pituitary sparing. Clinically, GH deficiency can result in short stature, bone loss, and metabolic abnormalities. Treatment with synthetic GH can allow children to maintain their expected growth percentile despite irradiation.

Other endocrine deficiencies, including decreased thyroid stimulating hormone (TSH), adrenocorticotrophic hormone (ACTH), follicle stimulating hormone (FSH), and luteinizing hormone (LH) appear to have a higher threshold. These effects are typically seen following doses greater than 40 Gy. It is important that children treated for tumors in the region of the hypothalamic-pituitary axis be followed closely for endocrine abnormalities, so that timely replacement therapy can be initiated.

15.6 Molecular Targets For Radiosensitization

15.6.1 Tyrosine Kinase Receptors

Tyrosine kinase receptors (RTKs) play a variety of roles in maintaining homeostasis from individual cells to entire organisms. They regulate cellular proliferation, survival, adhesion, and differentiation, and their function is tightly regulated (Porter and Vaillancourt 1998; Levitzki and Gazit 1995; Hunter 2000). RTKs include molecules with a ligand-binding extracellular portion, a transmembrane section, and an intracellular portion that contains the tyrosine kinase catalytic domain (Pawson and Scott 1997). This family includes the epidermal growth factor receptor (EGFR), platelet-derived growth factor receptor (PDGFR), vascular endothelial growth factor receptor (VEFR), fibroblast growth factor receptor (FGF), stem-cell factor receptor (SCFR), and nerve growth factor receptor (NGFR). Inactivating mutations that confer ligand-independent phosphorylation and activation of the kinases occur in various domains of the protein, including cytoplasmic juxtamembrane, extracellular, and kinase domains (Demetri 2001). Several human malignancies develop as direct consequences of tyrosine kinase activation, and such aberrations can influence prognosis (Taniguchi et al. 1999; Lasota et al. 1999).

Monoclonal antibodies and small molecules have been developed to inhibit RTKs by targeting specific extracellular or intracellular domains. Monoclonal antibodies block signaling through growth factor receptors by preventing binding of ligands (Drebin et al. 1985, 1986). Initial problems associated with rodent antibodies have been alleviated by advances in antibody construction (Fan and Mendelsohn 1998). Small molecule inhibitors block signaling through RTKs by competing with adenosine triphosphate (ATP) for its binding site in the receptor (Levitzki and Gazit 1995). Both of these agents when used in combination with ionizing radiation can cause radiosensitization of cancer cells.

15.6.1.1 EGF Receptor Family Inhibitors

The EGF receptor (EGFR) family consists of four different receptors: ErbB-1 (also known as EGFR), ErbB-2 (also known as HER2/neu), ErbB-3 (also known as HER3), and ErbB-4 (also known as HER4) (Klapper et al. 2000; Mendelsohn and Baselga 2000; Olayioye et al. 2000). EGFR, located on chromosome 7p12, plays a key role in oncogenesis of glioblastoma multiforme (GBM). It is the most commonly amplified oncogene in GBM, with amplification seen in 40 % of tumors (Wong et al. 1987; Ekstrand et al. 1991; von Deimling et al. 1992). One third of GBMs in which EGFR is amplified contain a mutant form, the EGFRvIII mutant, deletion of which in the extracellular domain results in constitutive tyrosine kinase activity (Ekstrand et al. 1992; Wikstrand et al. 1997). Mechanisms of EGFR activation include amplification, overexpression, and expression of a truncated constitutively active form.

Small-molecule inhibitors of EGFR target the ATP-binding site of the receptor (Fry et al. 1994; Klohs et al. 1997). Two such inhibitors, ZD1839 and OSI-774, both oral agents, have entered clinical trials for the treatment of gliomas. Monoclonal antibodies (mAbs) raised against the extracellular domain of the receptor can also inhibit EGFR signaling. Human/murine chimeric antibodies offer the advantage of reduced immunogenicity while preserving potency. MAb-C225 is an example of such an antibody whose administration delays tumor growth in a xenograft model (Goldstein et al. 1995).

15.6.1.2 PDGF Receptor Inhibitors

STI571 is a small-molecule drug that specifically inhibits the tyrosine kinases Abl, PDGFR, and Kit (Sawyers 2002). PDGFR-α and PDGFR-β are two distinct receptors that bind PDGF ligand. Clinical trials have documented the efficacy of STI571 in the treatment of chronic myeloid leukemia, a malignancy driven by

Table 15.2. Endocrine abnormalities resulting from radiation to the hypothalamus and pituitary gland

Hormone abnormality	Threshold dose
Growth hormone deficit	18–25 Gy
ACTH deficit	40 Gy
TRH/TSH deficit	40 Gy
Precocious puberty	20 Gy
LH/FSH deficit	40 Gy
Hyperprolactinemia	40 Gy

constitutive activation of Abl resulting from a chromosomal translocation called Bcr–Abl. Overexpression of the PDGF ligand and its receptor (PDGFR) are observed in all glioma grades (Maxwell et al. 1990; Hermanson et al. 1992, 1996) and is the rationale for using STI571 to treat them. Aberrant PDFR signaling in low-grade as well as high-grade gliomas suggests a role for this signaling cascade in the initiation and progression of this neoplasm. (Hermanson et al. 1996; Westermark et al. 1995).

15.6.1.3 VEGF Receptor Inhibitors

Tumor growth relies not only on uncontrolled cell proliferation and survival but also on the development of new blood vessels. Vascular endothelial growth factors (VEGF), are proangiogenic molecules that transmit their signals through Flt-1 (also known as VEGF-R1) and Flk-1/KDR (also known as VEGF-R2) receptors (Carmeliet and Jain 2000). Whereas VEGF ligands are secreted by tumor and stromal cells, VEGF receptors are expressed mostly by endothelial cells. As with other RTKs, small molecule inhibitors and antibodies directed against the receptor or ligand are used to block signaling through VEGF pathways. One pharmacologic agent, SU5416, selectively inhibits Flk-1/KDR and Flt-1 (Fong et al. 1999). A second molecule, SU6668, exhibits wider specificity towards other proangiogenic RTKs, including Flk-1/KDR, PDGF, and FGF receptors (Laird et al. 2000). Antibodies directed against VEGF or its recep-

tor have entered clinical trials (Presta et al. 1997). Phase I clinical trials employing VEGF inhibitors as single agents report disease stabilization but not objective tumor responses.

15.6.1.4 Farnesyltransferase Inhibitors

Intracellular signaling cascades triggered by activation of growth factor receptors use intermediate molecules to propagate their signals to downstream pathways. The Ras proteins are examples of such intermediaries that mediate many functions, including proliferation, survival, cytoskeletal organization, differentiation, and membrane trafficking. Ras cycles between an active guanosine 5'-triphosphase (GTP)-bound state and an inactive guanosine 5'-biphosphate (GDP)-bound state. Ras proteins are synthesized as cytosolic precursors and are converted to membrane-bound forms through post-translational modifications (Bourne et al. 1990; Downward 1996; Lowy and Willumsen 1993). Such post-translational modifications begin with the addition of a 15-carbon farnesyl moiety (a lipid) to a specific portion of Ras proteins called the CAAX box (A is an aliphatic amino acid and X is methionine or serine) of Ras (Rowinsky et al. 1999). This reaction is catalyzed by an enzyme called farnesyltransferase.

Farnesyltransferase inhibitors (FTIs) directly block the function of Ras but may also interrupt the effects of tyrosine kinase receptors that signal through Ras. Although gliomas rarely contain oncogenic forms of Ras, other alterations such as EGFR overexpression that rely on Ras signaling may be susceptible to targeting by FTIs. The precise mechanism of FTI action remains unclear and an enlarging body of evidence suggests that FTI activity is mediated in part through inhibition of farnesylation of other Ras family members, such as RhoB (Du et al. 1999; Reuter et al. 2000; Lebowitz and Prendergast 1998). Treatment of gliomas in vitro with FTIs results in decreased proliferation and induction of apoptosis.

15.6.2 Molecular Targeting Combined with Conventional Antineoplastic Treatment

Inhibitors of cell signaling are most likely to impact the treatment of human cancers when combined with standard forms of antineoplastic therapy such as chemotherapy and radiation. Such clinical impact will be maximized if novel inhibitors sensitize human malignancies to standard cytotoxic agents. Many studies, most commonly of cell lines in vitro or xenograft tumor models in rodents, indicate that treatment with signaling inhibitors augments tumor responses to radiation and chemotherapy (Jones et al. 2001). Molecular mechanisms implicated in radiosensitization associated with signaling inhibitors include effects on cell proliferation, survival, migration, invasion, angiogenesis, and DNA repair. The precise molecular mechanisms, however, remain elusive.

The strongest data for radiosensitization exist for agents that block EGFR signaling. EGFR overexpression correlates with resistance to radiation in vitro and in vivo (Pillai et al. 1998; Miyaguchi et al. 1998; Sheridan et al. 1997; Wollman et al. 1994). EGFR overexpression also correlates with radiographically measured radiation response of human GBM in vivo (Barker et al. 2001). In a model of human squamous cell carcinoma cells grown in mice, administration of MAb-C225 together with radiation resulted in complete regression of established xenograft tumors (Huang et al. 1999; Milas et al. 2000). Impressive efficacy of concurrent MAb-C225 and radiation has also been documented in intracranial tumors of human glioma cells grown as xenografts in athymic mice. Small molecule inhibitors of EGFR, such as ZD1839 and CI-1033, similarly sensitize human malignancies to radiation in cell lines in vitro and in animal models of human malignancies in vivo (Mendelsohn and Baselga 2000). These studies establish the rationale for current clinical trials examining concurrent administration of ZD183 and radiation in the treatment of adult and pediatric gliomas.

Similarly, FTIs reverse the radiation resistance of cell lines containing mutant Ras without affecting the radiosensitivity of cells expressing wild-type Ras (Jones et al. 2001). A critical unanswered question is whether FTIs will also preferentially radiosensitize cells with aberrant signaling cascades that rely on Ras as an intermediary. Direct evidence is lacking for radiosensitization by signaling inhibitors that target other RTKs such as PDGF and VEGF receptors. However, indirectly blocking VEGF signaling with anti-angiogenic drugs augments the cytotoxic effects of radiation in vivo (Gorski et al. 1999).

15.6.3 P53 Tumor Suppressor Protein

P53 regulates apoptosis, proliferation, differentiation, angiogenesis, and cell-matrix interactions in a tissue-specific manner and is mutated in over 50% of human cancers. For example, in vitro irradiation of hematologic malignancies, such as leukemia and lymphoma, produces rapid p53-dependent apoptosis. A clinical corollary of this laboratory observation is that radiation treatment of hematologic malignancies produces a rapid and durable response. Similarly, in many pediatric tissues, apoptosis plays a key role during organogenesis, and pediatric solid tumors, such as Wilms' tumor and neuroblastoma, exhibit significant apoptosis and excellent cure rates when treated with radiation. In contradistinction, in many adult solid tumor, such as astrocytoma, apoptosis plays a minor role and the balance of p53-mediated functions tilts toward proliferation and differentiation.

Although in glial neoplasms the role of p53 inactivation in mediating radiation resistance remains unclear (Nozaki et al. 1999), enhanced radiosensitivity of glioma cells occurs after reconstitution of p53 function (Lang et al. 1999). Two main approaches have been utilized to restore wild-type p53 function and overcome resistance to radiation: gene therapy and pharmacologic molecules that confer wild-type function on mutant forms of p53. Many impediments to gene therapy have arisen, including inefficient delivery and detrimental immune responses. Pharmacologic agents that impinge on p53 functions hold greater promise for translational clinical practice. Some mutated forms of p53 are amenable to treatment with either synthetic peptides or monoclonal antibodies that can restore wild-type p53 function.

15.7 Conclusion

Radiation is a key therapeutic modality in the treatment of brain tumors and plays a role in the multimodality approach to virtually every pediatric central nervous system malignancy. Efforts to increase the efficacy of radiation using IMRT, high-LET particles, BNCT, radiation modifiers, and altered fractionation have contributed to enhanced cure rates for pediatric patients. Nevertheless, great opportunities exist in improving prognosis for children with brain tumors while reducing long-term side effects of treatment. Novel pharmacological agents such as signaling inhibitors, particularly in combination with standard therapies such as radiation and chemotherapy, hold great promise for scientific and clinical breakthroughs.

References

Anteunis LJ, Wanders SL, Hendriks JJ et al (1994) A prospective longitudinal study on radiation-induced hearing loss. Am J Surg 168:408–411

Barker FG II, Simmons ML, Chang SM et al (2001) EGFR overexpression and radiation response in glioblastoma multiforme. Int J Radiat Oncol Biol Phys 51:410–418

Battermann JJ (1980) Fast neutron therapy for advanced tumors. Int J Radiat Oncol Biol Phys 6:333–335

Boldrey E, Sheline G (1966) Delayed transitory clinical manifestations after radiation treatment of intracranial tumors. Acta Radiol Ther Phys Biol 5:5–10

Bourne HR, Sanders DA, McCormick F (1990) The GTPase superfamily: a conserved switch for diverse cell functions. Nature 348:125–132

Brown JM, Giaccia AJ (1994) Tumour hypoxia: the picture has changed in the 1990 s. Int J Radiat Biol 65:95–102

Brown JM (1999) The hypoxic cell: a target for selective cancer therapy – eighteenth Bruce F. Cain Memorial Award lecture. Cancer Res 59:5863–5870

Carmeliet P, Jain RK (2000) Angiogenesis in cancer and other diseases. Nature 407:249–257

Catteral M, Bloom HJG, Ash DV et al (1980) Fast neutrons compared with megavoltage x-rays in the treatment of patients with supratentorial glioblastoma: a controlled pilot study. Int J Radiat Oncol Biol Phys 6:261–266

Chadha M, Capala J, Coderre JA et al (1998) Boron neutron-capture therapy (BNCT) for glioblastoma multiforme (GBM) using the epithermal neutron beam at the Brookhaven National Laboratory. Int J Radiat Oncol Biol Phys 40:829–834

Copeland DR, Fletcher JM, Pfefferbaum-Levine B et al (1985) Neuropsychological sequelae of childhood cancer in long-term survivors. Pediatrics 75:745–753

Demetri GD (2001) Targeting c-kit mutations in solid tumors: scientific rationale and novel therapeutic options. Semin Oncol 28 [Suppl 17]:19–26

Diaz AZ, Coderre JA, Chanana AD et al (2000) Boron neutron capture therapy for malignant gliomas. Ann Med 32:81–85

Donahue B (1992) Short- and long-term complications of radiation therapy for pediatric brain tumors. Pediatr Neurosurg 18:207–217

Downward J (1996) Control of ras activation. Cancer Surv 27:87–100

Drebin JA, Link VC, Stern DF et al (1985) Down-modulation of an oncogene protein product and reversion of the transformed phenotype by monoclonal antibodies. Cell 41:697–706

Drebin JA, Link VC, Weinberg RA et al (1986) Inhibition of tumor growth by a monoclonal antibody reactive with an oncogene-encoded tumor antigen. Proc Natl Acad Sci USA 83:9129–9133

Du W, Lebowitz PF, Prendergast GC (1999) Cell growth inhibition by farnesyltransferase inhibitors is mediated by gain of geranylgeranylated RhoB. Mol Cell Biol 19:1831–1840

Ekstrand AJ, James CD, Cavenee WK et al (1991) Genes for epidermal growth factor receptor, transforming growth factor alpha, and epidermal growth factor and their expression in human gliomas in vivo. Cancer Res 51:2164–2172

Ekstrand AJ, Sugawa N, James CD et al (1992) Amplified and rearranged epidermal growth factor receptor genes in human glioblastomas reveal deletions of sequences encoding portions of the N- and/or C-terminal tails. Proc Natl Acad Sci USA 89:4309–4313

Emami B, Lyman J, Brown A et al (1991) Tolerance of normal tissue to therapeutic irradiation. Int J Radiat Oncol Biol Phys 21:109–122

Fan Z, Mendelsohn J (1998) Therapeutic application of anti-growth factor receptor antibodies. Curr Opin Oncol 10:67–73

Fong TA, Shawver LK, Sun L et al (1999) SU5416 is a potent and selective inhibitor of the vascular endothelial growth factor receptor (Flk-1/KDR) that inhibits tyrosine kinase catalysis, tumor vascularization, and growth of multiple tumor types. Cancer Res 59:99–106

Fry DW, Kraker AJ, McMcMichael A et al (1994) A specific inhibitor of the epidermal growth factor receptor tyrosine kinase. Science 265:1093–1095

Goldstein NI, Prewett M, Zuklys K et al (1995) Biological efficacy of a chimeric antibody to the epidermal growth factor receptor in a human tumor xenograft model. Clin Cancer Res 1:1311–1318

Gorski DH, Beckett MA, Jaskowiak NT et al (1999) Blockage of the vascular endothelial growth factor stress response increases the antitumor effects of ionizing radiation. Cancer Res 59:3374–3378

Grau C, Overgaard J (1996) Postirradiation sensorineural hearing loss: a common but ignored late radiation complication. Int J Radiat Oncol Biol Phys 36:515–517

Grau C, Moller K, Overgaard J et al (1991) Sensori-neural hearing loss in patients treated with irradiation for nasopharyngeal carcinoma. Int J Radiat Oncol Biol Phys 21:723–728

Griffin TW, Davis R, Laramore G (1983) Fast neutron radiation therapy for glioblastoma multiforme – results of an RTOG study. Am J Clin Oncol 6:661–667

Halberg FE, Kramer JH, Moore IM et al (1992) Prophylactic cranial irradiation dose effects on late cognitive function in children treated for acute lymphoblastic leukemia. Int J Radiat Oncol Biol Phys 22:13–16

Hall EJ (2000) Radiobiology for the radiologist, 5th edn. Lippincott Williams and Wilkins, Philadelphia, p 588

Halperin EC, Burger PC (1985) Conventional external beam radiotherapy for central nervous system malignancies. Neurol Clin 3:867–882

Hermanson M, Funa K, Hartman M et al (1992) Platelet-derived growth factor and its receptors in human glioma tissue: expression of messenger RNA and protein suggests the presence of autocrine and paracrine loops. Cancer Res 52:3213–3219

Hermanson M, Funa K, Koopmann J et al (1996) Association of loss of heterozygosity on chromosome 17p with high platelet-derived growth factor alpha receptor expression in human malignant gliomas. Cancer Res 56:164–171

Huang SM, Bock JM, Harari PM (1999) Epidermal growth factor receptor blockade with C225 modulates proliferation, apoptosis, and radiosensitivity in squamous cell carcinomas of the head and neck. Cancer Res 59:1935–1940

Hunter T (2000) Signaling – 2000 and beyond. Cell 100:113–127

Jones HA, Hahn SM, Bernhard E et al (2001) Ras inhibitors and radiation therapy. Semin Radiat Oncol 11:328–337

Kalapurakal JA, Thomas PR (1997) Pediatric radiotherapy. An overview. Radiol Clin North Am 35:1265–1280

Klapper LN, Kirschbaum MH, Sela M et al (2000) Biochemical and clinical implications of the ErbB/HER signaling network of growth factor receptors. Adv Cancer Res 77:25–79

Klohs WD, Fry DW, Kraker AJ (1997) Inhibitors of tyrosine kinase. Curr Opin Oncol 9:562–568

Kondziolka D, Flickinger JC, Lunsford LD (2000) Stereotactic radiosurgery and radiation therapy. In: Bernstein M, Berger MS (eds) Neuro-oncology: the essentials. Thieme Medical, New York, pp 183–197

Kramer S, Lee KF (1974) Complications of radiation therapy: the central nervous system. Semin Roentgenol 9:75–83

Laird AD, Vajkoczy P, Shawver LK et al (2000) SU6668 is a potent antiangiogenic and antitumor agent that induces regression of established tumors. Cancer Res 60:4152–4160

Lampert H, Alegria A (1964) Treatment of post-poliomyelitis paralysis of long duration. Acta Neurol Latinoam 10:160–171

Lang FF, Yung WK, Sawaya R et al (1999) Adenovirus-mediated p53 gene therapy for human gliomas. Neurosurgery 45:1093–1104

Laramore GE, Diener-West M, Griffin TW et al (1988) Randomized neutron dose searching study for malignant gliomas of the brain: results of an RTOG study. Int J Radiat Oncol Biol Phys 14:1093–1102

Lasota J, Jasinski M, Sarlomo-Rikala M et al (1999) Mutations in exon 11 of c-Kit occur preferentially in malignant versus benign gastrointestinal stromal tumors and do not occur in leiomyomas or leiomyosarcomas. Am J Pathol 154:53–60

Lebowitz PF, Prendergast GC (1998) Non-Ras targets of farnesyltransferase inhibitors: focus on Rho. Oncogene 17:1439–1445

Levitzki A, Gazit A (1995) Tyrosine kinase inhibition: an approach to drug development. Science 267:1782–1788

Littman P, Rosenstock J, Gale G et al (1984) The somnolence syndrome in leukemic children following reduced daily dose fractions of cranial radiation. Int J Radiat Oncol Biol Phys 10:1851–1853

Loeffler JS, Siddon RL, Wen PY et al (1990) Stereotactic radiosurgery of the brain using a standard linear accelerator: a study of early and late effects. Radiother Oncol 17:311–321

Lowy DR, Willumsen BM (1993) Function and regulation of ras. Annu Rev Biochem 62:851–891

Maxwell M, Naber SP, Wolfe HJ et al (1990) Coexpression of platelet-derived growth factor (PDGF) and PDGF-receptor genes by primary human astrocytomas may contribute to their development and maintenance. J Clin Invest 86:131–140

Mendelsohn J, Baselga J (2000) The EGF receptor family as targets for cancer therapy. Oncogene 19:6550–6565

Merchant TE, Goloubeva O, Pritchard DL et al (2002) Radiation dose-volume effects on growth hormone secretion. Int J Radiat Oncol Biol Phys 52:1264–1270

Milas L, Mason K, Hunter N et al (2000) In vivo enhancement of tumor radioresponse by C225 antiepidermal growth factor receptor antibody. Clin Cancer Res 6:701–708

Miyaguchi M, Takeuchi T, Morimoto K et al (1998) Correlation of epidermal growth factor receptor and radiosensitivity in human maxillary carcinoma cell lines. Acta Otolaryngol 118:428–431

Mulhern RK, Ochs J, Fairclough D (1992) Deterioration of intellect among children surviving leukemia: IQ test changes modify estimates of treatment toxicity. J Consult Clin Psychol 60:477–480

Nozaki M, Tada M, Kobayashi H et al (1999) Roles of the functional loss of p53 and other genes in astrocytoma tumorigenesis and progression. Neuro Oncol 1:124–137

Olayioye MA, Neve RM, Lane HA et al (2000) The ErbB signaling network: receptor heterodimerization in development and cancer. EMBO J (19:3159–3167

Pawson T, Scott JD (1997) Signaling through scaffold, anchoring, and adaptor proteins. Science 278:2075–2080

Pillai MR, Jayaprakash PG, Nair MK (1998) Tumour-proliferative fraction and growth factor expression as markers of tumour response to radiotherapy in cancer of the uterine cervix. J Cancer Res Clin Oncol 124:456–461

Porter AC, Vaillancourt RR (1998) Tyrosine kinase receptor-activated signal transduction pathways which lead to oncogenesis. Oncogene 17:1343–1352

Presta LG, Chen H, O'Connor SJ et al (1997) Humanization of an anti-vascular endothelial growth factor monoclonal antibody for the therapy of solid tumors and other disorders. Cancer Res 57:4593–4599

Purdy JA (1999) 3D treatment planning and intensity-modulated radiation therapy. Oncology (Huntingt), 13 [10 Suppl 5]:155–168

Reuter CW, Morgan MA, Bergmann L (2000) Targeting the Ras signaling pathway: a rational, mechanism-based treatment for hematologic malignancies? Blood 96:1655–1669

Rowinsky EK, Windle JJ, von Hoff DD (1999) Ras protein farnesyltransferase: a strategic target for anticancer therapeutic development. J Clin Oncol 17:3631–3652

Rowland JH, Glidewell OJ, Sibley RF et al (1984) Effects of different forms of central nervous system prophylaxis on neuropsychologic function in childhood leukemia. J Clin Oncol 2:1327–1335

Sawyers CL (2002) Rational therapeutic intervention in cancer: kinases as drug targets. Curr Opin Genet Dev 12:111–115

Schell MJ, McHaney VA, Green AA et al (1989) Hearing loss in children and young adults receiving cisplatin with or without prior cranial irradiation. J Clin Oncol 7:754–760

Sheridan MT, O'Dwyer T, Seymour CB et al (1997) Potential indicators of radiosensitivity in squamous cell carcinoma of the head and neck. Radiat Oncol Invest 5:180–186

Sneed PK, Russo C, Scharfen CO et al (1996) Long-term follow-up after high-activity 125I brachytherapy for pediatric brain tumors. Pediatr Neurosurg 24:314–322

Suit H (2002) The Gray Lecture 2001: coming technical advances in radiation oncology. Int J Radiat Oncol Biol Phys 53:798–809

Syndikus I, Tait D, Ashley S et al (1994) Long-term follow-up of young children with brain tumors after irradiation. Int J Radiat Oncol Biol Phys 30:781–787

Taniguchi M, Nishida T, Hirota S et al (1999) Effect of c-kit mutation on prognosis of gastrointestinal stromal tumors. Cancer Res 59:4297–4300

Verhey LJ (1999) Comparison of three-dimensional conformal radiation therapy and intensity-modulated radiation therapy systems. Semin Radiat Oncol 9:78–98

von Deimling A, Louis DN, von Ammon, K et al (1992) Association of epidermal growth factor receptor gene amplification with loss of chromosome 10 in human glioblastoma multiforme. J Neurosurg 77:295–301

Waber DP, Tarbell NJ, Kahn CM et al (1992) The relationship of sex and treatment modality to neuropsychologic outcome in childhood acute lymphoblastic leukemia. J Clin Oncol 10:810–817

Walker DA, Pillow J, Waters KD et al (1989) Enhanced cis-platinum ototoxicity in children with brain tumours who have received simultaneous or prior cranial irradiation. Med Pediatr Oncol 17:48–52

Wara WM, Phillips TL, Sheline GE et al (1975) Radiation tolerance of the spinal cord. Cancer 35:1558–1562

Webb S (2000) Advances in three-dimensional conformal radiation therapy physics with intensity modulation. Lancet Oncol 1:30–36

Weil MD (2001) Conformal radiotherapy for brain tumors. Hematol Oncol Clin North Am 15:1007–1015

Westermark B, Heldin CH, Nistér M (1995) Platelet-derived growth factor in human glioma. Glia 15:257–263

Wikstrand CJ, McLendon RE, Friedman AH et al (1997) Cell surface localization and density of the tumor-associated variant of the epidermal growth factor receptor, EGFRvIII. Cancer Res 57:4130–4140

Willett CG (2001) Intraoperative radiation therapy. Int J Clin Oncol 6:209–214

Wollman R, Yahalom J, Maxy R et al (1994) Effect of epidermal growth factor on the growth and radiation sensitivity of human breast cancer cells in vitro. Int J Radiat Oncol Biol Phys 30:91–98

Wong AJ, Bigner SH, Bigner DD et al (1987) Increased expression of the epidermal growth factor receptor gene in malignant gliomas is invariably associated with gene amplification. Proc Natl Acad Sci USA 84:6899–6903

Yang TC (1999) Proton radiobiology and uncertainties. Radiat Meas 30:383–392

Subject Index